# MANAGING
# CLIENT
# CARE

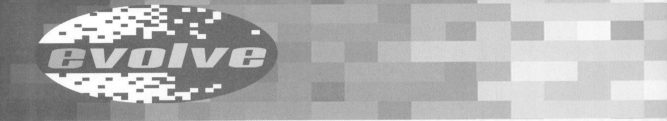

# The Latest *Evolution* in Learning.

Evolve provides online access to free learning resources and activities designed specifically for the textbook you are using in your class. The resources will provide you with information that enhances the material covered in the book and much more.

Visit the Web address listed below to start your learning evolution today!

▶▶ **LOGIN:** *http://evolve.elsevier.com/Wywialowski/*

Evolve Student Learning Resources for Wywialowski:
*Managing Client Care, 3rd Edition* offers the following features:

- **WebLinks**
  An exciting resource that lets you link to hundreds of Web sites carefully chosen to supplement the content of the textbook. The WebLinks are regularly updated, with new ones added as they develop.

- **Links to Related Products**
  See what else Elsevier Science has to offer in a specific field of interest.

*Think outside the book... evolve.*

THIRD EDITION

# MANAGING CLIENT CARE

**Elizabeth F. Wywialowski,** EdD, RN

*With illustrations by*
Bob Rich • West Haven, Connecticut

*and*

Ed Koehler • St. Louis, Missouri

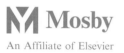

Mosby

An Affiliate of Elsevier

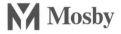

## Mosby

An Affiliate of Elsevier

11830 Westline Industrial Drive
St. Louis, Missouri 63146

**International Standard Book Number 0-323-02482-3**

*Acquisitions Editor:* Tom Wilhelm
*Developmental Editor:* Eric Ham
*Publishing Services Manager:* Melissa Mraz Lastarria
*Designer:* Teresa Breckwoldt

Printed in the United States of America

Last digit is the print number:   9   8   7   6   5   4   3   2   1

*In Memory of*

**"Mom and Dad"**

(Anna and John Wywialowski)

# Instructor Preface

*Managing Client Care* addresses the essential components of the client care manager role. Entry-level staff nurses and their employers are well aware of the need for staff nurses to manage client care effectively and efficiently, especially as efforts to control health care costs and maintain quality continue. To develop the appropriate content for a text that prepares staff nurses to manage client care, DACUM (developing a curriculum) studies were undertaken to identify the essential components of the entry-level staff nurse's role as a client care manager. A subsequent review of the findings of these studies revealed that in many instructional programs the curriculum content, teaching strategies, and time allotted to the client care manager role unintentionally fell short of what was needed. Other management/leadership textbooks that were available contained some of the needed information but omitted other major areas identified by the DACUM studies.

Retaining the integrity and intent of the earlier DACUM findings, the third edition of *Managing Client Care* focuses on the essential management competencies (skills) that are expected of entry-level staff nurses in today's evolving health care scene. The competencies are described in language that is common to staff nurses in the practice settings in which they are typically employed, such as acute and long-term care inpatient and ambulatory care settings. The interchangeable use of the terms entry-level staff nurse and client care manager in the text underscores the nurse's key role as a manager of client care.

A competency consists of a combination of the knowledge, values (attitudes), and psychomotor skills that are required to perform the desired observable or measurable behaviors. The term also refers to a general category of activities or duties required of a worker in an occupational category. This text uses a competency framework to present client care management concepts. The material is organized around the essential competencies required to fulfill the client care manager role. Such a competency-based approach is consistent with the trend of the health care system toward increased emphasis on quality improvement and measurable outcomes.

It is important to distinguish this competency framework from the traditional approach to organizing nursing textbook content, which is characterized by separate cognitive, affective, or psychomotor learning outcomes. In comparison, this text is organized around the competencies needed to manage client care, rather than the topics related to it. The competencies are arranged in order of increasing complexity, allowing students to learn less complex skills before attempting more complex skills. The competency framework may appear more complex in nature but actually is better suited to the measurement of outcome-based learning in today's increasingly complex nursing practice settings. Each chapter of the text addresses an essential competency of the client care manager role, focusing on the specific knowledge, attitudes, and technical skills that the learner needs to perform that competency.

Competency-based instructional programs differ from more traditional curricula in another way as well. Competency-based programs are consistent with current educational trends that focus on research-based criteria and accountability. Rather than emphasize predetermined content or a specified number of instructional hours, competency-based programs focus on behaviors that learners need to succeed in an occupational endeavor. They emphasize demonstrated performance of required skills and adherence to the criteria that are inherent in safe, reliable practice. Because competency-based instruction relies heavily on building more complex skills on previously learned, less complex ones, the client care management skills described in this text build on competencies that students will have acquired in their previous coursework, such as those needed to provide client care and to fulfill responsibilities as members of the discipline of nursing.

Competencies are also context specific—that is, a single competency will differ somewhat from practice setting to practice setting, because unique factors in each setting influence how, when, and why the nurse intervenes and what interventions are chosen. Thus the competencies will differ slightly among acute or long-term inpatient settings and community-based settings. Therefore each chapter defines key concepts in the context in which they are applied, providing a solid basis for clinical application. Principles and processes are discussed in a manner that clarifies their application in fulfilling nursing obligations in general and the duties of entry-level staff nurses in particular. Numerous examples are included throughout the text as illustration.

The third edition of *Managing Client Care* incorporates numerous changes that correspond with evolving management concepts, health care system issues, and research findings. The text is organized into four units. Unit I, "Understanding the Client Care Environment" (Chapters 1 through 4), addresses the competencies related to understanding the environment in which client care is delivered and the importance of prioritizing tasks. Additional information has been included addressing transformational leadership, technological changes associated with the information era and its effects on health care organizations. An introduction to disaster preparedness is also included. These competencies are fundamental to effective client care management, particularly in light of the rapid changes in American health care as a result of the effects of the global economy, organizational restructuring, the vested interests of organizations that finance health care services, the "information age," and terrorism. Unit II, "Managing Client Care" (Chapters 5 through 9), focuses on the competencies used to manage resources. To prepare learners to cope with the impact of economic scarcity in today's health care system, Chapter 5 was updated to explain how the staff nurse can conserve organizational resources while delivering safe, effective care. This chapter distinguishes among organizational, human, time, information, financial, and other resources and explains the staff nurses' role in managing all resources cost effectively. It also includes a section that explains the role of nursing research in providing cost effective, outcome-oriented nursing care. Chapters 6 through 9 are designed to help learners build on previously acquired competencies to develop interrelated management skills, including those needed to use common technological devices to reduce medication errors and increase client safety. Unit III, "Managing Others" (Chapters 10 through 14), addresses the essential skills needed to manage nursing work groups and contribute to multidisciplinary work groups involved in providing client care. Content was added to further address the principles of work assignment and delegation used to manage unlicensed assistive personnel who are employed more commonly to address the staffing shortage. Unit IV, "Professional Development" (Chapters 15 and 16 and the Epilogue), acquaints the learner with ethical and legal issues and promotes the development of professional integrity and career management skills. Throughout the book, new topic subheadings have been added, and many sections have been reorganized to facilitate the learning process.

Special features of the text are also designed to facilitate optimal learning and retention of chapter content. The eye-catching two-color design not only increases the visual appeal of the text but also highlights its pedagogic features, thus increasing its usefulness to the student. Features that appear in each chapter include: **objectives**, which outline the chapter's learning goals and help the student focus on key information; **key concepts**, which list important terms and concepts found in the chapter and help focus the student's attention on important content; **summary**, which condenses key chapter content in brief narrative form and facilitates review of important points; **application exercises**, which encourage the student to apply chapter content to real-life situations and think critically about them; and the new **critical thinking scenario** at the end of each chapter, which presents a brief narrative case study that incorporates principles discussed in the chapter and follow-up questions that encourage students to apply chapter concepts while thinking critically about the scenarios. Throughout the text are sample forms, worksheets, logs, checklists, and other "hands-on" learning tools that both familiarize students with forms they will likely encounter in the workplace and serve as convenient learning tools that guide practical application of chapter content. The entertaining cartoons that appear in every chapter add variety and humor while highlighting key points about client care management. In addition, the completely revised Instructor's Manual for *Managing Client Care*, Third Edition, has been moved online and can be found on the book's Evolve web site. The updated IM includes suggested learning activities, student worksheets and review sheets, performance checklists, and a detailed case study for each chapter, with follow-up questions designed to promote critical thinking and application of chapter content.

*Managing Client Care* was written with a twofold purpose: to prepare nursing students to make a successful transition from learner to practitioner, and to teach the competencies needed to manage the care of a group of clients effectively and efficiently in today's health care system. It is designed to serve as a client care management primer for nursing students who are about to enter the work force rather than an encyclopedia of comprehensive knowledge that staff nurses need to manage client care. This text provides a solid foundation on which staff nurses may begin their careers as client care managers, while encouraging them to put forth the continuous effort required to build on that foundation and remain competent throughout their careers.

# Acknowledgments

Writing *Managing Client Care* has taught me that as an author I need many hours of solitude to allow for concentration plus a great deal of mental energy—both to compose and to resist more leisurely temptations such as golf or nature walks. Without the encouragement, help, and support of many people, I could not have completed this book. I acknowledge them here with sincere gratitude.

My parents, who provided me my first caring experiences and later substantive insights into the demands of this process. They helped me gain insight into the need to limit altruism for the sake of self preservation and the need to care for oneself. They helped me learn that with self preservation comes dignity, character, and desire to do the job, "whether it be great or small," to the best of one's ability. With the increasing health care staffing shortages and health insurance company profits, the need to care for oneself has come into sharp focus. I have shared this priceless insight in an effort to help preserve the caring potential of our increasingly scarce health care workforce.

My dear friends and Registered Nurse colleagues, Lori Hayes and Carey Lee, who proofread and critiqued early drafts to ensure that the specific management competencies were addressed with clarity. They exemplify the very best in the profession and I am grateful for their contributions to the nursing profession and my professional development.

The Developmental Editor, Eric Ham, and Production staff at Mosby, whose enthusiastic support nurtured the book's timely publication. Their attention to detail will be appreciated by the readers.

The many nursing colleagues who confirmed information about the management competencies identified by the initial DACUM study participants and addressed in this book. Their input made writing this book worthwhile.

My friends and those in my family who repeatedly reminded me of my real priorities in life. They encouraged me when my enthusiasm waned and laughed heartily with me when situations made laughter impossible to resist. Each in his or her own way lovingly adjusted plans so that the time we could spend together inspired me to finish the book without delay.

**Elizabeth F. Wywialowski**

# To the Student

As an entry-level staff nurse in today's changing health care system, you'll need strong client care management skills more than ever before. The third edition of *Managing Client Care* not only provides the necessary conceptual knowledge but also offers practical strategies to help you apply the knowledge and perform the skills that are so vital to your success as manager of client care. This book may differ from other texts that you have used in that it is organized not according to topics but around the competencies that you'll need to fulfill the role of client care manager. A competency is a combination of the knowledge, attitudes, and psychomotor skills needed to perform desired observable or measurable behaviors.

Your text is divided into four units that reflect the key groups of competencies in client care management. Unit I, "Understanding the Client Care Environment" (Chapters 1 through 4), addresses the competencies that you'll need to understand the environment in which client care is delivered and to prioritize tasks effectively and efficiently. You'll find these competencies to be especially important because of the rapid changes taking place in health care today—changes that result from shifts in the global economy, organizational restructuring, the vested interests of health care financing organizations, and the "information age." Unit II, "Managing Client Care" (Chapters 5 through 9), focuses on the competencies that will allow you to manage resources effectively in this era of economic scarcity. It builds on competencies you will have acquired in previous courses to help you develop additional interrelated management skills. Unit III, "Managing Others" (Chapters 10 through 14), addresses the essential skills that will enable you to manage nursing or multidisciplinary work groups or interdisciplinary teams who are involved with you in providing client care. Unit IV, "Professional Development" (Chapters 15 and 16 and the Epilogue), acquaints you with important ethical and legal issues, offers strategies for nurturing your professional integrity, and sharpens your career management skills.

To help you make the most of your learning experience, try the following strategy after you complete each chapter: Stop and think about what the chapter conveyed. What does it mean for you as a client care manager? How does the chapter's content, and your interaction with it, relate to that of the other chapters you have already completed? How might you briefly summarize the content for a nonnurse friend? Reading the chapter, restating its key points in your own words, and completing the Application Exercises and Critical Thinking Scenario as suggested in the next section ("Learning Aids") will go far to help you make the content truly your own.

## LEARNING AIDS

The third edition of *Managing Client Care* features some important tools designed to help you learn about the principles of client care management and apply your new knowledge to the real world. Following is a description of some of these tools, along with suggestions about ways in which you can use these study aids to your best advantage:

The **objectives** describe the chapter's broad learning goals. Use them to guide you in choosing the general content areas on which to concentrate as you scan the chapter.

The **key concepts** provide a more detailed list of the chapter's important terms and concepts. You'll want to focus particular attention on them as you study the text more closely. The boldface, brightly colored type in which the key concepts appear helps you locate them easily, whether you're scanning the chapter for specific information or reviewing for an examination.

The **summary** condenses the chapter's key points into a brief narrative form. You might find it helpful to read the summary both before starting the chapter, as a "preview" of the material to come, and again afterward, as a way to increase your recall of the material you've just covered.

The **application exercises** contain questions that challenge you to apply the chapter's key concepts to real-life situations. Completing them will help sharpen your ability to think critically and to apply the chapter content that you've learned.

The **critical thinking scenario** at the end of each chapter is a brief case study that presents a situation you might encounter as a staff nurse. After the scenario are some follow-up questions that challenge you to apply chapter concepts to the scenario. Like the application exercises, the critical thinking scenarios will help sharpen your critical thinking and application skills.

The role of client care manager is a challenging and rewarding one. The skill with which you perform it directly affects the quality of care that clients receive, as well as the efficiency and effectiveness with which it is delivered. The author and all of the people who worked on this book have made every attempt to reflect these facts in the design and approach of *Managing Client Care*. We wish you much success in your career!

# Contents

# UNDERSTANDING THE CLIENT CARE ENVIRONMENT

# 1

# Introduction to Client Care Management

*When you complete this chapter, you should be able to:*

1. List components of client care management.
2. Describe the relationship of nursing roles and skills to the client care manager role.
3. Explain the differences between nursing management and nursing leadership.
4. Describe the primary purposes of health-care organizations compared with those of other human service organizations.
5. Describe four common types of organizational structures.
6. Explain the differences between formal and informal organizations.
7. Describe four common management theories of human motivation.
8. List two organizational changes anticipated in the future.

role
nursing role
core nursing roles
context
client care manager role
nursing management
nursing leadership
organization of a work group
autocracy
bureaucracy
adhocracy
matrix organizations

boundaryless organizations
learning organizations
formal organizations
informal organizations
human motivations
Maslow's hierarchy of needs
Theory X
Theory Y
Theory A
Theory Z
situational leadership
transformational leadership

This book is about client care management. It was written primarily for nursing students preparing to become entry-level staff nurses employed in inpatient and ambulatory care settings. Beginning staff nurses are expected to provide services that prevent diseases and promote and maintain health as well as to provide care for the ill or infirm. Throughout the text, the term *client* instead of *patient* is used to designate the recipients of nursing service. The term *patient* implies a passive role; it does not emphasize the individual's active participation in his or her health care. The term *client* is used to emphasize the professional nature of the relationship between nurses and the individuals they serve; it reflects the evolution of nursing as a profession, the client's needs as a consumer as the focus of the interaction, and the necessity of a working relationship that is rewarding to the consumer and the nurse.

This book discusses basic concepts of management related to the practice of nursing. It emphasizes the practical application of these concepts in settings in which beginning staff nurses are commonly employed. These inpatient or ambulatory care settings support the inexperienced nurse by providing structure (e.g., policies, protocols, procedures, and guidelines) and resources (e.g., supervision by more experienced nurses, preceptorships, and structured professional development programs). As the entry-level nurse has successful experiences and gains confidence and expertise, need for such support decreases, and eventually the nurse can practice in less structured or unstructured settings (e.g., public health or home-based care).

Entry-level staff nurses manage client care directly; for example, they directly observe or provide preventive or restorative services for clients. They manage care for a specified period, such as a shift, in contrast to nurses who manage care throughout a client's inpatient stay or for an indefinite period (e.g., a primary provider in a community-based setting). Entry-level staff nurses should not overlook or minimize their influence as critical decision makers in the use of available resources to provide cost-effective care. Nurses who supervise beginning staff nurses in first-line management positions, such as nurse managers, case managers, or unit managers, typically manage client care indirectly. The client care manager role is integral to nursing practice.

To succeed as a staff nurse, client care management skills are essential. Without these skills, entry-level staff nurses cannot effectively practice nursing in inpatient or ambulatory care settings. In the past, most nurses developed client care management skills after graduation from basic nursing programs, often through trial and error. Because client care management skills are essential, nursing students need to develop them before they begin practicing. Entry-level staff nurses are likely to find that developing these skills is an ongoing process.

## COMPETENCIES OF CLIENT CARE MANAGERS

What competencies (required skills) are expected of entry-level staff nurses as client care managers? To succeed as staff nurses, client care managers use organizational resources and routines while providing direct client care, use time productively, collaborate with the interdisciplinary work group, and use leadership characteristics to manage others within the nursing work group. More specifically, to manage client care, entry-level nurses:

1. Identify organizational resources and determine when they are needed.
2. Work within various nursing service delivery patterns.
3. Use position descriptions to establish the scope and limitations of their own and other nursing work group member practices.
4. Manage time purposefully and productively.
5. Prioritize client needs and related care.
6. Exhibit flexibility in providing care within available time constraints.
7. Show initiative, flexibility, and creativity as leadership qualities.
8. Think critically to make decisions required to solve client care problems.
9. Defend their own decisions.
10. Collaborate with other health team members.
11. Resolve conflicts within the work group.
12. Delegate appropriately.

## RELATIONSHIPS OF OTHER NURSING ROLES TO THE CLIENT CARE MANAGER ROLE

This book is based on information gathered from nurses practicing in acute and long-term inpatient and home care settings; it focuses on the management of client care. It covers skills expected of entry-level staff nurses employed in acute and long-term settings. The competencies discussed in this book were identified by entry-level staff nurses and their immediate supervisors, who indicated that these skills were essential for successful practice by beginning staff nurses. They arranged these skills and tasks in order of increasing complexity. Knowledge of this arrangement was used to organize the learning activities in this book to help nursing students learn less complex client care management skills before attempting more complex ones. Staff nurses as client care managers use agency resources to provide needed services effectively and efficiently.

A **role** is an expected typical behavior of a person with a specific status or social position. For example, parents are expected to behave in certain ways in the protection and care of their children. The role of an employee relates to the function, purpose, or tasks he or she performs for the organization. The practice of nursing is made up of several interrelated roles. A **nursing role** is a set of expectations that the nurse fulfills; it includes applying professional knowledge, exhibiting attitudes, and demonstrating behaviors common to the practice of nursing. **Core nursing roles** are roles that are common to all practicing nurses. They include being a provider of care, a member of the profession, and a manager of client care. Other common roles include communicator, client teacher, and investigator. Nursing educators and administrators have identified these common roles as a convenient way to describe components of nursing practice and plan instructional programs.

The process of learning to practice nursing is not universal, but there are common patterns. Learning to perform each nursing role usually proceeds from less complex to more complex activities.

## Role as Client Care Provider

In practice, the beginning staff nurse performs various aspects of each of the interrelated nursing roles identified earlier, depending on the client's needs and the resources available to meet these needs. In addition, the nurse uses various skills adapted to the setting, or **context** (i.e., he or she behaves in ways that are appropriate in the specific nursing practice environment). Each nursing practice environment is affected by its organizational systems, its primary purposes, routines, policies, and procedures. The nurse's practice environment significantly influences her or his activities. In the larger social context, the nurse is expected to adhere to various laws and codes of ethics.

## Role as Member of a Profession

Typically, nursing students learn to use the nursing process before they learn to teach clients about the complexities of self-care. While learning to apply the nursing process, students develop communication skills, identify legal and ethical issues, and adhere to codes of conduct. On the basis of their individual strengths and limitations, students learn to accept responsibility for self-directed learning early in their careers and when to seek assistance with client care. As they progress through their instructional activities, they learn about legal and ethical issues and various client needs and health problems throughout the life span. As they learn about ethical issues and legal constraints associated with various treatment options, they are expected to respond to client needs within the context of an agency's policies and procedures and the state laws influencing nursing practice. Fulfilling some of the role requirements as a member of the profession prepares the student for the client care manager role. The nursing student applies knowledge of legal and ethical issues to identify priorities for individual clients.

## Role as Client Care Manager

The **client care manager role** requires the nursing student to address the priorities of an assigned group of clients for a specified time. Only skills that are essential to client care management are addressed in this book. Basic nursing skills used in providing clinical care and fulfilling requirements as a member of the nursing profession are fundamental building blocks for developing client care management skills and for succeeding as an entry-level staff nurse. The nursing student learns management skills throughout her or his instructional program and may gain experience using a variety of strategies and timing. Often, depending on the amount of time available, nursing students gain "management" experience immediately before graduation.

When students advance beyond caring for more than one or two clients, they are typically required to demonstrate skills needed to manage nursing care for a group of clients. This progression suggests that in most nursing practice settings, client care management skills evolve from existing skills in less complex roles. In other words, some client care management skills depend on mastering less complex and interrelated roles. Accordingly, learners tend to learn client management skills after they acquire other, less complex nursing skills. The entry-level staff nurse may use client care management skills frequently while progressing in an instructional program.

All nurses do not learn the many nursing skills in the same sequence. Nursing procedures frequently used in practice are readily learned depending on the client's priority needs and the nature of the health-care setting. Some skills, such as cardiopulmonary resuscitation, may be learned early but are used infrequently and require regular reinforcement because a client's survival may depend on the nurse's immediate response. It is presumed, however, that students who are striving to develop client care management skills have developed the ability to carry out the following activities effectively: using nursing process skills to provide clinical care; communicating with clients, peers, and other work group members in face-to-face situations and through the agency's electronic information processing network; identifying specific agency resources; teaching clients and families about self-care; and adhering to the legal and ethical guidelines of nursing practice in various inpatient and structured community-based settings.

The client care manager role is generally more complex than the provider-of-care and member-of-the profession roles. It is not a combination of other roles. Rather, the client care manager role is different; it requires application of nursing knowledge with knowledge needed to fulfill other, less complex nursing roles. The client care manager role requires skills that enhance the performance of other nursing roles. Client care management skills entail applying knowledge and sensitivity to organizational variables in the health-care environment, coordinating the activities of other health work group members to meet client care goals, managing the efforts of others on the nursing work group, and managing one's career and personal lifestyle. It is crucial to take care of oneself at work and at home to prevent burnout and ensure survival.

Managers of client care are expected to allocate resources cost-effectively. They also supervise others providing direct care.

## NURSING MANAGEMENT COMPARED WITH NURSING LEADERSHIP

Sometimes the terms *nursing management* and *nursing leadership* are used as if they mean the same thing. They do not; nor are these terms mutually exclusive. Many effective staff nurses are both managers and leaders.

**Nursing management** refers to the judicious use of resources to achieve identified client goals. It implies responsibility for coaching, directing, and sometimes authoritatively controlling (Hillman, 1995, p. 115). **Nursing leadership,** in comparison, refers to the ability to influence others to respond in desired ways (e.g., to behave and relate to others in ways that encourage them to follow voluntarily). There is no single definition that suits all leadership situations (Yukl, 2002, p. 7), although many theorists agree that it is a social influence process. Leadership implies a persuasive power or influence that followers accept voluntarily without organizational authority. " . . . leadership is called forth by circumstances. The person rises to the occasion and the group falls behind" (Hillman, 1995, p. 154).

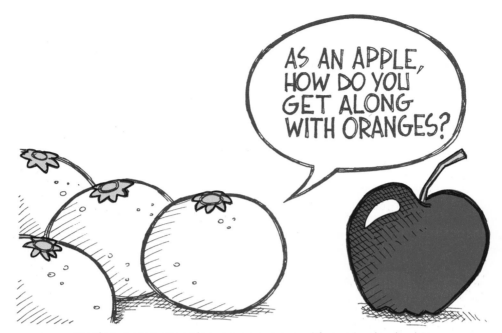

Nursing management is not synonymous with nursing leadership.

Nursing management is less difficult if the nurse has leadership ability to influence others to respond in desired ways. Nursing management implies more accountability to clients, however, in terms of the use of resources within the organizational context. All nurse leaders are not nurse managers, nor is every nurse manager a leader. Nurse managers need leadership qualities, however, to be effective and efficient.

Many health-care organizational charts show the level of first-line nurse managers (i.e., nurses supervising direct care providers). The formal organization of different functional units varies widely. Consequently the staff nurse's location on the agency's formal organization chart may or may not be specified. Staff nurses directly managing client care might be shown on unit level organization charts. The organizational sanction (i.e., approval or okay) of the management role of the staff nurse is often clarified by its position description. How the organization divides the work to be done (i.e., client care) is included in its approved descriptions of work group relationships. These relationships are discussed further in Chapter Three.

Leadership, by comparison to management, is an earned, informal position. General characteristics that the leader uses to influence followers and the quality and features of informal interrelationships between the leader and followers (e.g., trustworthiness, truthfulness, knowledge, openness of communication, charisma) contribute to the leader's earned influence.

## ORGANIZATIONS

The organizations within which client care managers work exist because the work to be done cannot be accomplished by one person. Groups of people are divided according to the type of work and how and when it needs to be done. The **organization of a work group** evolves to provide for the interdependencies of various subgroups or divisions of the work to be done. It is designed to help these groups meet their overall common goals. The organizational structure divides the work and reflects how decisions are made within the structure. Because health-care organizations evolve in response to client needs, the more complex the client care, the more complex the organizations designed to provide it are likely to be. Entry-level staff nurses need information about their organizational systems to direct available resources and communicate effectively with other team members to address client needs. With the increasing use of information technology in the provision of health care, staff nurses need to understand how it affects the context of their practice. They also need to know how information technology is changing the boundaries of health-care organizations (Howard, 1995, pp. 89–96). These organizational changes related to information technology affect nursing practice daily and will continue to do so in the future.

## Common Types of Organizational Structures

Nurses usually practice within more than one of the common types of organizations: autocracy, bureaucracy, adhocracy, and matrix organizations. Any type of organization of itself is neither good nor bad. Rather, the effectiveness of the organization depends on the interaction of several variables, including the following: the needs of the organization's clientele, the needs of the workers as they attempt to meet client needs, the manner in which the organization responds to change, the stability of the environment, and the manner in which the organization uses information and technology to address its clientele's needs (Imparato and Harari, 1994, pp. 154–185). An effective organization is dynamic, continuously learning and changing, and seemingly chaotic at a glance. It is not likely to be static, orderly, or sequential in logical decision making. Nurses, as participants in health-care organizations, manage clinical care by applying professional knowledge; using clinical data, computers, and other information technology; and collaborating with nursing and other interdisciplinary work group members, including licensed and unlicensed staff, to satisfy clientele needs in a timely manner.

### Autocracy

Although not often recognized, nurses are employed in autocratic organizations. In an **autocracy,** decisions are made at the highest level often by one person and communicated and implemented at subordinate levels as the work of the organization is divided. Historically a monarchy would typify an autocracy. This type of organization is common in military groups or in departments where urgent decisions are commonly needed. The positive gains of timely decisions may make an autocracy the organizational type of choice. It is dependent on the strengths and

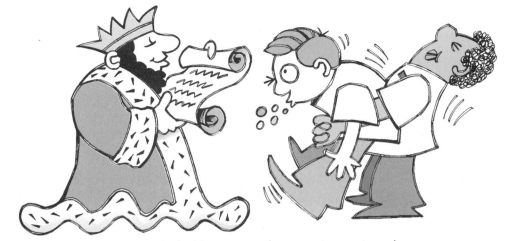

Autocratic decisions are made to meet urgent needs.

biases of the decision maker, who might not be close enough to the situation to consider all essential variables.

### Bureaucracy

In the past, most nurses were employed in bureaucratic organizational structures. This type of organizational structure divides the work along centralized departmental or functional lines. Figure 1-1 depicts the linkages or relationships of a **bureaucracy**. Most of the decision-making authority is vested in the upper levels of the organization. In bureaucratic organizations, many nurses experience difficulty responding to the diverse needs of clients because they lack the autonomy or authority to make the decisions required for quality nursing care in a timely manner.

### Adhocracy

As greater emphasis is placed on customer-oriented service, more attention has been given to an organizational structure known as a decentralized organization or an **adhocracy**. This type of organization provides for decentralized decision making and considerable employee participation. Figure 1-2 depicts the typical linkages or relationships of an adhocracy. Some nurses who practice in environments characterized by frequent changes in technology, skilled personnel, and client needs often experience less frustration in adhocracies because they participate in decision-making processes. Adhocracies often provide opportunities for staff nurses to participate in decisions that affect client care processes and incorporate factors that heavily influence quality.

Many factors, such as the trends discussed in Chapter Two, affect the purposes, goals, and mission of health-care organizations. These factors cause changes in health-care organizations and have an impact on nursing roles and practice. With the increased competition and emphasis on cost-effectiveness and customer satisfaction, nurses providing direct care to clientele are expected to make decisions that

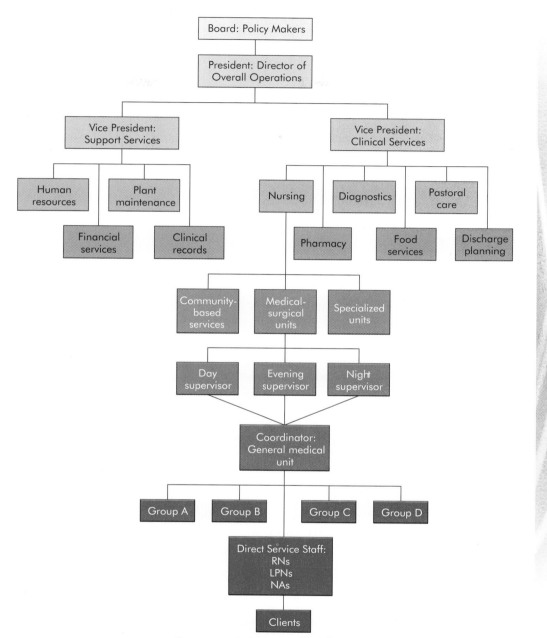

FIGURE 1-1 Bureaucratic (or centralized) organization.

affect the processes and outcomes of the services provided. Decentralized organizations that support professional authority and accountability for clinical decision making also promote increased quality of care and customer and nurse satisfaction. Even the most decentralized organization has components of centralized decision

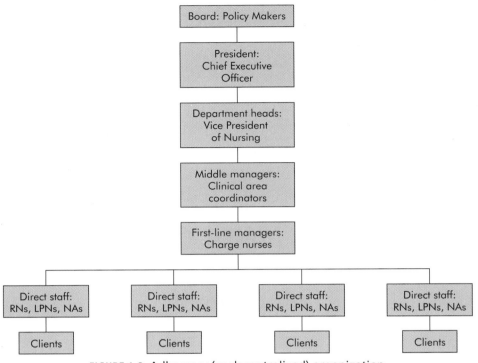

FIGURE 1-2 Adhocracy (or decentralized) organization.

making, however, for overall strategic planning, formulation of organizational philosophy and mission, and resource allocation.

A major advantage of the trend toward more decentralized health care organizations is that direct care providers (of all disciplines) have an opportunity to apply their professional skills to personalize the services provided. Correspondingly the direct care providers accept responsibility and accountability (i.e., they are answerable) for clinical decisions made and implemented (i.e., client outcomes and cost-effectiveness). These decisions must be data-driven and based on research and professional findings associated with continuous quality improvement efforts.

Modern health care is complex and multifaceted. Providing quality, cost-effective health care requires cooperation of several disciplines; consequently, decentralized organizations evolve "collaborative teams" (Marshall, 1995, pp. 112–124). Another advantage of the trend toward decentralization is that effective decentralized health-care organizations support open communication and collaboration between direct care providers in the interest of quality client care. Health-care organizations that focus attention on the process of service delivery (i.e., interactions involved in providing the service) and the outcomes satisfy more customers than organizations that do not (Schneider and Bowen, 1995, pp. 19–53).

A major disadvantage of the expansion of decentralizing organizations is the tendency to overassign direct care providers with time-consuming tasks that decrease their time and energy to provide care. For example, centralized staffing, in which a few people focus on adequately staffing every unit for the entire organization, has often proved to be more cost-effective than decentralized staffing, in which direct staff are expected to obtain shift-by-shift replacements. Another major disadvantage of decentralization, perhaps of greater overall significance, is that sufficient resources must be allocated to ensure that the knowledge and skills of the direct service staff are current because the quality of care depends on it. Many firmly held convictions might need to be softened, and new ones developed, in support of mutual trust and open communication required of a collaborative work group member (Marshall, 1995, pp. 140–162, 175–176). With the increased emphasis on cost-effectiveness, the quantity of services may be emphasized to the detriment of quality, with consequent decreased customer satisfaction. Less staff time may be spent on service components that typically consume more time or resources and are directly related to quality care (e.g., individualizing care, teaching clients and significant others, or providing for continuity). Indirect costs incurred to maintain staff competency and equipment also may be neglected to the detriment of quality care.

As the trend in health-care organizations continues toward greater decentralization, staff nurses need to collaborate and coordinate efforts of an interdisciplinary work group. Entry-level staff nurses will be expected to provide direct care and coordinate the resources required to provide all direct care needed by the nursing and interdisciplinary work groups in a cost-effective manner. Figure 1-3 depicts a service organization (Schneider and Bowen, 1995, p. 7) and describes the organizational position of a client care manager in the evolving decentralized health-care organization.

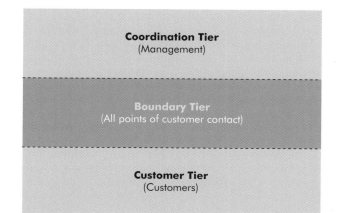

**FIGURE 1-3** Client care manager's position in a three-tiered service organization. The *coordination tier* is made up of interdisciplinary management. The client care manager is located within the *boundary tier*, the direct-service level where all providers have direct contact with clients. The *customer tier* is made up of health-care clients. (From Schneider B, Bowen D: *Winning the service game,* Boston, 1995, The Harvard Business School Press, p. 7.)

## Matrix

As the complexity of health care continues to demand highly skilled workers in specialized work units, **matrix organizations** may be used to organize functional work groups. Matrix organizations allow a manager with special skills to guide workers who report directly to another manager. Figure 1-4 depicts a typical pattern of relationships within a matrix organization. A matrix organization allows a work group to solve special problems while the original organizational structure is retained. Nurses practicing in highly complex environments, such as research centers, might practice within a matrix organization.

## Boundaryless

While the trends to be described in Chapter Two materialize, organizations are challenged to "do more with less." Concurrently the nursing profession is confronted with an increasing "shortage" of nurses. Both of these demands cause organizations to change in an effort to increase efficiencies and performance with existing resources. To survive, organizations will leverage (i.e., use their power) over resources, including nurses, to maximize gain. To the extent that the organization increases flexibility, integration, and innovation in meeting its customer needs, it is more likely to increase its efficiencies (Jennings and Haughton, 2002, pp. 237–249; Ashkenas et al., 2002, pp. 304–319) and survive.

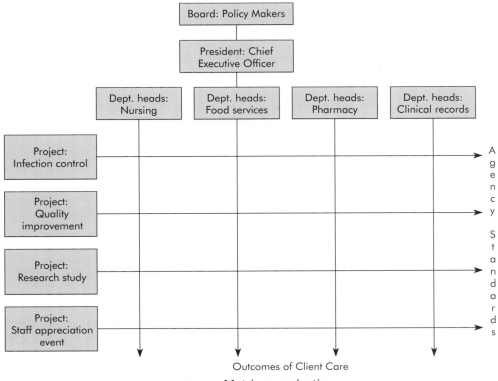

FIGURE 1-4 **Matrix organization.**

What is a boundaryless organization like? The organizations discussed in this chapter so far have had vertical and horizontal boundaries illustrated by lines. That is, they depicted relationships of different persons according to the hierarchy of decision making and work to be done (i.e., functions or departments). **Boundaryless organizations** have, if any, blurred (widened, fuzzy, permeable, gray rather than black) lines as well as additional boundaries that were not previously depicted. These additional boundaries include external and geographic dimensions. The *external boundaries* relate to the relationships between the customer, other organizations, and the health-care organization. The external organizations might include community organizations that provide various health-related or non–health-related services. External boundaries affect the health of clients and the services available to meet their needs, such as Internet information sources or agencies that provide clients with insight into their special health needs (e.g., American Heart Association, senior centers, or community centers). *Geographic boundaries* are boundaries related to physical space and distance. As the use of information technology increases globally, distance will become less influential as to the pace of the health-care provision process because the information can be transmitted in much shorter periods of time. The required amount of time to communicate will be much less. Regional differences will continue to play an important function; to the extent possible, technology will be used to market and communicate with clients.

Most importantly, the boundaryless organization will differ from the types of organizations previously described in that it will focus on the efficient leveraging of resources to promote the process of care and desired outcomes. Its emphases include removing restrictions, real and imagined, to create new patterns of collaboration, learning, and effective and efficient work. Boundaryless organizations depend heavily on the intellectual capacity of their people (i.e., professional staff and individuals providing services directly to clients). This type of organization is discussed further in Chapters Two and Three.

### Combined Structures

Combinations of organizational structures are usually used, although to the casual observer the current health-care scene may appear like chaos. These combinations typically attempt to maximize the advantage and minimize the disadvantages of each type of structure to meet best the purposes and goals of the organization.

As the rate of change accelerates in the informational era, **learning organizations** are expected to increase in number. This type of organization is expected to unravel how best to use the commitment of its people and their ability to learn at every level of the organization. It focuses on *systems* (interrelationships of functional units) versus *linear* (direct line authority) thinking, language that work groups working together find useful, and evolving commitment based on shared visions and common values (Senge, 1994). Learning organizations are designed to maintain a competitive edge by understanding "dynamic complexity" (Senge, 1994, p. 365) to develop needed solutions to increase effectiveness and productivity. Learning organizations are the bridge between traditional and boundaryless organizations.

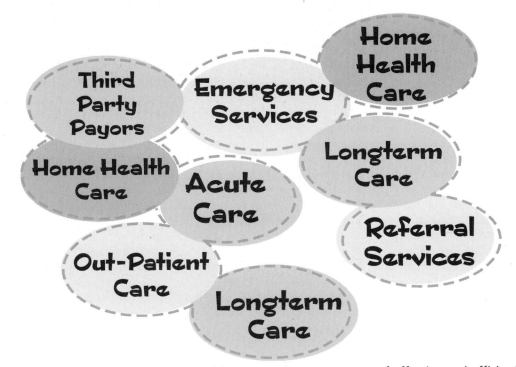

Lines of boundaryless organizations blur to enable new patterns of effective and efficient work.

## Formal and Informal Organizations

The preceding discussion concerned **formal organizations**. These structures can be diagrammed or illustrated to depict the work division and decision-making or care processes. The formal structure of an organization is often presented in materials describing the governance and administrative processes in effect for the organization.

In contrast, **informal organizations** evolve from the many human variables within work groups. Informal organizational structures are not diagrammed or officially approved. They may evolve from informational sources, from power positions based on useful knowledge but lacking formal organizational authority, or from spontaneous human responses to issues within or outside the organization. Often, informal organizations evolve around daily communications between members of work groups. Two common types of information groups are the "networks of practice" (located externally) and "communities of practice" (located internally) within the formal organization (Brown and Duguid, 2002, pp. 137–143). The *networks of practice* are groups of workers who share knowledge to help each other solve practice problems, although they are likely working in different organizations. Membership in a district special interest nursing organization is a customary entry into a network of practice. The *communities of practice* are groups of employees who share learnings gained during the course of their practice within the group (i.e., cli-

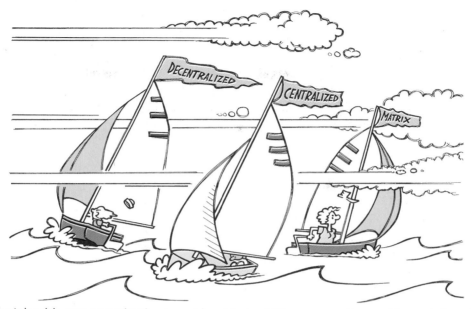

Today's health-care organizations must be able to shift course easily to withstand the winds of change.

nicians who work within the same functional or departmental unit). It is vital for beginning staff nurses to become engaged socially in their community of practice to benefit from the other practice experiences of colleagues. Preceptorships and mentors are examples of customary entries into a community of practice.

The "rumor mill" is typically a part of the informal organization. Although often described negatively, the rumor mill provides information reflective of the concerns of the work group. This information might be used to help anticipate some of the formal organization's changes.

Informal organizations help maintain meaningful communications among their members. Astute client care managers use critical thinking skills to maximize benefits afforded by the informal organization.

## HUMAN MOTIVATIONS

Historically, early studies of work organizations involved manufacturing industries. These studies were designed to learn about the **human motivations** of workers or the reasons employees responded to work situations as they did. By using this information, managers tried to increase the effectiveness of their organizations. Consequently, many of the organizational and management theories adopted by service organizations were more suited to manufacturers than to health-service providers.

Several theories contributed to the evolution of current management styles. Some of these theories are described to provide insight into the motivations of human behavior in work organizations.

## Maslow's Hierarchy of Needs

**Maslow's hierarchy of needs** is a theory of human motivation that many nursing students learn. Basically, managers following Maslow's theory believe that workers have a hierarchy of needs that drive them to make choices in a predictable manner. According to this theory, physiologic needs must be satisfied first for survival. Safety needs are the next level in the hierarchy; workers strive to meet safety needs when their physiologic needs are satisfied. The safety level includes physical and psychological needs. Next, the worker needs to feel love and to belong. Workers who gain a sense of love and belonging reach the next level and strive to gain a sense of self-esteem. When workers perceive that their contributions are valued and feel positive about themselves, they are likely to seek self-actualization. Self-actualization, the highest level need, depicts the workers' sense of fulfillment associated with their accomplishments.

Although Maslow's theory describes a positive approach to the motivation of workers, studies testing this theory revealed that satisfied needs are not motivators. Rather, unsatisfied needs, such as the need for self-actualization, were more consistent motivators. Studies also found it difficult to show that everyone has the same need hierarchy (Miner, 1980, pp. 28–37; Terry, 1992, pp. 261–263). Given its positive and negative aspects, Maslow's theory might be used to design a management strategy for motivating coworkers.

## Theories X and Y

**Theory X** has been quoted frequently as a set of the early assumptions about people that a manager might use to manage workers. In the early 1960s, McGregor, summarizing common management approaches in use at the time (Terry, 1992, p. 512), described the three major assumptions about employees that reflect Theory X. Managers assume that:

1. Employees avoid work because they dislike it.
2. They must control, direct, coerce, and threaten employees to make them strive toward organizational goals.
3. Employees lack ambition; they prefer to be directed, to avoid responsibility, and to seek security through work.

McGregor sought to stimulate more humanistic management practices and offered **Theory Y** as an alternative to Theory X. Assumptions underlying Theory Y reflect a more optimistic view of employees, as follows:

1. Employees do not dislike work; rather, they view physical and mental work as a natural part of life.
2. Employees are self-motivated to achieve goals to which they are committed.
3. Employees remain committed to goals for which they are rewarded when achieved.
4. Employees seek and accept responsibility under favorable conditions.
5. Employees are innovative in solving job-related problems.
6. Human potential is underused in most job settings (Terry, 1992).

McGregor succeeded in stimulating interest in developing participative management methods.

## Theory A

Other popular human motivating theories that are increasingly advocated are Theory A and Theory Z. **Theory A** describes the traditional American management style for work organizations of "typical American firms," including:

1. Short-term employment.
2. Predominantly downward communication patterns.
3. Emphasis on decision making of individuals versus work groups.
4. Rapid evaluation and promotion.
5. A segmented concern for employees (emphasizing hierarchic instead of functional work groups involved in mutual goal setting).

In the evolving global economy, many organizational analysts have advocated a change from the use of Theory A to the use of Theory Z to remain competitive.

## Theory Z

**Theory Z** describes the beliefs underlying the Japanese style of managing. Theory Z emphasizes:

1. Long-term employment.
2. Open communication patterns.
3. Harmonious work group or consensus decision making.
4. Slow evaluation and promotion.
5. Holistic concern for employees.

Although there is considerable popular support for this style of management, there is reason to question whether it is suitable for organizations that require significant amounts of individual flexibility and creativity (Dubrin et al., 1989, pp. 638–643). These concerns may be difficult to resolve for people who are culturally rewarded for individual achievement and when creativity and flexibility are crucial employee characteristics. Americans typically are rewarded for individual achievements, with less acknowledgment of the group efforts involved in the accomplishment. Health-service organizations depend highly on creative and flexible employees. As described earlier, the changing health-care environment and organizations are being challenged to maximize the potential of scarce human knowledge and resources. The manager's strategy needs to fit the context and one's own needs as well as the needs of others.

Another theory advocated over time throughout history is to "work with human nature" instead of against it. If the manager wants to stimulate behavior that is consistent with what people would do naturally, success is more likely. If the desired behavior is contrary to human nature, the behavior is less likely to change. The manager needs to accept the reality of human nature, both the positive and the negative potentialities, rather than acting on the basis of what one wishes human nature to be. The manager's task is to identify strategies that bring out the best in oneself as well as one's colleagues, while minimizing the worst of both (Sample, 2002, p. 105).

## Situational Leadership

Perhaps a more adaptable approach to human motivation that incorporates many of the variables important to client care managers is situational leadership. This theory of management incorporates the needs of the work group and their responses to the tasks to be done. The leader adopts a management style corresponding to the developmental level of the work group (Blanchard, 1995, pp. 22–25).

The goal of **situational leadership,** according to Hersey and Blanchard (1982, p. 312), is to "help people understand and share expectations in their environment so that they can gradually learn to supervise their own behavior and become responsible, self-motivated individuals." This theory incorporates the individual employee and work group needs, types of work tasks, and leadership styles. It advocates that managers attend to these variables in the work situation before identifying desired leadership behaviors to promote organizational effectiveness. This theory assumes that, just as there is no perfect organizational structure that fits every work group, there is no motivational theory that fits every employee.

The entry-level nurse might have the good fortune of having a situational leader when beginning an inservice orientation program. The situational leader would incorporate the entry-level nurse's needs and learning style with the resources available within the specific work group. If the work group is high in task orientation, a specific plan would be developed for successfully completing these tasks, incorporating the developmental needs of the entry-level staff nurse and the work group. If the work group is well established and developed with high esteem and task mastery, the situational leader would encourage the group's involvement,

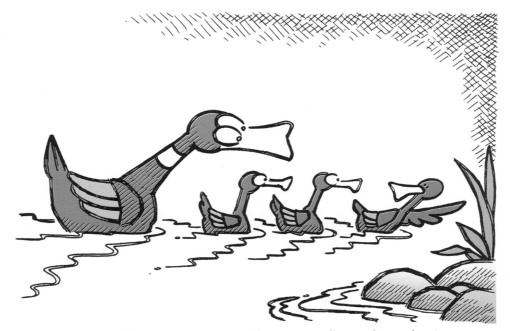

A situational leader adopts a management style corresponding to the workers' responses.

including the entry level nurse's input, in designing and implementing the inservice orientation program. In either instance, the situational leader would attend to the needs of individuals and the group, the nature and urgency of the work to be completed within the type of practice setting, and the available resources. The amount of supporting, mentoring, coaching, and directing depends on the identified needs rather than the preferred style of the leader.

Figure 1-5 depicts the major components of the concept of situational leadership. It describes the four major styles of leadership that might be adopted by a leader, based on the needs of a specific group. The diagram shows that the leader would provide varying amounts of supportive or directive behavior to the group, according to the developmental level of the group and the success of its members in completing tasks and offering support to one another. The less developed the followers, the more directive the leader would need to be, while emphasizing emotional support less, in efforts to help the group succeed. Less experienced followers (i.e., followers less confident of competence but enthusiastic and open to learning) need more clear, specific direction and close supervision; more experienced followers (i.e., followers who feel more confident and competent) would benefit from supportive leadership behaviors, such as coaching and mentoring, to reinforce confidence and competence as a group. As groups grow in competence in accomplishing tasks and confidence in their abilities to succeed, situational leaders need to delegate and direct less and support by mentoring and coaching instead.

Much has been learned through systematic study of managerial thought and human motivation. In the past, theories of human motivation often evolved from the study of industrial settings. As the industrial era is replaced by the informational era, new theories of human motivation will be tested. As appropriate organizations evolve to support customer-oriented client care managers, more useful theories of human motivation might be developed. At present, management theories advocate sensitivity to human needs and close attention to environmental variables and contexts.

## Transformational Leadership

**Transformational leadership** is a style of leading that is increasing in popularity. Perhaps its popularity is related to the evolution of organizations during the "informational era," when there is more social instability. Change has become known as the only constant. Transformational leaders offer followers supportive social characteristics including moral values, such as "honesty, fairness, responsibility and reciprocity" (Yukl, 2002, p. 241). Transformational leaders successfully influence others to gain the commitment of followers to work toward shared goals.

Although transformational leaders are charismatic, this is not sufficient for being transformational. Their distinguishing characteristic is their ability to gain the trust of followers who become motivated to do more toward shared goals than the followers were expected to do. The social influence of transformational leaders motivates their followers to reprioritize self-interests so that they work for the sake of the organization as a greater priority.

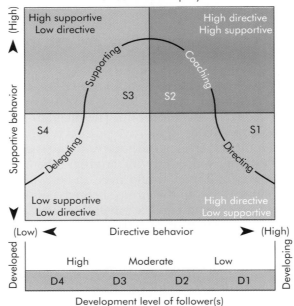

The Four Leadership Styles

FIGURE 1-5 **Situational leadership.** (Reprinted with permission from Ritvo RA, Litwin AH, Butler L: In *Managing in the age of change,* Burr Ridge, IL, 1995, Richard D. Irwin, p. 23.)

Transformational leaders use four categories of behavior to motivate their followers: (1) idealized influence (i.e., behaviors that stimulate followers to identify with the leader); (2) intellectual stimulation (i.e., behaviors that help followers to learn about the problems faced and how to view them differently to solve them); (3) individualized consideration (i.e., supporting, encouraging, and coaching followers); and (4) inspirational motivation (i.e., communicating an appealing vision and using symbols that mobilize followers' efforts while modeling desired behaviors) (Yukl, 2002, pp. 254-267). After considerable research study, transformational leaders were found to do more than other types of leaders to empower followers and develop self-confidence in the followers' abilities to create self-managed teams successfully (Yukl, 2002, p. 261). This style of leadership is particularly adapted to chaotic contexts; it also seems to be effective over the long-term.

The beginning staff nurse could benefit from knowledge of transformational leaders. These leaders may be found in any organization at any level. By using knowledge of transformational leadership, the client care manager can determine whether the leader merits followership.

## LOOKING TO THE FUTURE

The study of the science of management in the context of organizations is evolving slowly. As the practice of nursing remains an art, so does managing. Successful

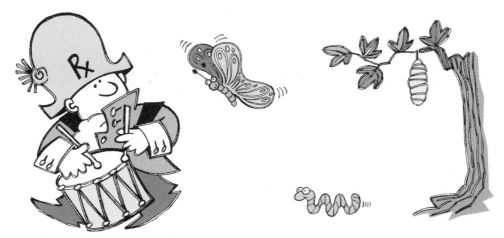

Transformational leaders motivate followers to grow to meet organizational needs.

organizations in the future increasingly will deemphasize shape or will be more unstructured. Change remains constant. To achieve internal stability with less structure, more attention will be paid to facilitating the process and building relationships inherent in fulfilling the organization's higher purpose that will never be permanently defined (Ashkenas et al., 2002, p. 307). Organizations that can learn and adapt to succeed in providing measurable success, while focusing on bottom-line results, will be more able to sustain internal stability, maintain customer and employee satisfaction and openness over time, and survive in an era of rapid change (Ashkenas et al., 2002, p. 310).

As workplaces, these organizations will use cultural and work group diversity as a strength instead of a response to personnel mandates. Organizationally, employee profiles will reflect pluralism of society; that is, the organization's work group will be selected strategically so as to be more like the population of the customers they aim to serve. As an economic strategy, diversity of the work group will be an asset for marketing services to its clientele (Imparato and Harari, 1994, pp. 186–203).

## SUMMARY

The client care manager role is an essential component of the practice of entry-level staff nurses. Current elements of the client care manager role, as defined in this book, initially were delineated by entry-level staff nurses and supervisors of such nurses. These nurses were employed in acute care, long-term, and community-based settings.

Client care management skills depend on the prior development of other inter-related nursing roles and skills. Client care management skills needed by entry-level staff nurses include the ability to use organizational routines and resources, provide direct client care, collaborate with the interdisciplinary work group, manage time purposefully, and use leadership qualities to manage others in the nursing work group.

Nursing management is not the same as nursing leadership, and these terms are not mutually exclusive. Nursing management refers to the judicious use of resources to achieve client goals. Nursing leadership implies influence, without organizational authority, that followers accept voluntarily.

Common types of organizational structures within which nurses might work are autocracy, bureaucracy, adhocracy, and matrix organizations. Boundaryless organizations are becoming more common in health care. The different types of organizational structures have varied patterns of work division and decision making. More focus on individual and organizational learning is expected in response to change associated with the informational era. Informal organizations coexist with formal organizational structures and are worthy of attention.

Managers' beliefs about the motivation of human behavior affect the people they manage. Maslow's hierarchy of needs theory has been popular, but it has been difficult to show that everyone in an organization has the same needs, as Maslow's theory stipulates. Theories X, Y, A, and Z have been used to help managers maximize the effectiveness of human resources, primarily in industrial settings. Situational leadership theory incorporates individual and work group needs, types of work tasks, and leadership styles. Transformational leadership is believed to empower followers effectively and assist in addressing shared organizational goals. To date, there is no motivational theory that fits every employee. As service-oriented organizations evolve to support client care managers, suitable theories will evolve to help them respond in a sensitive manner to their fellow employees and clients.

Change is a constant. Future organizations are expected to be less structured, emphasize results, leverage scarce human resources, and build satisfying relationships with their customers. Diversity of the work group will be viewed as an asset and used to increase organizational assets.

## APPLICATION EXERCISES

1. As you completed each nursing course, you developed nursing knowledge and skills to fulfill your core nursing roles. List the management skills you have already developed and skills you will need to develop to be a successful staff nurse.
2. Compare characteristics of nurse managers and leaders that you prefer with characteristics favored by your peers.
3. You have completed various client care assignments in a large medical center located in an urban area in the past. Now you are assigned to practice your client care management skills in a long-term care facility in a suburban community that has a capacity for 60 clients. Describe how the context of the long-term care facility will influence your nursing practice.
4. Review the organizational chart of your assigned agency. Describe the type of formal organization it is, including more than one, if accurate. Describe how the organizational boundaries promote or inhibit the staff nurses' autonomy and accountability for clinical decisions.

## APPLICATION EXERCISES—cont'd

5. In groups of two or more, critique Theory A, Theory Z, and "work with human nature" management theories. Choose the theory that you would want your manager to use. Give your reasons for your choice. Describe whether you would use the same theory and state your reason.

6. In groups of two or more, debate the pros and cons of transformational leadership as a strategy for motivating employees. Would you want your employer to use it?

## CRITICAL THINKING SCENARIO

An ideal world is without bias in the past, present, or future. The real world abounds with potential for subtle, unintentional bias toward persons perceived to be different. This learning exercise is designed to help the learner begin to sort some of the complexity of providing health care in a culturally diverse real world.

Imagine that you have recently been employed as an entry-level nurse in a busy community-based care setting. Your primary function is to provide for primary and secondary prevention (i.e., preventing diseases through promotion of positive health practices and assisting with the early detection of disease through teaching about diagnostic procedures). Many of your clientele have gender, ethnic, and spiritual beliefs different from your own; are without private health insurance; and are underemployed. Your coworkers are white, second-generation, middle-class Americans residing in suburban areas; they often express frustration with the "lack of motivation" of your clientele. You are the most recent addition to your health-care team.

1. What would you do to gain a better understanding of your clientele?
2. How would you learn about the primary purpose and values of the organization?
3. Who or what would you try to change? How?

## REFERENCES

Albrecht K: *Moving toward an internal service culture*, Northwood, IL, 1990, Jones-Irwin.

Ashkenas R, Ulrich D, Jick T, Kerr S: *The boundaryless organization: breaking the chains of organizational structure*, ed 2, San Francisco, CA, 2002, Jossey-Bass.

Blanchard, KH: Situational leadership II: Chapter Two. In Ritvo RA, Litwin AH, Butler L: *Managing in the age of change: essential skills to manage today's diverse workforce*, Burr Ridge, IL, 1995, NTL Institute: Irwin Professional Publishing.

Brown JS, Duguid P: *The social life of information,* Boston, MA, 2002, Harvard Business School Press.

Dubrin A, Ireland JRD, Williams JC: *Management and organization,* Cincinnati, OH, 1989, South Western Publishing.

Hersey P, Blanchard KH: *Management of organization behavior: utilizing human resources,* ed 4, Englewood Cliffs, NJ, 1982, Prentice-Hall.

Hillman J: *Kinds of power: a guide to its intelligent uses,* New York, NY, 1995, Currency-Doubleday.

Howard, A (editor): *The changing nature of work,* San Francisco, CA, 1995, Jossey-Bass.

Imparato N, Harari O: *Jumping the curve: innovation and strategic choice in an age of transition,* San Francisco, CA, 1994, Jossey-Bass.

Jennings J, Haughton L: *It's not the BIG that eat the SMALL . . . it's the FAST that eat the SLOW,* New York, NY, 2002, HarperCollins Publishers.

Marshall EM: *Transforming the way we work: the power of the collaborative workplace,* New York, NY, 1995, AMACOM, a division of the American Management Association.

Miner JB: *Theories of organizational behavior,* Hinsdale, IL, 1980, The Dryden Press.

Sample S: *The contrarian's guide to leadership,* San Francisco, CA, 2002, Jossey-Bass.

Schneider B, Bowen DE: *Winning the service game,* Boston, MA, 1995, The Harvard Business School Press.

Senge PM: *The fifth discipline: the art and practice of the learning organization,* first paperback edition, New York, NY, 1994, Currency Doubleday.

Terry JV: *International management handbook,* Fayetteville, AR, 1992, The University of Arkansas Press.

Wurzbach ME: Rumors, *Nurs* 85(11):89–91, 1985.

Yukl GA: *Leadership in organizations,* ed 5, Upper Saddle River, NJ, Prentice-Hall, 2002.

# 2

# *Understanding the Context of Health Care*

*When you complete this chapter, you should be able to:*

1. Describe trends of societal change that influence health-care delivery systems.
2. Describe the interrelationship of economic and technologic trends.
3. Describe the interrelationship of political and technologic trends.
4. Describe trends that promote increased community-based, outpatient care.
5. Describe the agencies commonly involved in the health-care continuum.
6. List agencies commonly involved in providing seamless client care.
7. List three different ways that client care managers use informatics, including the Internet, to provide timely care.
8. Describe how client care managers can influence changes in delivery of health-care services.

## KEY CONCEPTS

trends
informational era
Internet
external support systems
health-care continuum
types of health-care agencies
  public

private
proprietary
nonprofit
types of services
  institutionally based services
  community-based services

## TRENDS AFFECTING HEALTH CARE

This chapter is designed to help client care managers use knowledge of trends to help them identify forces underlying or causing the changes with which they are being asked to cope. These "drivers of change" (Jennings and Haughton, 2002, pp. 29–42) help the client care manager to anticipate how client perceptions are changing and ultimately to develop strategies that increase client satisfaction and effectiveness of services provided.

Nursing practice, similar to any other activity, cannot be analyzed out of context (i.e., without background knowledge of the setting). Background knowledge of the context includes enough historical background to enable the nurse to gain perspective of the trend. Factors surrounding the practice of nursing include societal, demographic, economic, global, political, technologic, and financial trends and professional organizational needs. **Trends** (patterns of change) in these areas affect health care and influence the evolution of nursing practice in certain directions. Some primary societal changes are discussed. The nurse uses knowledge of trends when discussing the desirability of various options with clients and when interacting with various health-care agencies on the client's behalf. The client care manager uses knowledge of trends to help anticipate future developments of the health-care system.

This chapter helps entry-level staff nurses understand the context of health care by applying knowledge of current trends, actively participate in making desired changes in health-care delivery, and help clients use health-care options available to them. Examples of how these trends affect health-care delivery are provided.

## Primary Societal Trends

Several futurists (predictors of future trends) have described primary trends in terms of major societal changes. At the turn of the 21st century, many predictions were made, some of which are materializing. The interdependencies of global existence will persist. The rates of increase of population growth of rich countries are decreasing, whereas those of poor countries continue to increase (Ikenberry, 2001). These trends continue to occur, increasingly on a global level. Although globalization may help to stabilize world politics, instability will persist with continued economic inequality. Consequently, work with nongovernmental agencies will grow in importance in reducing social tension and violence. Earlier, Toffler described in detail the transformation of the industrial era into the **informational era**. This change, he explained, would entail an increased focus on contexts, relationships, and holism (Toffler, 1980, p. 30). Later findings supported Toffler's predictions (Naisbitt and Aburdene, 1990). Although slow to progress, the increasingly more open borders associated within the context of globalization will promote not only global economic policies, but also global security, environmental, education, and health-care policies (Johnson, 2001). This growth of global policies is aimed at reducing the source of terrorism and increasing the number of potential partners in sustaining a civilized society. Progress will slow with the complications of increasing global complexity; a much-needed recognition of our common humanity may continue to be disguised by regional differences and consequently delay progress in addressing common human needs (Johnson, 2001).

As the informational era continues, differences in cultures and the contexts surrounding them are communicated almost instantaneously by technology. The need for negotiation and collaboration is increasingly stark given increasing incidents of violence. When negotiation and collaboration occur, it is directed at reducing violence and terrorism and promoting human survival.

### Technology

The road of technology development of the past is not the same as the road ahead (Dertouzos, 2001, pp. 195–217). Rather than making technology that is difficult for most people to use, technology needs to be designed better to serve people. Increasingly more people are able to afford the technology and learn how to use it and use many types of technologic innovations to promote self-sufficiency and exercise autonomy in making decisions affecting themselves. Computers as vehicles for processing and transmitting information are transforming work, the workplace, and lifestyles. Information technology is being used to reduce dependence and interdependence on others and increase speed of access and analyses. Technology has enabled the mass media to provide a great variety of information in many diverse forms, not only in the workplace, but also at home for personal use. The use of the **Internet** is discussed later in this chapter.

Drucker (1999) described the multidimensional aspects of the real revolutionary impact of the informational era. He indicated that its impact is not solely the ability to transmit important information. He reflected on the rapid growth of e-commerce (i.e., business transactions occurring through the Internet instead of slower traditional means) and its influence on the worldwide distribution of goods and services. Giving several historical examples of similar changes related to the Industrial Revolution, Drucker (1999) predicted that e-commerce will be the basis for the emergence of unpredicted industries and the abruptness with which they will emerge. The e-commerce industries will not change the nature of the processes inherent in the business; rather the resulting routinization of processes will save time and ultimately costs of the products or services. Examples of e-commerce-based industries are biotechnology and salmon fish farming (Drucker, 1999). Drucker (1999) also indicated that information technology is revealing a significant difference between how children learn and how schools teach. This trend needs to be integrated into designing meaningful health education materials.

As the informational era proceeds, more people use computers to manage and transmit information at work and in their personal lives; concurrently, they need to apply critical thinking skills to decipher useful from inaccurate information. Individuals who use various print and electronic media to obtain information do so to meet personal information needs and interests. Significant efforts are being made to lessen the number of individuals who do not use technology to decrease the economic gap between the "haves and have-nots": Witness the willingness of large computer hardware and software vendors who provide computer equipment at reduced cost to elementary and secondary schools.

### Individual Choice

Evolving technology is increasing individual choices. Adherence to a common schedule is less emphasized than during the industrial era. More individuals are taking an active role in decision making about the use of their time and resources. In keeping with these trends, more clients expect to be included in decisions affecting their health care to enable them to commit to making necessary changes in their daily living without making unnecessary changes that do not match their patterns and timing of daily activities. Clients expect to make choices about health-care options that conform to their specific individual lifestyles.

In response to demands of their increased participation in the workplace, the emerging roles of women continue to alter the divisions of work within the family. In addition, the traditional nuclear family is being replaced by many diverse family structures and roles. Family caregiving patterns are changing as family structures and roles shift (Aburdene and Naisbitt, 1992, pp. 216–244). That is, smaller family size and extended families are making varied choices on how they use their resources to provide traditional (versus highly complex and technical) home care.

### Change

As the evolution of the informational era continues, the pace of change is expected to increase, placing greater demands on managers of organizational resources. Due to the pacing of change, implementing change will allow less time for planning and advanced training. Rather, the planning will need to be done and carried out immediately before effecting the change. Computerized information management systems and use of reference resources are examples of changes that will occur frequently.

Constant change is related to the dynamics of the global context and other external health-care and social agencies (Dienamann and Van de Castle, 2002, pp. 303–319). Staff nurses increasingly will use a variety of information technology to manage client care. To manage information effectively, client care managers, as knowledge workers, need to be computer literate. They need to access multiple sources of information using available technology at the work site. Instead of relying on printed references, client care managers will rely increasingly on computer databases to obtain and print information from the organization's intranet or the Internet. In addition to integrating clients in decision making required for their care, the nurse needs to access current information that is constantly changing at an accelerating pace to provide personalized health education. This information may be available within local electronic libraries and information resources or client health education centers or databases to which the agency subscribes. Although many client care managers perceive the constancy of change as a persistent stressor, it also can be a stimulus for personal and professional growth that leads to increased productivity and reward.

### Holism

The nature of organizational structures is changing to reflect increased emphasis on the need to provide coordinated care. As information technology is leveraged as a resource, more health-care organizations will become integrated vertically and horizontally. The hospital as an entity or corporation is being replaced by an integrated health system. Integrated health systems will remove boundaries between types of providers and types of cooperating agencies so that communication of needed information can occur apparently seamlessly. Increased use of information technology networking will increase the efficiency of transmitting information to a variety of providers in more than one agency to address financial pressures to decrease (or not to increase needlessly) length of stay (Rodeghero, 1999, p. 37). Nurses increasingly will use relational databases from several agencies composing the total health-care enterprise to gather information to plan and provide holistic care, or they might use several related databases to gain knowledge needed to answer important clinical questions (Thede, 2002, p. 79). Health-care systems, as business organizations, increasingly serve several purposes rather than a single primary function, and consequently they need to organize resources differently. Acute care health agencies frequently provide services to the sick and injured as inpatients, episodic outpatient care (i.e., short-stay surgery), and health promotion services designed to prevent and detect diseases. Typical health-care agencies are restructuring their organizations to provide primary care designed for health promotion and maintenance; secondary care, emphasizing the diagnosis and treatment of disease; and traditional tertiary care, focusing on the treatment of disease complications. This restructuring often is related to the various types of financing mechanisms.

Corporations, including health-care systems, are held legally accountable for the products and services they produce and for their positive and negative impact on the environment. Health agencies, as legal entities, are expected to use technology and human resources to improve the quality of the communities and environments in which they are located. The public expects these agencies to promote the well-being of the community, while providing services to individual clients. Hospitals are expected to provide care for ill individuals and to promote the health of community residents. Consistent with the trend toward greater holism, health-care agencies are involved locally, regionally, and nationally to promote positive images as providers of health services instead of predominantly illness-oriented care.

### Environmental Issues

Closely related to public perception of corporate interconnectedness is the increased emphasis on preserving environmental integrity. Wastes, including those that are toxic to people and the environment, are increasing in volume. The public is aware of the growing difficulties in safely disposing of wastes. More people are changing their lifestyles to reduce wastes to preserve a safe environment. Environmental goals include safe water, air, and food chains for future generations. Many people are willing to pay more for purified water and food grown and preserved naturally without chemicals to maintain their health and that of the environment. Emerging basic values held by increasing numbers of people are resulting in greater commitment to integrate nature in human activities, rather than striving to dominate it (McGinn, 2002, pp. 75–100).

Health-care agencies are expected to comply with laws regulating the management of toxic waste in the interest of public safety. Client care managers are expected to incorporate knowledge of these trends when managing wastes within the work environment and when assessing client needs and identifying options to meet them. Client care managers are expected to dispose of toxic, infectious, or otherwise dangerous wastes in a carefully prescribed manner and to assist their coworkers to do the same.

### Evolving Community Populations

The environmental health movement is intricately involved with the increased interdependencies and complexities of multinational corporations. People involved with these multinational corporations are more mobile and culturally diverse than in the past. Widespread global migration will stimulate changes in ethnic and racial composition of American communities (Briggance and Burke, 2002, p. 61). As a result, the lifestyles and health-care needs of the evolving community populations will be increasingly culturally diverse. Client care managers need to apply knowledge of diverse cultures to communicate with a wide variety of people or develop "cultural competence." Another strategy to help address ethnically diverse clientele is to develop a health-care work force that reflects the proportional ethnic representation in the population served (Briggance and Burke, 2002, p. 64).

## Demographic Trends

Several demographic trends influence population needs for nursing services. Common types of demographic changes are presented.

### Cultural Diversity

Perhaps one of the most profound demographic trends is that of the increasing numbers and proportions of people of color (i.e., Asian Americans, African Americans, and Latinos), projected to compose 85% of the U.S. population within the next 20 years (Baker, 1995, p. 170). This cultural change will have an impact on the ethnic backgrounds of clientele and the health-care work force. Client care managers will apply knowledge of the key issues inherent in a culturally diverse society to avoid miscommunications, misinterpretations, and misunderstandings between clientele and health-care providers. When the health-care work force becomes increasingly culturally diverse, the need for cultural competence is likely to be more apparent.

### Aging Population

The proportion of elderly persons living in the United States is increasing as it is globally (FutureScan, 2001, p. 1). This trend is related to many factors, including the types of health services available throughout the life span and the declining birth rate associated with contraceptive use (Engelman et al., 2002, pp. 137–142). As the U.S. population ages, long-term care may consume a greater portion of the health-care budget (Estes, 1990, pp. 4–8).

### Continued Population Shift

The U.S. population continues to shift from rural to metropolitan areas. Concentrating populations in environments with increased pollution increases risks to health.

These risks continue to stimulate political interest in reducing pollution and maintaining a safe environment. This population shift is likely to increase the need for nursing services to promote and maintain health and care for sick people.

### Risk Factors and Personal Choice

Another major trend related to demographics is that many factors contributing to common health problems of the U.S. population reflect individual lifestyle choices and are preventable. Personal choice will continue to influence individuals to change exercise, diet, and stress reduction strategies to reduce risk factors under their control (Gardner and Halweil, 2000, pp. 59–78). Nursing services will need to assess risk factors of clients and how they are being addressed to help individuals change their lifestyles.

## Economic Trends

Economic interests shape the evolution of technology and health care. The types of health-care services delivered continue to be limited by multiple factors, most notably cost constraints. Many health-care services require highly skilled providers and complex equipment and supplies. Clients and providers need to consider the costs, benefits, and financing of health care within the context of the global economy. Health-care services compete with other types of human needs and services, such as education, transportation, public safety, and security. As the "war on terrorism" continues, health-care services as a component of human services will continue to play a key role in providing safety from violence (Renner, 2002, p. 172).

Economic trends probably will continue to dominate the evolution of the health-care system. Cost-effectiveness issues are stimulating the evolution of prospective health-care financing mechanisms. Health insurance options made available to employees include health promotion and maintenance services, in addition to the traditional diagnoses and treatments for diseases (Curtin, 1992, pp. 7–8). Consequently, greater emphasis is being placed on primary care provided in community-based settings, in addition to the traditional acute care settings (Curtin, 1990). The working relationships between health insurance programs and health-care agencies depends on clientele. This type of interrelationship works to continue the bonding of health-care agencies with businesses and industries in the community. Although the cost-effectiveness of disease prevention has been discussed for decades in nursing, it is being recognized slowly by the entire medical community, with an emphasis on holism long espoused by nursing. This trend is consistent with the values held by nurses about the need to provide client-centered care (Gillette, 1988, pp. 10–11). Although increasing dissatisfaction with health maintenance organizations is well established, there is no concrete evidence that it is mobilized sufficiently to force change contrary to the vested interests of the health insurance industry.

## Global Trends

Economists speak of marketing goods and services in a global economy. There will continue to be movement of business production outside of the United States, resulting in increased unemployment. With the emergence of a global marketplace, economic forces will continue to exert substantial influence on health-care programs. Consequently, employers will continue to monitor the "bottom line" (total overall amounts) of profits, and the insured are likely to be paying larger deductibles, while insurance premiums and the number of uninsured increase. These trends are likely to continue.

## Political Trends

The cost of health care has increased faster than the cost of living. As the cost of health care increases, fewer people can afford it. Economic interests are intertwined with political relationships. Because there are many vested interests in the systems that provide quality health care and pay for it, political conflicts have arisen in many areas. Individuals have been required to use a larger proportion of their resources to pay for health care. Many employers providing health insurance benefits to their employees have argued that the increasing costs of health-care benefits have increased the costs of their products or services and that this business expense has interfered with their ability to compete in the global economy.

With increased political pressure and monetary limits, government-sponsored programs will continue to pay less of the total costs of health care. For individuals with limited incomes, increased out-of-pocket costs will require some to choose between food or health care. Consequently, individuals without adequate health

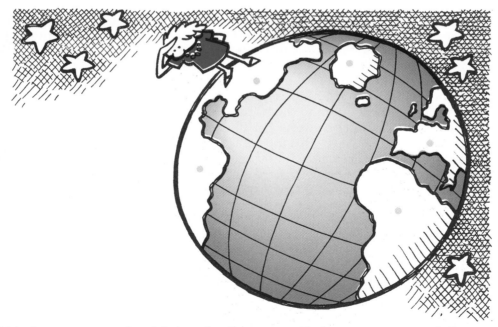

With the emergence of a global marketplace, economic forces exert greater influence on health-care programs.

insurance may wait longer to access care and risk using more costly inpatient services because they are more likely to be included in publicly funded insurance programs.

As the pace of change in the informational era accelerates and health-care costs increase, financing health care is likely to remain a political issue. In the future, related issues, such as living wills, assisted deaths, and personal responsibilities for maintaining health, will remain common topics of political discussion (Nornhold, 1990, pp. 35–41). Individual expectations to participate in decisions affecting health care continue to persist.

As the American population ages and more people become entitled to health care financed by the government, quality health care will grow as a social concern. As demographic changes are integrated into the political system, legislation will be enacted to address issues in accordance with the basic social values of the public. Increased public participation in decisions at various governmental levels is likely to result in greater interest in satisfying political and social human needs. People with vested interests are more likely to express their perceptions and needs in an attempt to influence political decisions affecting them. Despite the fact that health care is highly valued, the public has placed limits on health-care costs, although on the personal level, individuals desire optimal care. As costs have increased, individuals pay more of the actual cost of health care, rather than relying on government or private insurance programs.

Client care managers need to be aware of the effects of current legislation on their nursing practice and on the quality of care afforded individuals throughout the health-care continuum. As professionals and citizens, they are expected to communicate their concerns to their employers and elected political representatives (i.e., as the "shortage" of nurses grows, the use of mandatory overtime [where legal] also increases, which contributes to the increasing "shortage"). Health-care financing trends will be described in more detail later.

## Technologic Trends

The evolution of technology is driven by economic benefits (i.e., technology that increases cost-effectiveness, quality of care, or customer satisfaction is likely to gain quick acceptance). Consequently, much information is gathered and used to analyze aspects of a corporation's products or services to determine technologic approaches to reducing costs. In accordance with these trends, it should not surprise client care managers to see many cost-cutting technologic innovations designed for use in various health-care settings (Lower and Nauert, 1993, pp. 42, 44; Matz and Gary, 1993, p. 96FF). More technology will be rented instead of sold so that the support services needed to maintain it are provided (Hall, 2000, pp. S14–S15).

Information technology is used in health care to gather and transmit information in a timely manner to various providers, between health-care agencies, and within various departments of agencies. Nurses will continue to use computerized information systems to gather information and communicate with others (Simpson, 1993, pp. 30, 32). This communication of essential and confidential

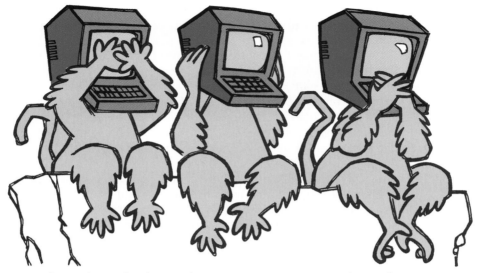

Information technology such as computers cannot perceive truth or error.

information will continue to be integral to providing cost-effective nursing services. Considerable effort will be needed to ensure that this information is accurate and that access is limited to approved users. In addition, computerized information systems will continue to be used to analyze patterns of care, with an emphasis on costs, benefits, and effectiveness (Kennedy, 2002, pp. 94–108).

Nurses need to remember that the technology used in health care increases the complexity of care. They must use it properly (as any equipment) and realize that it cannot and will not replace their professional skills, knowledge, and judgments. Information technology provides additional tools to help nurses practice their profession, but it cannot perceive truth or errors. Nurses need to rely on their own analyses of available data in the health-care context to help them determine its relevance to a client's care. They *must* use critical thinking and clinical decision-making skills to evaluate client responses.

## Government Involvement

Health-care financing mechanisms are tied closely to government regulations. Government agencies have assumed greater responsibility for the cost of health care for high-risk groups, such as the very young, the elderly, the poor, and the unemployed. Consequently, government payment for health care increasingly uses prospective payment mechanisms, which pay a specified amount for specific categories of care, such as diagnosis-related groups (DRGs) or resource utilization groups (RUGs), regardless of actual costs. Because government payments now are limited, health-care agencies attempt to control their costs by controlling the clients' length of stay. In some cases, cost-effective quality care may be compromised. By focusing on shortening lengths of stay, many health-care organizations unintentionally deemphasized individual client needs (Smeltzer, 1990, pp. 1–10). Government programs have generated increased regulations as a primary method of maintaining quality care. Public acceptance of care that is regulated increasingly by the government has declined because providers of care and individual clients have decreased opportunities to participate in decisions affecting care. Political support for further changes in financing health care is increasing.

As mentioned earlier, the number of elderly persons continues to increase, and this trend is expected to continue. Increasing government involvement in financing health care seems inevitable due to spiraling costs and the increase in the number of high-risk individuals, such as the elderly, who tend to be politically active. Considerable effort will be required to address the needs for costly illness care, while providing health promotion and maintenance services that are expected to be less costly in the long-term.

Perhaps the most widely known methods of government financing of health care are the Medicare insurance programs, Parts A and B, which are administered through the Social Security Administration. Medicare sometimes is referred to as the *Title XVIII program*. It is a health insurance program for disabled or elderly persons and their dependents. Medicare Part A pays for some acute and convalescent care. Medicare Part B provides benefits to pay for physician and other treatment services, such as those provided in ambulatory care departments or medical clinics. The financing mechanisms of Medicare have been influential in increasing the number of health-care clinics and treatments offered on an ambulatory basis. Printed materials about Medicare programs can be obtained from local post offices or local offices of the Social Security Administration.

As the population of eligible Medicare participants has increased, the costs of health care have increased, but the percentage of total health-care costs paid by Medicare has decreased. Individual annual deductibles also have increased since 1967. The amount of payment for services varies and is determined by fiscal intermediaries, which are large insurance companies that have contracted with the federal government to manage reimbursement. As a result of these decreases in Medicare payments, many people obtain private supplementary insurance to help pay for the actual costs of their health care.

Closely associated with the Medicare insurance program is Medicaid, a health insurance program for financially needy people of all ages. Medicaid sometimes is referred to as the *Title XIX program*. Part of the Medicaid insurance program is state funded. To be eligible for Medicaid, a client must meet stringent financial requirements and typically must apply at authorized local welfare agencies. Given the high costs of health care, it is common for clients to become eligible for Medicaid after experiencing extensive injuries or catastrophic illnesses that require expensive treatment. Further information about eligibility requirements usually can be obtained from social service staff employed by various health agencies or local social welfare departments.

To receive payment from either Medicare or Medicaid, health-care agencies are required to meet a wide variety of "conditions of participation," such as requirements for life safety, staffing, quality assurance programs, and types of services

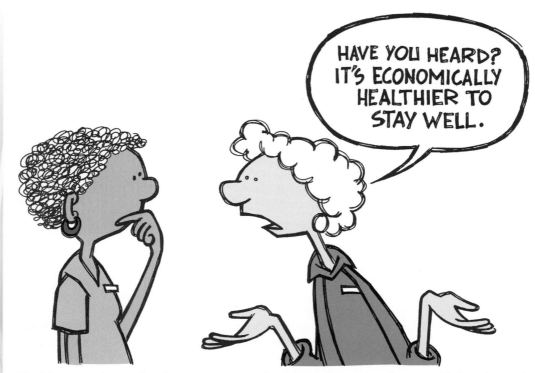

Health promotion and maintenance are preferable to the current focus on high-tech, costly illness care.

provided. These conditions are detailed in the *Federal Register*, a government publication of federal regulations. In addition, states have their own criteria for licensing health-care agencies; these agencies often are required to meet two different standards of care due to differences in state and federal requirements. In such cases, they often attempt to meet the higher standards to obtain maximum reimbursement for services.

## Professional Organizational Trends

As previously described, recipients of health care expect to participate in decisions affecting them. The providers of health care also want to participate in the development of a system that addresses their needs.

As the complexities of health care increase, the variety of providers and caregivers and the number of corresponding professional organizations are increasing. These organizations help socialize health-care providers into their various professional roles (sets of expected behaviors for meeting societal needs) by developing position or policy statements on various issues that describe responses for their members.

Each profession has one or more representative organizations. The American Nurses' Association is the national professional organization for nurses. There also are numerous specialty nursing organizations. Each professional organization attempts to (1) guide the profession in meeting societal needs and (2) safeguard the interests of its members. The American Nurses' Association has established standards of nursing practice that apply to nursing practice in any setting. Some specialty organizations also offer certification. Specialty organizations represent various areas of specialized or advanced nursing practice. Specialty organizations have established standards of practice in critical care, rehabilitation, orthopedics, and operating room nursing. Not all members of specialty nursing organizations are certified. Individuals who are certified (having met established criteria of nursing knowledge, skill, or experience) are expected to meet established standards of specialty nursing practice. Client care managers also are expected to meet the general standards of practice delineated by the American Nurses' Association.

To guide their profession, members develop standards of care and codes of conduct, which are made available to the public. Although membership in a professional organization and adherence to standards of care and codes of conduct are voluntary, these criteria often are used as guidelines to evaluate safe practice.

To ensure that their interests are addressed, care providers participate in shaping the health-care system through the political activities of their organizations. Professional organizations function as advocates of health-care providers and ultimately influence the evolution of the health-care system. Professional organizations also influence health-care legislation.

## Trends and Their Effect on Health Care

The health-care delivery system has been affected powerfully by the transformation of the industrial era to the informational era. Change is dynamic (versus linear) and continuous. Concerns about individual choice, participation in decisions affecting oneself, and sensitivities to the contexts in which health care is provided are some primary social trends. The world has become a global market driven by changing technology and characterized by complex political interdependence. Clusters of various trends lead to societal changes that affect health-care systems (Figure 2-1). Given the nursing focus on the whole person over the individual's life span and the need to minimize costs, health promotion and maintenance are preferable to the current focus on high-tech, costly illness care.

### EXTERNAL SUPPORT SYSTEMS

**External support systems** include all the agencies that provide health-care services to clients separately or in collaboration with a specific health-care agency. Nurses are expected to use knowledge of external support systems to help clients meet their health-care needs. Community-based health-care agencies are key elements of a client's health-care system. In the informational era, external support systems have numerous and varied interrelationships. These interrelationships, evolving around who is paying, who is providing, and who is receiving benefits,

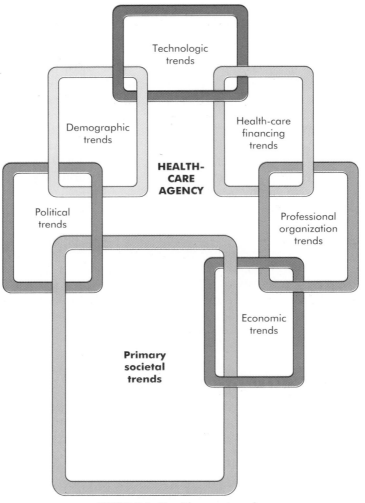

FIGURE 2-1 Health-care trends.

depend on which agencies are involved and, increasingly, on how clients finance their health care (i.e., the client frequently chooses one of several options of health insurance programs on the basis of age, family composition, costs, and preferences of primary care providers and inpatient facilities).

The nurse is expected to assess individual health needs and help the client select satisfactory options from the array of available services. Due to the rising costs of care, paid increasingly by individuals, clients need information and referrals to less costly services to meet their health needs. Although the mass media provide the public with general information about available community resources, the nurse is expected to make appropriate specific referrals for needed care. Entry-level staff nurses are not expected to "know everything"; rather, they are expected to use resources that are available within a health-care organization, recognize limitations in their knowledge, and ask for help from others (i.e., consult with nursing case managers, advanced practice nurses, social workers, or community health nurse discharge planning coordinators).

Clients expect to be involved in decisions affecting their lives and health care. Before their admission, many clients know how long they will be hospitalized. Often they are not aware, however, of the various options likely to meet best their health needs or of the consequences of selecting them. Nurses are expected to evaluate regularly individual client progress toward desired goals related to changing or discontinuing health services. Clients expect feedback about their progress, and they expect to participate in their discharge planning. Either the clients or their families should assume responsibility for making arrangements for continued care with help from health-care providers.

Nurses are expected to take initiative and be creative in helping clients address their health needs. Nurses use information from various sources to help clients select the options best suited to their health and insurance needs. The client and the nurse assume responsibility for satisfying health-care needs within the limits of cost and available resources. It is crucial to understand that the nurse's primary function is to assist the client to identify health needs and what is needed to address them. Secondarily, the nurse may help the client decide how the needed services will be financed.

## HEALTH-CARE CONTINUUM

The **health-care continuum** is the range of all health-care services, from services that promote and maintain health or optimal well-being to services that support services requisite for a peaceful death. Figure 2-2 depicts the health-care continuum. The characteristics of health-care systems reflect (1) common strategies used to access publicly funded health-care programs, (2) the many public and private agencies used throughout the health-care continuum, and (3) the nature of individual clients' needs. Each health-care agency is likely to have numerous printed reference materials, electronic databases, and human resources available to help nurses maintain current sources of information about the evolving availability of services. Health-care agencies design and revise service programs to address various needs throughout the health-care continuum on the basis of available resources.

### Common Access Strategies

The entry-level staff nurse uses knowledge of agencies involved in the health-care continuum to initiate referrals and make discharge plans. The type and purpose of an agency affect the eligibility or admission requirements clients must meet to receive the agency's services. The client's options for care often are affected by the increasing governmental financing of health care and by the availability of health insurance benefits. Although this strategy remains (ethically) controversial, for many agencies the financing mechanisms of health care dictate who receives which services.

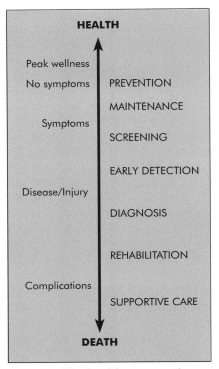

FIGURE 2-2 The health-care continuum.

The staff nurse is expected to use knowledge of various agencies and financing mechanisms to plan and evaluate client care. Sometimes a health care agency provides a community resource directory as a reference. This information is used to determine the client's needs, plan priorities of care, and estimate the client's length of stay, if hospitalization is needed on the basis of available community options. The nurse is expected to use available community-based options to provide cost-effective efficient client care rather than costly inpatient services whenever feasible.

The context or setting (e.g., acute, long-term, community-based care) of a health-care agency is influential in shaping nursing practice. The primary purpose of an agency is determined by the type of agency (i.e., inpatient, acute, long-term, primary care) and the types of clients it serves. The context affects not only what the nurse does, but also how it is done, as influenced by available organizational resources. Acute care settings are different from long-term care settings in terms of staffing, equipment, and supplies. Another important variable related to the context of an agency is its relative location on the health-care continuum.

The next section focuses on the predominant functions of common types of agencies. There is considerable overlap, however, in the functions of various agencies. Because many health-care organizations are multipurpose, an agency might declare that it promotes and maintains health and treats illnesses of clients. Each agency has one or two predominant functions that dictate their clients' eligibility requirements and the type of care delivered. Various methods of paying for services also affect the context of care and the focus of the practice setting.

## Types of Agencies

Basically, there are two major **types of health-care agencies**: public and private.

### Public Agencies

Various levels of government authorize **public agencies.** They are controlled and managed financially by the level of government legally authorizing them, whether it is federal, state, or local. Federal health agencies are governed or controlled by the U.S. government. They may be administered through the Department of Health and Human Services. Perhaps the most widely known federal government health-care agencies are federal hospitals, such as the National Institutes of Health and Veterans' Administration health-care facilities. Other federal health agencies include those that provide services to military personnel or Native Americans.

State-regulated government health-care agencies (often supported partially by federal funds) are typically available to clients with special needs. These special needs include acute illnesses and mental or developmental disorders. Individuals with various developmental disabilities, injuries, or diseases that interfere with their ability to hold paid employment can apply for assistance from state divisions of vocational rehabilitation. Vocational rehabilitation counselors assess individual needs for special treatment, education, training, and financial assistance. Social service staff employed by various health agencies usually can provide information needed to refer clients to vocational rehabilitation programs.

Other state government agencies are involved in health care indirectly. Nurses need to know which state agencies license and maintain registries of qualified health-care providers. These state agencies help ensure that health-care providers meet mandatory licensing requirements. The primary function of these regulatory agencies is to protect the public. The state licensing agencies collaborate closely with the state departments that maintain legal definitions of nursing that must be followed within a state. These legal definitions of required minimum practice are in contrast to the standards of nursing practice delineated by professional organizations describing desired professional practice for various disciplines. The staff of these licensing agencies consults about various situations that might result in unsafe practices. Information about licensing requirements and practice is contained in state statutes and administrative codes. These resources are usually available in the reference section of local libraries.

Frequently, legal standards of professional practice at the state level differ significantly from the standards detailed by the professional organizations described earlier. The legal definitions for safe practice must be followed within a state. In contrast to the standards of nursing practice delineated by professional organizations, which are the same nationwide, these legal definitions frequently differ from state to state.

In a similar manner, the operation of different types of health-care facilities is determined by specific state regulations, which are described in state statutes or administrative codes. If this information is needed but unavailable within the health agency, it is usually available in local public libraries. These regulations guide organizational operations and define the legal parameters of nursing practice within the various contexts where nurses work. Practicing nurses need to know these parameters. Client care managers employed in long-term care agencies are expected to know the specific limits of the various "levels of care" that are provided within the context of state definitions and regulations.

Local public agencies are supervised by locally elected officials who may serve on governing boards. These agencies frequently are county acute and long-term care facilities that receive their primary direction from elected officials; they may receive federal and state funding. An example of a public agency is a county health department that provides therapeutic home care services (largely funded by Medicare and Medicaid programs) and preventive programs designed to meet the various health promotion needs of residents in the specified area. Client care managers are expected to be aware of the availability of county health department options and the eligibility requirements for these services.

Closely related to the county health department are locally controlled county long-term care (inpatient) facilities and departments of social services, housing, and recreation. In addition, community-based facilities and programs are frequently available for special populations (e.g., Offices of Aging, Aid for Dependent Children). Depending on individual client needs, client age, and agency requirements, the client care manager may collaborate with these agencies to enable the client to meet basic human needs.

Schools often provide limited health or support services. It is necessary to be knowledgeable about differences in schools and the age groups they typically serve. Local elementary, secondary, and postsecondary schools provide different types of health-care services to support the health-care programs of children, adolescents, and adults. These agencies are instrumental in helping clients meet their developmental needs or occupation goals.

At the other end of the age spectrum, the county or area Office of Aging often provides a wide array of supportive services to older people. These support services include information and referral; nutrition programs, including home-delivered meals; socialization activities; recreation; chore services; assistance in completing forms to obtain health insurance benefits; and special transportation for medical appointments. Although information about these agencies is frequently available in local community resource manuals, social service or other support staff may be excellent sources of current information within a health-care agency.

### Private Agencies

In contrast to public agencies, **private agencies** have voluntary governing bodies. They are not governed or administered by government employees. Private agencies are not directly publicly funded, although fees for their services might be paid by publicly funded insurance programs. Clients served by private agencies may use Medicare or Medicaid insurance benefits to pay for services received. In addition to meeting specific "conditions for participation," private agencies are required to meet state licensing requirements and regulations corresponding to the classification of their governing authorities. Private agencies provide health-care services needed throughout the health-care continuum, as do public agencies.

Private agencies can be classified further as being for profit or not for profit. For-profit or **proprietary agencies** have financial gain as one of their primary purposes. Not-for-profit or **nonprofit agencies** receive tax exemptions but cannot transfer funds acquired in excess of expenses to owners or governing bodies.

Common private health agencies provide two **types of services:** institutionally based or community-based services. Traditional **institutionally based services** are provided on a 24-hour daily basis in settings such as hospitals or nursing homes. Traditional **community-based services** are provided on an intermittent basis in settings such as homes or neighborhood health clinics. As health-care agencies have become more organizationally complex and competitive, more acute and long-term health-care institutions have developed programs to provide community-based services that for limited periods may provide 24-hour daily care. In addition to traditional inpatient services, an increasing number of acute care facilities provide episodic (intermittent illness–oriented) primary health care, emergency care, and follow-up ambulatory care. Comparable services often are provided in proprietary medical clinics or physicians' offices at comparable or lower cost. These acute care facilities also provide inpatient services, including 1-day or extended-stay programs that are similar to traditional hospital treatment but of a shorter duration. Sometimes the needed equipment, staffing, or cost determines to whom and where the services are provided. In other situations, the specific requirements of health insurance programs may influence the client to select one setting over another to reduce personal costs.

Depending on the variety of agencies in the region, some acute care facilities also provide other supportive programs, such as screening tests, health education programs, telephone reassurance services, and self-care support group assistance. Some health agencies provide health maintenance services to market or promote a positive image within the community. These contacts with the public also are used to promote access to other hospital services. In accordance with evolving demographic trends, acute care facilities are involved in providing services needed by chronically ill people. For the most part, these services are of limited duration for specified diagnostic and treatment purposes.

Long-term care facilities sometimes provide a wide variety of services to chronically ill people, in addition to the traditional 24-hour daily care. Typically, however, their primary purpose is to provide health and social services to people who reside in the facilities for varying and often indefinite periods. In addition, long-term care facilities might provide day-care, home-care, or respite-care programs to reduce the high costs of institutionalization.

## Nature of Clients' Needs

Ideally the client's health and social needs determine participation in selected health-care options. More frequently, however, cost reduction efforts undertaken by public or private insurance programs dictate which programs clients participate in or which services they receive. Emphasis is placed on costs and the clients' sources of payment in many current health-care contexts. Consequently, nurses need information about various options, about the client's rationale for choices, and about the risks and advantages of selected options. In addition, nurses are expected to document accurately services rendered to meet the requirements of third-party payers, such as insurance programs. In this confusing and demanding routine, nurses incorporate advocacy activities to help their clients obtain and pay for needed care.

## CHANGE PROCESS AND HEALTH CARE

Historically, health care was not perceived as a business or industry as it currently is (Schneider and Bowen, 1995, p. 1). Is this change desirable? What has promoted this change? How can a client care manager exert influence on the evolution of health care to serve its primary purpose best (Bruhn, 2001, pp. 47–58)? The process of change is increasingly complex and broader in scope. Leadership skills needed to guide change would incorporate awareness of global competition, of the increasing pace of change, and of the need for reorganizing with a sharp focus on customer needs (Becher, 2001, pp. 164–179). Box 2-1 lists guidelines for change.

Client care managers need to understand that the process of change involves many factors, vested interests or values of stakeholders, and organizations with multiple implied and explicit purposes. Entry-level staff nurses are less likely than more experienced staff nurses to need to unlearn "old ways" before making desired changes. It is helpful to gain and maintain perspective on the process of change and common effects on those experiencing it (Manion, 1995, pp. 41–43). With the rapid pace of change, appreciating the emotional demands of multiple changes might lend support and recognition of progress and accomplishments. This strategy would help the initiators of change and those experiencing change to maintain perspective.

Accordingly, changing social trends girded by technologic advances and demographic changes affect the political issues in financing health care. Organizations, providers of care, and customers (clients), as stakeholders (persons with vested interests) in health-care reform, advocate changes that fit their particular needs and perspectives. In periods of rapid change, it becomes crucial that the primary purposes of health-care organizations are communicated explicitly to all of the stakeholders so that intelligent strategies can be developed to maximize benefits for all concerned. Progress in meeting stated purposes must be measured, and indications for additional changes must be identified.

Change in the health-care system is dynamic, not linear (i.e., progressive, straightforward). Health-care reform cannot be stopped any more than the trends forcing change can be reversed. As the demands for health promotion and maintenance increase consistent with increasing productivity, the focus of health care will shift accordingly, if slowly. Concurrently, individuals entitled to treatment of complex diseases also will demand resources. As in the past, the protection of individual rights long held dear will persist, with broad cultural support adding complexity.

BOX 2-1

## Guidelines for Change

1. Start with a positive attitude about the challenge of change. There is something in every organization that wants to stay the same. Change is tougher than it looks; yet the future depends on it.
2. Identify the stakeholders in the change, paying attention to those who are observers/critics and those who are likely to be participant supporters. Help all of the stakeholders see how the change benefits them. Focus on client needs as clients perceive them.
3. Communicate all the facts and how-to's to those affected as the key strategy for managing fear and the unknown. Emphasize relationships; rehearse changes before implementation when feasible.
4. Ask for constructive input from stakeholders; communicate and celebrate progress with the change process.
5. Reinforce the change process incorporated in the organization's mission, values, culture, and everyday operations. Help others understand how the desired change fits.
6. Emphasize an openness about change. Participate in evolving a learning workplace that teaches how to "go with the flow" and uses change to its maximum benefit for quality care for clients.
7. Invite everyone to participate in the change process; make an effort to include all stakeholders in bringing about the desired changes—win/win results for all involved (McFarland et al., 1993, pp. 220–222).

Client care managers assume influential positions in health-care programs and services. Client care managers need to articulate strategically concerns about trends that affect the health needs of clients and the day-to-day operations of health-care organizations (The Price Waterhouse Change Integration Team, 1995, pp. 4–6). Not to articulate concerns when opportunities are provided within the external political systems or internal health-care organizations is to approve (by lack of resistance) what other stakeholders decide. Client care managers will need to evolve cost-effective systems for delivering care when care is needed versus accepting that financing mechanisms can best decide who has access to needed care. The change process is complex, dynamic, and ignored by stakeholders only at great risk.

## SUMMARY

Knowledge of trends with an awareness of historical perspective helps the client care manager to anticipate change. The transition from the industrial era to the informational era has entailed many societal changes that have affected the health-care system. Characteristics of the informational era include increasing emphasis on self-help, individual choice, and representative participation in decisions affecting oneself. Consistent with these changes, organizational structures are increasingly complex, interconnected, and interdependent on other organizations on a global level.

Economic interests are influencing technologic and political trends. Within the health-care arena, government regulations and financing mechanisms are shifting emphases from individualized quality care to reduction of costs by decreasing reimbursement and consequently length of stay. Through professional organizations, providers of care continue to establish standards of care used as guidelines for providing services.

The context of health care shapes nursing practice. Entry-level staff nurses use their knowledge of the various types of health-care agencies available to help clients plan for follow-up care and to provide continuity of cost-effective and efficient care. The agencies that commonly comprise the external health-care system are likely to be multipurpose in nature and to receive funding from several sources. These agencies are designed to address the needs of clients of various ages throughout the health-care continuum. Staff nurses are expected to use information about these agencies to help clients select options for providing continuity of care. They are expected to have access to current information about available services from many different sources in and outside of the agency in which they practice. To plan seamless care within boundaryless or less structured organizations, the staff nurse must identify available options within the limits of the client's financial resources.

Client care managers are stakeholders in health-care reform. As such, they need to communicate their concerns to influence the nature of the changes in the interests of the clients they serve and in their own practice interests as well.

## APPLICATION EXERCISES

1. Compare the changes occurring within the health-care system related to the informational era with the changes previously associated with the industrial era.
2. Describe how changing social roles of women affect human resources available to the health-care system and recipients of its services.
3. Your client is a 3-year-old boy who was admitted with fractures likely caused by child abuse. The client's parents are currently unemployed and have no health insurance. What types of agencies need to be involved in providing follow-up after the client is released from your agency?
4. Your client is an 87-year-old woman who was admitted because of dehydration and malnutrition. She is unable to describe her daily routines or her caretakers. She vaguely describes a nephew's family. Which types of agencies might be involved in providing follow-up care and protective services?
5. Discuss whether Medicare is more likely to be involved in financing institutionally- or community-based services? Give reasons for your answer.

## CRITICAL THINKING SCENARIO

Imagine that you are an entry-level staff nurse assigned to a busy surgical inpatient unit for people with various types of cerebrovascular diseases; in addition, you are assigned to "cover" the corresponding outpatient clinic one afternoon a week. You notice that about 50% of the clients scheduled for follow-up visits in this clinic do not keep their appointments. The clerical staff schedule appointments and receive telephone calls directly from clients (who leave messages as to whether they expect to keep or cancel their appointments or request rescheduling).

1. What would you do to gain insight into the needs of your clientele in the outpatient clinic?
2. How would you learn about the explicit and implicit purposes of the outpatient clinic services?
3. Whom or what would you try to change and how? Give reasons for your plan for change.

## REFERENCES

Aburdene P, Naisbitt J: *Megatrends for women,* New York, NY, 1992, Villard Books.

Baker OV: Meeting the challenge of managing cultural diversity. In Ritro RA, Litwin AH, Butler L (editors): *Managing in the age of change: essential skills to manage today's diverse workforce,* Burr Ridge, IL, 1995, Irwin Professional Publishing.

Becher EC: Improving the quality of health care: who will lead? *Health Affairs 20*(5) 164–179, 2001.

Briggance BB, Burke N: Shaping America's health care professions: the dramatic rise of multiculturism, *West J Med 176*(1):62–64, 2002.

Bruhn JG: Being good and doing good: the culture of professionalism in the health professions, *The Health Care Manager 19*(4):47–58, 2001.

Curtin L: Designing new roles: nursing in the '90s and beyond, *Nurs Manage 21*(2):7–9, 1990.

Curtin L: Signs of things to come, *Nurs Manage 23*(7):7–8, 1992.

Dertouzos M: *The unfinished revolution: human-centric computers and what they can do for us,* New York, NY, 2001, HarperCollins, Publishers.

Dienamann J, Van de Castle B: The impact of health care informatics on the organization. In Englebardt SP, Nelson R (editors): *Health care informatics,* St Louis, MO, 2002, Mosby.

Drucker P: Beyond the information revolution, *The Atlantic Monthly,* October, 1999.

Engelman R, Halweil B, Nierenberg D: Rethinking population, improving lives. In Flavin C, et al (editors): *State of the world 2002,* New York, NY, 2002, WW Norton & Company.

Estes CL: Long-term care is mainstream: why separate it from acute care? *Perspect Aging 19*(4):4–8, 1990.

FutureScan: Global trends, but falling birth, fertility rates. *Growth Strategies.* 930: 1–2, 2001.

Gardner G, Halweil B: Nourishing the underfed and overfed. In Brown L. et al (editors): *State of the world 2000*, New York, NY, 2000, WW Norton & Company.

Gillette E: Caring, common sense, and computers, *Point of View/Ethicon 25*(2): 10–11, 1988.

Hall M: ASPs in the catbird seat, *Computer World 34*(46): S14–S15. 2000.

Ikenberry JG: Global trends 2015: a dialogue about the future with nongovernment experts, *Foreign Affairs*, May/Jun, 2001.

Jennings J. and Haughton, L.: *It's not the BIG that eat the Small ... it's the FAST that eat the SLOW*, New York, NY, 2002, Harper Business.

Johnson D: Global trends 2015: *A dialogue about the future with nongovernmental experts by US Central Intelligence Agency, Office of Public Affairs, Washington, D.C. 20505*, May/Jun 2001. Website: www.odci.gov/cia/publications/global trends 2015/index.html.

Kennedy M: Supporting administrative decision making. In Englebardt SP, Nelson R (editors): *Health care informatics*, St Louis, MO, 2002, Mosby.

Lower MS, Nauert LB: Charting: the impact of bedside computers, *Nurs Manage 23*(7):40–42, 44, 1993.

Manion J: Understanding the seven stages of change, *Am J Nurs 95*(4):41–43, 1995.

Matz LB, Gary G: Patient outcomes measure home health care accomplishments, *Nurs Manage 24*(5):96Y, 96Z, 96DD, 96FF, 1993.

McFarland LJ, Senn LE, Childress JR: *21st century leadership: dialogues with 100 top leaders*, Los Angeles, CA, 1993, The Leadership Press.

McGinn AP: Reducing our toxic burden. In Flavin C, et al (editors): *State of the world 2002*, New York, NY, 2002, WW Norton & Company.

Naisbitt J, Aburdene P: *Megatrends 2000: ten new directions for the 1990s*, New York, NY, 1990, Avon Books.

Nornhold P: 90 Predictions for the '90s, *Nurs 90 20*(1):34–41, 1990.

Raymond C: Global migration will have widespread impact on society, scholars say, *Chron Higher Ed 37*(2):A6, 1990.

Renner M: Breaking the link between resources and repression. In Flavin C, et al (editors): *State of the world 2002*, New York, NY, 2002, WW Norton & Company.

Rodeghero, JA: Benchmarking Physicians' Practices: Trends toward the millennium, *J Health Care Finance 25*(4):15–37, 1999.

Schneider B, Bowen D: *Winning the service game*, Boston, MA, 1995, Harvard Business School Press.

Simpson RL: Client/server technology: a new way to manage information, *Nurs Manage 24*(5):30, 32, 1993.

Sinclair VG: Potential effects of decision support systems on the role of the nurse, *Comput Nurs 8*(2):60–65, 1990.

Smeltzer CH: The impact of prospective payment on the economics, ethics, and quality of nursing, *Nurs Admin Q 14*(3):1–10, 1990.

Thede LQ: Understanding databases. In Englebardt SP, Nelson R (editors): *Health care informatics*, St Louis, MO, 2002, Mosby, pp. 55–80.

The Price Waterhouse Change Integration Team: *Better change: best practices for transforming your organization*, Burr Ridge, II, 1995, Irwin Professional Publishing.

Toffler A: *The third wave*, New York, 1980, Bantam Books.

U.S. National Center for Health Statistics, Public Health Service: *Charting the nation's health trends since 1960*, DHHS Pub. No. (PHS) 54–1251, Hyattsville, MD, 1985, Department of Health and Human Services.

# 3

# *Supporting the Organization*

## OBJECTIVES

*When you complete this chapter, you should be able to:*

1. Describe how all departments of a health-care agency work together to meet its stated purposes.
2. Use communication protocols to foster effective working relationships with health care providers.
3. Participate in establishing nursing policies or procedures.
4. State reasons nurses need to accept and support client care goals.
5. Participate in continuous quality improvement and assurance processes.
6. Describe common types of nursing service delivery patterns.
7. Describe how information technology and boundaryless organizations contribute to seamless health care.
8. Discuss preventive actions that need to be taken to avoid drug administration errors.
9. Explain the scope of practice and responsibilities of entry-level nurses, using position descriptions.
10. Describe the use of classification systems to identify client needs and allocate nursing resources to meet them.

## KEY CONCEPTS

integrated health delivery system
agency
  seamless health care
  stated purposes
  organizational chart
  policy
  procedure
  interdepartmental policies
  departmental philosophy
  philosophy

explicit knowledge
tacit knowledge
communication protocols
telephone etiquette
electronic information transmission
continuous quality improvement
  (CQI) (quality assurance) processes
  processes
  products
  medication errors

patterns of nursing service delivery
  case method
  functional nursing
  team nursing
  modular nursing

primary nursing
  case management method
  alternative practice model
  position description
  classification system

## MEETING CLIENT AND AGENCY GOALS

As indicated in Chapter Two, the nurse uses knowledge of current trends affecting health-care delivery to understand the context of nursing practice. Consistent with these trends, any agency involved in the provision of health care is likely to be a component of a group of cooperating agencies commonly described as an **integrated health delivery system**. Due to this evolution of health care, especially its complexity and costs, the need for cooperation and coordination results in groups of agencies working together under the auspices of one governing body. This chapter is designed to help the staff nurse understand the major components of the client care manager's role in supporting the existing organization of the health-care **agency** and its evolution consistent with current trends. Supporting the agency in this way helps it achieve its goal of meeting client needs through the provision of coordinated care (i.e., **seamless health care** as perceived by clients). Departmental functions, methods used to promote interdepartmental communication, common methods of organizing nursing services, and methods of communicating with varying levels and agencies external to the organization are discussed.

As a client care manager, the nurse is in a pivotal position to help clients meet their needs. The responsibility of coordinating services needed by clients places the nurse in an influential organizational position and requires timely and effective communications. Often these communications involve service providers working in comparable horizontal levels of the organization. The success of the health-care organization depends on the nurse's effective coordination of clinical client care services. At the same time, the nurse contributes to the success of the integrated delivery system's effectiveness in providing coordinated cost-effective services. As a knowledge worker, the nurse is expected to use various types of information technology equipment to transmit information to various departments internally and externally to other related agencies within the health continuum (Lang, 2001b, pp. 539–553).

The nurse who does not support the internal organization does not serve clients well. The goals of the health-care organization need to be distinguished, however, from individual client health-care goals.

Although not the only factor, financial considerations continue to influence client choices heavily in selecting health-care agencies. The nurse is expected to know the various **stated purposes** and limits of the health-care agency in meeting individual client needs. The client care manager works with clients to determine the nature of these needs, where on the health-care continuum these needs can be met best, and how the client's goals relate to agency purposes. Often the beginning staff nurse works with more experienced nurses and interdisciplinary work group members to obtain accurate information in a timely manner. Without this information, the nurse is unable to identify and discuss service options and alternative strategies with individual clients. The nurse uses this information to determine care priorities and discharge plans and to help clients select specific options on the basis of the nature of their individual health needs, personal resources, and financial considerations. In today's evolving integrated delivery system contexts, clients need experiences to convince them that they are nursing's first priority. Health-care systems and the profession of nursing exist to serve clients; clients do not exist to serve health-care organizations. In modern health-care settings, the nurse is expected to focus primarily on client goals, in accordance with the American Nurses Association (ANA) Code for Nurses. This nursing responsibility includes providing client care and mobilizing organizational resources when needed. At times, client care wrongly becomes secondary to maintaining staff routines. Priorities should not be misaligned in such a way that nursing staff adhere to nursing unit schedules first and place client needs second. Client advocacy frequently requires the nurse to communicate with representatives of various levels of the internal organization and departments to obtain accurate information required to clarify client options. As an advocate, the nurse pursues client goals until they are met through coordination of organizational resources. In advocacy activities, the timeliness of the nurse's activities is crucial.

## Identifying Agency Objectives

An agency's stated purposes are reflected in its philosophy, its programs, and the services it provides to meet them. They usually can be found in administrative or personnel manuals. Vision or mission statements that describe general beliefs, key concepts or ideas, values, and purposes often are used to help employees gain perspective of the agency's purposes. Consistent with trends affecting the increasing complexity of health care, consumer and health-care provider satisfaction guide the evolution of processes used. Although a variety of processes can be used, ultimately the results achieved in satisfying client needs are paramount (Grinstead and Timoney, 1994, pp. 4–7).

Frequently, agencies inform their employees of their strategic plan (i.e., the primary functions, values, and anticipated general approaches) for achieving their stated purposes in specified periods of time. Subsequently, various divisions or departments, using the strategic plan, develop time-limited goals to aid staff in making changes needed to meet agency objectives.

Each health-care agency within an integrated delivery system has stated and assumed objectives concerning its governance and fiscal management. These objectives directly relate to the agency's clients. It is important to know whether the agency is "for profit" or "not for profit" and whether the agency's organizational system is predominantly centralized or decentralized. This information is used to establish the agency's routines and policies and to develop procedures to resolve potential ethical issues on behalf of clients.

## Policies and Procedures

Written descriptions of departmental roles and functions are a reflection of the agency's formal **organizational chart**. Each department develops a system of meeting its responsibilities that varies with the department's functions and size. The system is maintained by policies and procedures written to guide staff.

The formal organizational chart often is illustrated in administrative manuals. This chart describes the formal divisions of the organization's work into departments. As mentioned in Chapter One, the organizational chart depicts lines of authority and patterns of decision making used by the organization to accomplish its goals. It describes some of the relationships of various departments to each other. As health organizations become more boundaryless, less emphasis is likely to be placed on a single agency's organizational chart, and more emphasis is likely to be placed on the relationships of various components of the integrated delivery system and other health-related community resources. Crucial functional relationships will more likely be depicted so that employees will understand the integrated health system, its governance, and patterns of decision making. Organizational charts relate primarily to administrative functions; clinical decision making typically involves more horizontal organizational integration to obtain needed coordinated care.

A **policy** is a general description of the required agency approach to achieving agency goals in an expedient manner. An admission policy commonly describes an agency's intent not to discriminate on the basis of age, race, creed, disability, ethnicity, or gender. Another policy might be that admission documentation be completed within 24 hours. A **procedure** describes a specific process needed to complete a task, such as a procedure for inserting a sterile urinary catheter or the steps to follow in preparing a client for a myelogram.

Typically, **interdepartmental policies,** as expressed in administrative manuals or written policies, describe how the various divisions of staff relate to each other to accomplish the agency's goals. These policies are the highest level and are broad in scope.

Nurses usually can access their **departmental philosophy** and associated policies and procedures in reference manuals located on each nursing unit. The nursing department's **philosophy** describes the beliefs, values, assumptions, purposes, and goals of the nursing staff that contribute to meeting the agency's goals. Nurses review these materials to learn about their client care coordination responsibilities. As new technology and equipment are introduced, revisions in policies and procedures are communicated to staff, often verbally and in writing, through printed or electronic messages. Sometimes, criteria or standards of accrediting agencies stimulate revisions. At other times, revisions in federal or state regulations associated with publicly funded health-care programs stimulate revisions in nursing policies and procedures. As a basis for coordinating client care activities, nurses are expected to know current policies and procedures of the nursing department and where to locate information about other policies that affect client care.

## WORKING WITH OTHER DEPARTMENTS

### Knowledge

To coordinate client care activities, the nurse uses information about departmental functions and services and interdepartmental policies and procedures. This type of knowledge is called **explicit knowledge**; it can be accessed easily from manuals, books, or electronic databases (Lang, 2001a, p. 48). This information enables the nurse to request needed services on the client's behalf and to communicate concerns to other departments when clients present special needs not addressed by agency routines. For example, the nurse needs to know the various types of nutritional services provided by the dietary department to enable the client to receive a general or therapeutic diet. It is important that the nurse follow procedures when requisitioning diets to enable the dietary department's subsystem to follow through efficiently. The nurse also communicates special nutritional needs to the nutrition department if the client has food intolerances, preferences, allergies, or restrictions related to health needs or other therapies, such as drug therapy. In addition, the nurse is expected to inform the client of special dietary programs required for diagnostic tests and to help the client adhere to them.

Another type of knowledge that the client care manager needs to use is **tacit knowledge** (Lang, 2001a, p. 48). Tacit knowledge refers to know-how and skills that nurses carry inside their heads and is not accessed or shared easily. When tacit knowledge is shared, it typically is done through social relationships and interpersonal interactions with colleagues and peers. Tacit knowledge is a form of extremely valuable insight and is dynamically changing as diverse perspectives converge into the complex care provided clients. Frequently, beginning nurses develop tacit knowledge during internships or while working with more experienced nurses or mentors. This type of knowledge becomes more readily recognized, valued, and rewarded; it is crucial to learning to manage client care effectively and efficiently in a specific practice context.

Within the context of clinical client care management, the nurse is expected to know the primary functions of each department. He or she is expected to follow interdepartmental policies and procedures to provide services to individual clients. The nurse is expected to understand nursing responsibilities related to preparing the client for surgical procedures and prescribed therapies. This nursing function might require explicit and tacit knowledge. Policies may not always be written, and written documents may not always be current or thorough, but nurses are expected to know what the policies and procedures are and adhere to them to support the organization's division of work and ensure that the client's needs are met satisfactorily. With the increasing use of information technology, many of the policy and procedure references can be accessed through the agency's computerized databases. In addition, the nurse is expected to know the client's priorities in treatment and to determine if and when policies and procedures require modification to address those priorities. Considerable tacit knowledge is used to perform these functions.

## Clarification

If information about agency policies and procedures (e.g., whether or not to withhold medications before a diagnostic study) is not adequate to enable the nurse to meet client needs, clarification must be obtained. It may be necessary to contact the department where the study is to be performed as well as the client's attending physician for clarification. These efforts should be documented in the client's clinical record to avoid duplicating clarification efforts and to provide for follow-through to prevent unnecessary delay in the client's diagnostic procedures or treatment programs.

## FOSTERING EFFECTIVE COMMUNICATION

An essential part of the staff nurse's role in managing client care is to relay accurate information about client needs, responses, and plans to various members of the nursing and interdisciplinary work groups. Nursing staff are available throughout the client's inpatient stay. The nurse also often coordinates client care in the ambulatory or community-based settings. Consequently the client care manager accepts responsibility for coordinating the client's care with nursing work group members so that the client is prepared and available to other departments as scheduled. When these goals cannot be met, the nurse is expected to communicate with others in a timely manner to ensure that the client's needs ultimately are satisfied. The nursing student is expected to have developed an adequate knowledge base and basic verbal and communication skills before being assigned the responsibilities of a client care manager. As indicated earlier, whether by telephone, face-to-face, handwritten, or electronic messages, the nurse assumes responsibility for communicating client care information accurately and in a timely manner to the nursing work group and to involved multidisciplinary work group members.

## Communication Protocols

**Communication protocols** include customary manners of addressing others face to face, by telephone, through e-mail, or through handwritten messages. These protocols are designed to meet the needs of each party involved and include common considerations of courtesy, information, and follow-through. Applying basic principles promotes effective communication by increasing the likelihood that messages sent will be received and comprehended as intended. The entry-level staff nurse uses knowledge of the communication process in each of the core roles.

Communicating without using common courtesies reduces effectiveness by decreasing the receiver's ability to listen actively and to receive accurately messages sent. To communicate effectively, the sender designs the message so that it can be understood readily by the receiver, using appropriate words, tone of voice, and gestures. Proper medical terminology can be used to increase accuracy, but, in practice, paraphrasing medical terminology can increase the receiver's comprehension of the message. Because words are symbols that often have different meanings in different contexts, feedback is needed, and the communication process should be repeated as often as necessary to ensure that messages sent were perceived accurately.

### Written Communication

Common communication mistakes result when words or their abbreviations are used as if they have the same meanings for senders and receivers when, in fact, they do not. Nursing staff members with different educational credentials or experiential or cultural backgrounds are at risk for communication mistakes because they might not be using a common language. Errors also may occur when members of different disciplines use words that have different meanings in different fields.

Common nursing situations require staff nurses to anticipate multidisciplinary communication needs to ensure effective coordination. Nurses often discuss client needs face to face with members of the multidisciplinary work group and request services of other departments by electronic means to meet special client needs. To communicate effectively, the nurse must determine what information is needed by other departments. Before communicating with other work group members, the nurse tries to anticipate what basic information other departmental staff members use to address the client's needs. Often the nurse must collect and organize the information beforehand. Sometimes the agency provides a form or structured blank message to help identify and organize the needed information. After the information is communicated, the nurse documents it to avoid duplication of nursing effort and to provide a record for follow-through.

To the extent possible, clients are expected to assume responsibility for making decisions about their diagnostic and treatment programs; clients need to know what the plans are and the expectations placed on them. The staff nurse is expected to assume responsibility for assisting the client to follow through on the multidisciplinary treatment plan.

### Face-to-Face Communication

Staff nurses need to communicate effectively with coworkers in face-to-face situations. Observing behavioral cues and seeking feedback to monitor the perceptions of receivers in face-to-face situations promotes effective communication.

Some nurses find face-to-face communications difficult and prefer other ways of relaying information (e.g., in writing, by computer, or by telephone). In face-to-face situations, the nurse must be sensitive to the receiver's circumstances. If the recipients do not perceive the messages as important because of competing demands for their time, they may not be ready or able to receive them when the client care manager sends them. Frequently a receiver's response to the information, instruction, or request initially may not be favorable. Alternatively a nurse who is feeling rushed might not seek needed feedback to ensure that the message received was interpreted accurately. In face-to-face communications, the sender can gather feedback by monitoring the receiver's behavior. Sensitivity to the receiver's responses often increases communication effectiveness.

If the nurse is ambivalent, uncertain, or anxious, face-to-face communications are less likely to be effective. Sometimes a nurse's behavior (e.g., lack of eye contact, tone of voice, or nonverbal gestures) can be inconsistent with or override the actual verbal message. The nurse needs to be sensitive to the messages sent verbally and behaviorally.

As a nurse gains nursing experience, the need to continue to improve communication skills becomes obvious. As client care manager, the nurse should strive to communicate through words and actions the attitudes and messages that accurately convey the nurse's expectations of others.

*Telephone Etiquette*

Nurses frequently use the telephone to communicate with various departments in a timely manner and to help clients communicate with their families or support systems. It is important to use telephone etiquette to convey information effectively and efficiently. **Telephone etiquette** consists of following guidelines that take into account the needs of senders and receivers. Using telephone etiquette promotes positive working relationships between departments and staff. When coordinating effort with other departments, the nurse is expected to follow communication protocols and telephone etiquette. Box 3-1 presents guidelines for telephone etiquette.

The nurse's telephone communication skills improve with practice. Box 3-2 shows a performance checklist for monitoring telephone etiquette in common clinical situations. This checklist describes behaviors expected of nurses in the client care manager role.

*Electronic Information Transmission*

Given the fast pace of client care, frequently information about the client's current status is needed by other health care providers. Electronic databases help to make this information accessible, but it needs to be entered in a timely manner to maximize its usefulness. Current information about individual clients and their responses to treatment increasingly is being compiled in electronic health records for **electronic information transmission**. Other common names for the

---

**BOX 3-1**

## Guidelines for Telephone Etiquette

Be alert: A cheerful, wide-awake greeting sets the tone of any conversation and communicates that you are ready to help.

Be natural: Use common terms. Avoid slang and jargon.

Be expressive: Speak at a normal pace and loudness, but vary the tone of your voice to add life and emphasis to what you say.

Be distinct: Pronounce your words clearly and carefully. Always speak directly into the telephone receiver. Do not have anything in your mouth while you are speaking.

Be pleasant: Show that you want to help. Personalize your conversation by using the person's name. Try to visualize the caller and speak to her or him—not to the telephone.

Be attentive: Listen politely. Do not interrupt the speaker.

Follow up: Determine whether the caller wants to leave a message or if another staff member could return a call. Summarize what you will do.

Be courteous: Use "please," "thank you," and "you're welcome" when appropriate.

BOX 3-2

## Telephone Etiquette Performance Checklists

### Talking with peers and colleagues
**Criteria:**
Answer the telephone promptly.
Speak clearly and distinctly and at a moderate rate.
   Identify agency.
   Identify unit.
   Identify self.
Establish purpose of telephone call.
Determine if you are an appropriate respondent.
Ask questions to verify message.
Answer questions appropriately.
Offer help by describing specific options.
Promise specific actions in follow-up.
Document message if indicated.

### Receiving information from other departments
**Criteria:**
Answer the telephone promptly.
Speak clearly and distinctly and at a moderate rate.
   Identify unit.
   Identify self.
Listen carefully to establish purpose of telephone call.
Determine if you are able to respond as needed.
Ask questions to verify message.
Offer to help by stating choices to caller.
Promise specific actions as follow-up.
Document message or describe nursing implications of message received.

### Sending information to other departments
**Criteria:**
Gather information needed to make telephone call: anticipate questions.
Call desired telephone number.
Verify identity of respondent.
State purpose of call.
Deliver information.
Ask questions to verify respondent's receipt of information.
Allow respondent to react to the information.
Answer questions accurately.
Promise specific action as follow-up.
Document telephone call if indicated.

electronic client records are *electronic medical records, computer-based patient record,* and *computer-based health record* (Hunter, 2002, p. 211). Clients need nurses to enter nursing information into the record in a timely manner so that it is available to the multidisciplinary work group to enable them to provide services in an effective and efficient manner.

Just as any communication mode is imperfect, so is the electronic method. The client care manager increasingly will use various information technologies to document services provided consistent with a client's plan of care. The client care manager needs to make a special effort to ensure that the data are entered in the intended client record and are accurate and timely. Although nurses have a history of providing individualized care, the evolving electronic technologies may not be conducive to capturing these nursing concerns. These nursing concerns remain important, however, and need to be documented and addressed. Changes in client care related to diagnostic, drug, health education, and family concerns need to be recorded to help other disciplines respond to these changes in a timely and effective manner.

Although the electronic method of information documentation and transmission automatically records time, date, and name of client, it is incumbent on the nurse to ensure that proper identification of client and nurse are made and that security measures are maintained. To ensure that protocols are followed, it is recommended that the nurse seek more experienced supervision when using these methods to ensure the client's safety, to ensure accuracy and timeliness of information entered, and to ensure that security is maintained until confidence and adequate comfort levels are reached. The electronic equipment is "fast and dumb," whereas the nurse is required to be "accurate, clear, and unambiguous" in the interest of safe care.

## ACTING AS A LIAISON BETWEEN ADMINISTRATION AND THE HEALTH-CARE TEAM

Members of the nursing department include vice-presidents of patient care, directors of nursing, assistant directors of nursing, staffing coordinators, shift supervisors, clinical area coordinators (sometimes known as nurse managers), nursing specialists (e.g., infection-control nurses or enterostomal therapists), and lead nurses (sometimes known as team leaders or nursing work group leaders). Sometimes, more frequently in long-term care settings, coordinating client care requires the nurse to act as a liaison between administrative, multidisciplinary, and nursing work groups. Liaison activities help client care managers remain sensitive to evolving client needs by requiring them to listen to concerns expressed by others on the clinical staff and the client. By relaying information to administrative staff, the client care manager is assured that administration is aware of the clinical staff's concerns. Direct service staff input is communicated to supervisory staff, who relay it to administration (staff with decision-making authority within the agency for the allocation of resources and the development and implementation of policies and procedures). Through these liaison activities, administrative staff maintain awareness of issues that clinical staff are attempting to address. In this way, the client care manager's participation in liaison activities facilitates client advocacy.

In acute care settings, client care managers often communicate concerns directly to their immediate supervisors within the organization. They often relate to supervisors who have varying administrative responsibilities and may be referred to as shift supervisors or clinical area coordinators. In acute care settings, the nurse frequently has more (vertical) organizational levels through which to communicate to relay concerns to administrative staff than in long-term or community-based settings.

Conflict may occur between nursing work groups and overall organizational goals (e.g., the nursing group may want to delay a client's discharge to ensure adequate preparation and recovery, whereas the agency's goals are to avoid financial loss of an extended stay). The entry-level nurse strives to adhere to the nursing code of ethics, which emphasizes putting the client's needs first, while attempting to resolve problems caused by the extended stay. Strategies for conflict resolution are discussed in greater detail in Chapter Seven. Resolving ethical dilemmas is discussed further in Chapter Sixteen.

## Supporting the Goals of Client Care

Indirectly, satisfying organizational needs promotes individual client interests. Sometimes in long-term care settings, the administrative staff allow gaps to develop, however, in communicating their expectations to direct service staff (e.g., nursing assistants) or in giving feedback about effectiveness. Direct service staff (staff who work directly with clients) depend on the organization's division of work for guidance in performing their duties. When the nature of the services that clients need changes, staff need administrative help to make the corresponding changes. Staff often modify their responses to client needs when demands of the external health-care system change; for example, the pain experienced by terminally ill clients can be controlled by using new technology and drugs, allowing these persons to return to their homes sooner. Frequently, these changes result from new legislation, health-care financing methods, technology, or regulatory requirements. As discussed in Chapter Two, these changes affect the types of clients served as well as the methods and equipment used to meet their needs. If direct staff is not informed of changes in a timely manner, they may perceive the lack of communication as a lack of support or interest. In most cases, the goals of the agency and the work group do not change, but the policies and procedures used to meet them do. As liaison, the client care manager is expected to explain the need for these changes to direct service staff and communicate their expressed concerns to administration. These communications often help direct service staff to make the desired changes in procedures and provide administration with feedback about the staff's success in making them. If direct service staff as stakeholders feel their input is heard and important, they are more likely to make the necessary changes sooner.

As a liaison between the work group and administrative staff, the entry-level nurse needs to accept and believe in the agency's general goals and individual client care goals. If the nurse does not accept them, both sets of goals are devalued. It is crucial that the nurse seek clarification of goals that are vague or seem to be in conflict. Conflicts in goals may arise with the emergence of ethical issues related to various treatment or nontreatment plans, culturally diverse client value systems, or priorities established on the basis of costs. When the nurse becomes aware of conflicting goals, putting them in writing can help the staff appreciate and focus on agency and individual client goals. When conflicts between client care plans and organizational goals arise, the nurse communicates with administrative staff through supervisors to seek organizational support, clarification, and needed resources.

The component of the client care manager role that involves liaison activities helps the staff nurse to coordinate organizational resources on behalf of clients. In addition to acting as a liaison between the work group and administrative staff, the entry-level nurse may be involved in quality assurance or continuous quality improvement processes to support organizational development.

## Participating in Continuous Quality Improvement Processes

Consistent with the evolving patterns of complexity and integration of client care systems, "service logic" or coordination models of care are being developed (Klingman-Brundage et al., 1995, p. 22). Efforts to unify service to develop a system to provide seamless care need to integrate organizational, provider, and customer viewpoints. In addition, emphasis is placed on improving the processes involved in the provision of care to increase the reliability of results. To unify these care processes, the scope of the staff involvement widens to include other disciplines and functional areas so that clients perceive seamless care as continuous rather than riddled with gaps and overlaps. These models of care integration strive to promote effective group work and collaborative interactions between clinical staff on behalf of individual clients. **Continuous quality improvement (CQI) (quality assurance) processes** are activities designed to monitor and ultimately to improve the quality of care provided. Quality improvement efforts are continuous. They are an ongoing component of implementing the agency's philosophy and are shaped by the specific practice environment or context. Client care managers use quality indicators often identified in the agency's standards of care that also guide nursing practice.

CQI efforts are integral to the nurse's practice. Nurses use standards of care to determine desired client outcomes consistent with the agency's stated philosophy and purposes. Leadership staff describe the components of quality care with input from direct service staff. Direct service staff experience the process of caregiving and become aware of the adequacy of staff, equipment, supplies, and timeliness of communication. They also witness when desired client outcomes are met or unmet (Schneider and Bowen, 1995, pp. 19–53). Clinical staff are important stakeholders in the quality of care provided. Consequently, input and feedback from direct service staff are integral to CQI activities. As client care managers gain experience as interdisciplinary work group members, they are expected to provide some of the input and feedback required to maintain or improve the quality of nursing services provided.

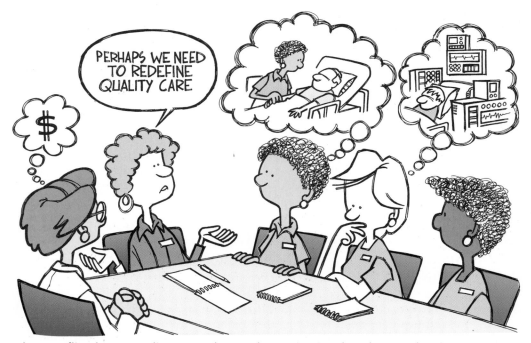

When conflicts between client care plans and organizational goals arise, the nurse communicates with administrative staff to seek organizational support and needed resources.

Two forces external to the agency influence CQI processes related to nursing practice in most acute care, most community-based care, and some long-term care facilities: the ANA standards of practice and the Joint Commission on Accreditation of Healthcare Organizations (JCAHO) criteria, which are believed to depict standards of quality care. Both are influential in stimulating CQI activities.

The standards of nursing practice established by the ANA are of primary importance in the design of CQI programs. These standards, established by nurses for nurses, represent expected standards of nursing practice or performance criteria. These standards of nursing practice apply in any context (ANA, 1991, pp. 3–5). They emphasize the nurse's use of the nursing process to meet individual client healthcare needs. Nursing peers use these standards as performance criteria to evaluate the quality of their practices. The judiciary system also may use them in settling legal disputes.

Entry-level nurses are probably familiar with these standards because educators frequently use them to orient and enable students to acquire the attitudes, knowledge, and skills needed for nursing practice. They are described in most texts used by nursing students learning the fundamentals of nursing. Ideally, entry-level nurses have integrated these standards thoroughly into their personal nursing philosophies and theories and use them routinely in providing care to individual clients.

The ANA also has collaborated with specialty nursing organizations to establish standards that address specialty practice or populations with special needs and advanced nursing practice. Similar to the general practice standards, specialty standards are used as performance criteria by nursing peer review organizations in various inpatient and community-based health-care settings.

Another important external force influencing CQI programs is the criteria for accreditation used by the JCAHO. The JCAHO is a private agency that incorporates medical and nursing practice standards in its criteria for CQI efforts. Health-care agencies voluntarily request review by the JCAHO to receive accreditation or verification that the health-care agency's operations exemplify quality health care. The JCAHO established criteria for all health agency department operations, including nursing. JCAHO accreditation is used as one requirement for reimbursement by some third-party payers (e.g., Medicare) because it is used as a measure of the quality of care provided.

## Components of CQI Programs

CQI programs focus on three primary components: (1) organizational structure, (2) process, and (3) results or client outcomes. Structure refers to the agency's establishment of representative committees and their purposes and related activities. Examples include CQI departments and unit CQI committees. Agency support may include providing staff with the time, equipment, supplies, and operational decision-making authority to make effective use of these committees.

CQI **processes** are the activities of these committees. The committees design special data collection, analyses, and follow-up recommendations to help the organization improve the quality of care being provided. For example, a group of staff nurses working on a surgical unit, concerned about the incidence of postoperative complications, might collect data on the number of postoperative wound infections. On the basis of their analysis of these data and interpretation of their findings, they would recommend indicated remedial actions to be taken to prevent or reduce the number of postoperative wound infections.

Frequently, these committees review records and other readily available organizational data to identify key issues and problems. In addition, committee members act as key resource persons to help nurses manage clients' special needs to achieve desired outcomes. The CQI committees work closely with administrative and clinical staff to revise policies, procedures, standards of care, and standards of practice to improve the quality of care so that it meets various standards.

A CQI process includes all the steps of the problem-solving process, from informing involved persons to eliciting the cooperation needed to follow through. The client care manager is expected to participate in CQI programs. The manager is expected to provide input about issues, concerns, and problems encountered in providing care; to understand the standards of care involved in the issues identified; to participate in collecting the necessary data; and to revise practices when indicated.

To perform these responsibilities, the nurse must understand the structure, processes, and outcomes of CQI programs used by the agency. By participating, the nurse can provide input for data generation, collection, and analyses needed to improve the quality of care the agency provides.

Often, if the CQI process relies heavily on historical data to evaluate desired client outcomes, a retrospective approach is being used. To meet these data requirements, an entry-level nurse is asked to use specific guidelines to document desired client outcomes and the plan of care. The nurse should not wait until CQI and quality assurance processes reliant on retrospective review reveal problems, however. If specific problems are experienced or witnessed, remedial action is called for, using a proactive, client advocacy approach. Clients with similar needs are likely to benefit from a review of records by direct staff, using a systematic method of data collection to improve the quality of care in an immediate and direct way. This type of review typically benefits clients served later as well.

The **products** of CQI programs are described in terms of the agency's standards of care or desired client outcomes. Documentation of discharge plans and client outcomes frequently is used to measure the results of CQI efforts. Often CQI activities contribute to the revision of nursing policies, procedures, interdisciplinary standards of care, and standards of practice used by staff nurses.

## Medication Errors

CQI efforts have not been sufficiently successful in providing quality care or even safe care (Institute of Medicine, 1999). Research findings indicate that there is yet no coherent strategy for improving the quality of health care and practices (Becher and Chassin, 2001, p. 164). The issue of **medication errors** brought to the public's attention verifies the need for external monitors and checks on health-care quality control and indicates that the health-care industry remains unable to regulate itself sufficiently to protect the public (Evans, 2001, p. 96). Subsequent to multiple media revelations that approximately 7% of all recipients of care in hospitals also received medication errors, several politically heavyweight groups responded to legislate safe care. The vested interests did not claim responsibility; rather, they requested (and received) further funding to remedy the errors and provide further monitoring. The emphasis on the need to remedy the unsafe practices was bolstered by the increased health-care costs attributed to the errors. Consequently, standards for (1) automated drug ordering systems, (2) drug packaging and labeling, (3) product trade names, and (4) expanding electronic databases on the reporting of adverse drug errors were formulated (Wechsler, 2000, p. 22). Instead of CQI programs, laws mandating reporting of errors and remedial actions were needed. In the interest of protecting clients from existing delivery systems, client care managers need to continue to reflect on the processes being used to meet client needs and observe results, paying attention to whether these processes increase or avoid complications.

Criteria in established standards of care may relate to diagnosis-related group (DRG) guidelines and the availability of client and community resources. If CQI programs truly address the issue of quality, they include clients' perceptions of the care they received, using indicators of quality care chosen by the recipients of such care (Klingman-Brundage, 1995, p. 22; Schneider and Bowen, 1995, pp. 19–83).

## Establishing Nursing Standards

Historically, many nursing departments organized policy and procedure committees that sought input and feedback from staff nurses. More recently, greater emphasis is being placed on shared governance and corresponding shared accountability for quality assurance between administrative and clinical nursing staff. Specifically, shared governance includes organizational concepts that support professional practice, including standards of practice and care, quality assurance, and professional development and review (Porter-O'Grady, 1992, p. 65). Commonly evolving health-care organizations have a nursing department with a philosophy and corresponding formal organization that relies on staff nurse input to maintain policies and procedures affecting practice (Porter-O'Grady, 1992, pp. 32-33). Shared governance organizational structures provide for shared accountability (Porter-O'Grady, 1992, pp. 30-36). This trend in formal nursing organizations reflects the transfer of the autonomy, authority, and control of nursing practice to direct care providers and the evolution of nursing as an established profession. Typically, representatives of direct service nursing staff serve on committees whose purposes are to revise policies, procedures, and standards of care and practice when approaches to care change. Frequently, these committee members (direct care providers) attempt to help other staff nurses adhere to policies by acting as resource persons to interpret the policies accurately when questions arise. In addition, entry-level staff nurses attend in-service programs and conferences to learn about these revised policies in efforts to maintain a current knowledge base.

As the pace of change in organizations and complexity of care increase, client care managers should anticipate that electronic information systems will be used to communicate revisions in procedures. Revisions are likely to be more frequent and aimed at consuming less staff time to implement changes required to improve care. Clinical staff time is a scarce, highly valued agency resource. When customers (clients from various agencies within the integrated delivery system) increasingly are involved as partners in evaluating care processes, continuous efforts to improve quality of services provided also will be more likely to succeed. Although nursing has long advocated relating to clients as partners in their care, this approach continues to evolve as a reflection of an innovative corporate service strategy. Concurrently, clinical staff in integrated delivery systems who learn to manage knowledge by applying what is learned to daily operations are likely to be more competitive than staff who do not (Brailer, 1999, p. 16).

## NURSING SERVICE DELIVERY PATTERNS

The nursing service delivery patterns used by the evolving client care–focused systems vary with the formal organization, the nature of the client population served, and the resources available. These service delivery patterns also reflect the evolution of nursing as a profession.

History provides valuable insight into the evolution of various organizational settings (Hannan and Freeman, 1989, pp. 17–27). In a similar manner, insights into the evolution of nursing service delivery patterns may help entry-level nurses to understand their varied and continued use in current organizational settings. In addition, by gaining knowledge of various types of nursing service delivery patterns, client care managers may be better able to anticipate changes in response to health-care trends.

There are many different combinations or modifications of nursing service delivery models in use in various settings where nurses practice. Five distinct **patterns of nursing service delivery** in current use are:
1. Case method
2. Functional nursing
3. Team nursing
4. Primary nursing
5. Case management

These models are discussed with reference to their historical context and factors that promoted their evolution. No single pattern of service delivery is inherently good or bad. Rather, each method must be considered within the context of the organization and the goals to be achieved with the available resources. Each pattern of service delivery is evaluated according to its effectiveness, cost-effectiveness, and efficiency in meeting client needs and should be viewed within the context of its historical development and relationships to some of the key forces that shaped its evolution. Similarly, future nursing service delivery models are likely to incorporate features of these models depending on the health organization's and client's needs.

Comparing these patterns of service delivery out of context is like comparing a horse and carriage, Model T Ford, street car, gasoline-powered compact car, electrically powered van, and supersonic passenger plane. All of these vehicles are means of getting from one point to another. None of these forms of transportation is good or bad in itself. Rather, each form is evaluated best within its context, considering the extent to which it meets passenger needs and goals with available resources. There are situations in which the horse-and-carriage method of transportation is highly valued and popular. Similarly, Model T Fords, streetcars, gasoline-powered compact cars, electrically powered vans, and supersonic passenger planes can meet diverse passenger needs. Their popularity has been influenced by their history and perceived effectiveness within the context of the contemporary transportation industry.

The use of each pattern of nursing service delivery is discussed briefly in the context of its historical development. Most current nursing departments use an adapted combination of several of these models to provide care within institutional or community-based practice settings. Many factors influence which pattern of service delivery is used (e.g., nursing needs of the client population and the availability of nursing and other multidisciplinary work group or interdisciplinary team skills required to meet them).

## Case Method

The **case method** of nursing service delivery was used by private duty nurses in the early stages of modern nursing. This method involved one nurse providing nursing care for an ill client (Donahue, 1985, pp. 338–343). Figure 3-1 illustrates this pattern of nursing service delivery. The nurse worked collaboratively with the client, family, and physician to monitor the client's condition and provide for the client's basic needs and comfort. The nurse usually was compensated directly by the client or fam-

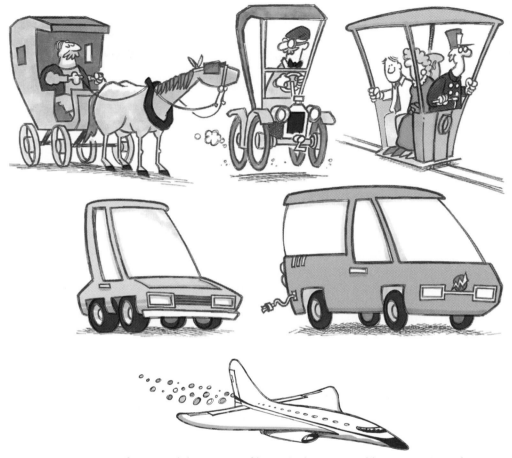

Comparing patterns of service delivery out of historical context is like comparing a horse and carriage, Model T Ford, streetcar, gasoline-powered compact car, electrically powered van, and supersonic plane.

ily. Typically the nurse performed all of the nursing work at the bedside without involvement of a health-care organization. The public perception of nurses was based on the experiences of individual clients and families; there were no mass media.

The major advantage of this method was its efficiency because there was no need to communicate to many staff members over several shifts each day for a number of days. The nurse was familiar with client and family needs because she consistently provided the care. In addition, the nurse was accountable to the client and family because she was paid directly by them. The nurse worked closely with the client and family; there typically was no need to assign nursing care to others.

The major disadvantage of this method was its cost. Within the current health care scene, case method ratios of 1:1 are used in a variety of settings, such as trauma and emergency centers.

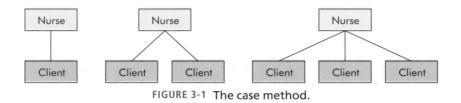

FIGURE 3-1 The case method.

## Functional Nursing

**Functional nursing** came into common use in the early 20th century (Donahue, 1985, pp. 441-446). Figure 3-2 illustrates this pattern of nursing service delivery. Historically, as sanitation concerns grew, there was an increased need for nurses to provide the proper care and environment for ill and injured persons in inpatient settings. Functional nursing emphasized the tasks of care. Its pattern of work division was consistent with the patterns of the common military and manufacturing organizations of the industrial era. The nursing staff performed tasks of care in a routine manner; the primary emphasis was on the type of task, and less attention was paid to the nature of the client's needs. One member of the nursing staff would provide drinking water, another would perform personal hygiene tasks, another would administer medicines, and another would give treatments. Typically the leader of the nursing work group responsible for a specific time period (e.g., an 8-hour shift) would assign available nursing staff according to their qualifications, their abilities, and the tasks to be completed. The nursing work group leader also coordinated the individual client's care during the specified period. The head nurse

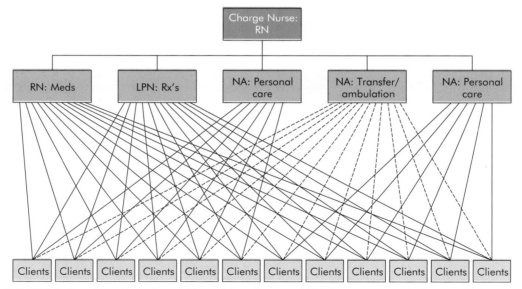

FIGURE 3-2 Functional nursing. RN, registered nurse; LPN, licensed practical nurse; NA, nursing assistant.

(manager of the nursing unit) was responsible for coordinating the client's care for the duration of the client stay. Organizationally the emphasis was on the treatment of diseases or injuries from a medical point of view. It was difficult and not perceived to be important for nurses to evaluate client progress. Nursing documentation of client responses to care was sketchy and not highly valued by the organization. The health-care organizations of this era emphasized custodial tasks and delegated medical procedures rather than client care plans. High priority was given to completion of delegated medical functions.

A major advantage of the functional method of care was the correspondence between the pattern of work division and the tasks to be done. Staff assignments also corresponded to their qualifications. More clients could be provided basic care with fewer staff.

A major disadvantage of the functional method was that nursing knowledge and skills were not well used. Consequently, clients did not receive the benefit of available nursing skills to satisfy needs.

## Team Nursing

**Team nursing** (one-leader nursing work groups) came into vogue in the 1950s (Donahue, 1985, pp. 446–447). Figure 3-3 illustrates this pattern of nursing service delivery. Several trends supported its popularity. Health care increasingly came under the influence of third-party payers, and more private insurance programs were financed by employers. As a result, the emphasis gradually shifted from custodial services and medical procedures to treatment and goal-directed approaches to care.

Many nursing practice acts included expectations that nursing practice include disease prevention, promotion of health, and restorative care for the ill or injured. Nursing leaders articulated the need for autonomy in the practice of nursing as a profession. The need for nurses to obtain formal preparation in institutions of higher learning was recognized more frequently. Organizational leaders supported this trend by advocating formal nursing preparation to meet requirements for licensure, but the number of nurses who received such training remained small.

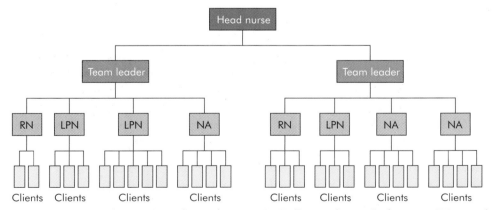

FIGURE 3-3 Team nursing. RN, registered nurse; LPN, licensed practical nurse; NA, nursing assistant.

During this period, health-care organizations were confronted with a persistent shortage of qualified nurses. Organizational structures were designed to divide nursing work by geographic subdivisions of a hospital (formerly called *wards*). The head nurse assumed responsibility for the overall effectiveness of the ward and the primary responsibility for coordinating client care with other disciplines and organizational departments. He or she usually assigned nursing "work" according to the qualifications of the staff available to provide care for groups of patients. The registered nurses (RNs) were assigned to lead the work group, develop nursing care plans, coordinate efforts of the work group in implementing care plans, provide care requiring complex nursing skills, and assist the work group in evaluating their effectiveness. Documentation of client outcomes was often incomplete. The use of nursing care plans as references for change-of-shift reports gained popularity as a communication tool to promote continuity of care, but, faced with the multiple demands of communication, coordination, and evaluation of client progress, RN work group leaders frequently noted that it was difficult to keep the plans current.

Depending on available staff, nursing work group member assignments changed with every shift on a daily basis. Many nurses believed that, compared with the functional method, the nursing team method decreased fragmentation of care. Some nurses accepted greater responsibility for clinical decision making. As clients progressed in their treatment programs, some nursing staff were uncertain about which decisions could be made by various work group members.

RNs typically were assigned as team leaders. As team leaders, they were expected to assess client needs, develop plans, assist and supervise other work group members carrying out the plans, and revise the plans according to the clients' progress. The nursing work group leader was accountable for meeting the client needs that could be met within a specific time period and communicating with other nursing staff and other disciplines and departments to provide for continuity of care. Often nursing team leader functions were similar to those of the head nurse; the head nurse coordinated the 24-hour nursing care for the duration of client stays and accepted responsibility for the overall effectiveness of the nursing work groups and nursing unit.

A variation of the team nursing method of service delivery in which the geographic location of clients in the physical setting largely determines nursing assignments sometimes is called **modular nursing**. In this approach, nurses were assigned varying numbers of clients. In addition, they supervised other nursing work group members assigned to care for the same clients. The number and qualifications of staff per nursing module depended on the number of clients and complexity of client needs. A clinical coordinator, head nurse, or supervisor usually was responsible for assignment of staff to each module of clients (Young and Duncan, 1990, p. 97). As the nursing work group leader, the RN provided specific directions, assigned client care in each group, and evaluated the effectiveness of the group's efforts. Modular nursing used characteristics of the floor plan to divide the work involved in providing care for a group of clients. It was intended to reduce nursing efforts (frequently the amount of walking) needed to care for a large number of clients.

A major advantage of team nursing is that the method of work division enables the nurse to apply nursing knowledge broadly and influence the care provided to more clients than he or she could care for alone. Typically a nursing team, more accurately described as nursing work group, consisted of an RN, licensed practical nurses (LPNs), and nursing assistants, depending on the number of clients and the complexity of needs to be addressed. This method of organization gave the nurse some autonomy in designing care plans to benefit the client. Team nursing popularized *client-centered care*, while addressing the persistent shortage of highly skilled nurses.

A major disadvantage of team nursing was that many nursing staff were not prepared adequately to function as a team member or leader of a work group. Consequently, each nursing work group assigned to clients needed to adapt to each group's ways while providing increasingly complex client care. The increased need for communication and supervision of lesser skilled (prepared) staff placed additional demands on the team leaders.

With the increased pressures to decrease numbers of licensed staff to provide care for clients with increasingly complex needs, some efforts have been made to use unlicensed assistive personnel using a team method. Client care managers have needed to delegate tasks (versus nursing functions) properly to work group members. This approach frequently has not succeeded in providing efficient quality of care due to the amount of education and communication required by existing licensed staff and unlicensed assistive personnel.

## Primary Nursing

As the informational era began to establish itself, the complexity and cost of health care increased. High-tech equipment began to be used to process large amounts of data. In the search for cost-effective solutions, greater emphasis was placed on systematic study of health-care issues. Similar ways of processing health-care data and managing information were used by many public and private organizations. Complex health-care issues, caused in part by competitive forces of the emerging global economy, were studied more systematically to identify solutions.

The private insurance mechanisms for financing health care needed by employees became increasingly diverse. Government agencies became more involved in financing health care for high-risk populations. Concurrently, regulations affecting health-care organizations increased. These regulations reflected the interests of various professional organizations, primarily those of medicine. As special political interest groups, these organizations advocated that their standards of practice be implemented. Organizational structures of health-care agencies became more decentralized, reflecting the increased complexity of health care and interdependencies of external agencies.

**Primary nursing** evolved as a predominant method of service delivery in acute-care health agencies to conserve scarce nursing resources (Marram et al., 1974, pp. 51–53). Nursing knowledge and skills were needed to communicate with various multidisciplinary work group members about complex issues involved in client care. Figure 3-4 illustrates this method of nursing service delivery.

Many nursing work groups in acute care and community-based settings attempted to use the primary nursing method in response to increasing use of technology and acuity of client needs. Stimuli for these changes included the needs

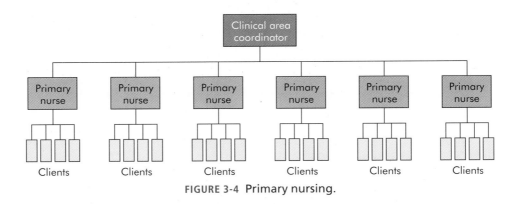

FIGURE 3-4  Primary nursing.

to monitor client responses closely, to use nursing knowledge and skills cost-effectively, and to communicate between providers to eliminate costly gaps and overlaps in client care.

To accommodate changes in the division of work involved in providing complex client care, organizational changes were needed. Decentralized organizational structures enabled nurses to interact readily with interdisciplinary work group members with a greater flexibility in the corresponding horizontal level of the organization. As a result, nurses could participate more readily in clinical decision-making processes on behalf of individual clients. The primary nurse was assigned to provide direct client care, which included personal hygiene, dependent nursing functions delegated by physicians, and independent nursing functions. These independent nursing functions included assessing client status, planning care with clients, teaching clients and families, evaluating client responses within the context of desired standards, and coordinating care with multidisciplinary work groups and other organizational departments. Some clients and families reported that they could identify more readily with the primary nurse accountable for their care. Many nurses believed that, under the primary nursing system, fragmentation of care was reduced, while efficiency increased. Because health-care organization goals emphasized cost-effectiveness, the length of institutional stays decreased, particularly in acute care settings.

The primary nurses provided client care, including the assessment of needs, mutual goal setting with clients, and revising the care plan based on the individual client responses. Primary nursing made greater use of the nursing skills acquired in basic educational programs. Proponents of this method of service delivery believed the quality of care was higher compared with other popular methods. Increased nurse satisfaction was believed to reduce the costs of staff turnover and of higher nurse-to-patient ratios (Freeman and Coronado, 1990, p. 556).

Some primary nurses continued to express frustration with time limitations and the need to update nursing care plans as communication tools when the primary nurse was not on duty. In addition, the acuity levels (quantity and complexity of nursing needs) of client conditions frequently involved marked changes in relatively short periods, requiring corresponding revisions in care plans. Many plans written by primary nurses described common routines or standard approaches and did not account for the possibility of dramatic changes in client responses.

Primary nurses were assigned to provide care for individual clients for the duration of stay from admission to discharge rather than to perform tasks needed during a specific work period. These staff nurses began to demonstrate use of their professional nursing knowledge and skills; they used assertive communication skills to support their clinical decision making within nursing work groups and their corresponding multidisciplinary work groups.

Although not explicitly described in the primary nursing model, the nursing work group often identified a nursing work group leader from among the primary nurses. This nursing work group leader's functions changed according to the nursing work group's needs; frequently the nursing work group leader provided direct care and coordinated the specific nursing work group's efforts during a specific shift or period. The nursing work group leader, usually a primary nurse, shared accountability with other primary nurses and the nurse manager for coordination, continuity, and effectiveness of care.

Often during a 24-hour period in an acute care setting, the client received several different methods of nursing service delivery. Most commonly, a pattern of primary nursing service delivery was used on the day shift. A team nursing model was used during the evening shift. A functional method was followed on the night shift due to the organization's allocation of scarce nursing resources to meet client needs. In the long-term care setting, as acuity levels rose, more modified "team" nursing models were used to maximize effectiveness of available staffing. Similarly, in community-based settings, modified primary nursing and team nursing approaches were used to provide efficient, complex care. Emphasis on cost-effectiveness and corresponding client acuity levels increased the demand for highly skilled nursing staff to direct the client's nursing care on the basis of the client's responses to treatment of multiple disease processes and complex needs for health promotion and maintenance.

Two major advantages of primary nursing were the increased coordination of care by skilled nurses on a continuous basis and the increased accountability of the nursing work group to clients and families. Communication between nurse and client usually improved. Care plans were used more frequently to provide for identified client needs.

A major disadvantage of primary nursing was the number of nurses needed to implement the model. As the acuity level of client needs increased, lower ratios of nurses to clients were needed. Nursing shortages increased due to a variety of causes, and the number of available nurses was far short of the number needed. Consequently, increased numbers of lesser skilled staff were employed to assist the RN staff. Features of primary nursing and team nursing were combined to address the emerging nursing shortage and increased acuity of client needs. Care maps or critical pathways were developed to help with the coordination and documentation of complex multidisciplinary client care.

## Case Management

The **case management method** of nursing service delivery emphasizes the assignment of one nurse to plan, direct, and evaluate a client's care throughout the client's stay. Case managers typically did not provide direct care. Some believed that case managers helped to organize nursing staff and divide their "work" to meet client needs in an effective (quality) and efficient (cost-effective) manner. In dividing the work, primary consideration is given to the complexity of client needs, including health promotion and treatment of illness. The availability of nursing expertise and the number of nursing staff are crucial to the design of practice models using a case management pattern of service delivery.

Various methods of case management became popular in the late 1980s, not because of dissatisfaction with the primary nursing model, but rather as a deliberate response of health-care organizations to provide cost-effective complex care. Health-care organizations tried to retain qualified, highly skilled nurses to manage complex care often provided by an interdisciplinary work group for clients who could not receive adequate care in other, less costly settings. Today case management often is used in combination with care pathways or critical paths to guide clients and their corresponding multidisciplinary work groups.

The case management pattern of nursing service delivery required organizational changes that were determined by internal and external forces. A variation of the case management method is the **alternative practice model,** in which primary nurses prepared at the baccalaureate level worked with associate nurses prepared at the associate degree level. This model provided staff nurses with two or more organizational options for nursing practice. This approach to staffing supported the evolution of two levels of nursing practice.

In 1983, most nurses employed in institutional care settings were prepared at the diploma or associate degree levels (ANA, 1985, p. 7). Many nursing leaders believed that nurses needed more higher education to practice proficiently. At the same time, research findings indicated a need for organizational structures that promoted nurse satisfaction with practice (Jacobson, 1990, pp. 24–26; Kramer, 1990, pp. 67–74). The nurse shortage and the demand for adequately prepared nurses to meet complex client needs in a cost-effective manner continued. Greater emphasis was placed on efficient and effective use of available nursing resources to satisfy complex client needs. The case management method provides nurses with practice options designed to increase work satisfaction and effectiveness that reflect the agency's response to scarce nursing resources, external financing mechanisms, and the agency's purpose. The emphases on increasing cost-effectiveness and efficient use of high-tech equipment, highly skilled staff in acute care settings, and increased use of long-term care and community-based settings continue.

The emerging patterns of nursing service delivery reflect different nursing practice options that use different levels of nursing skills available within the agency. The actual division of work in various case management models incorporates elements of primary nursing. Case management models incorporate "a multidisciplinary care process method" (Olivas et al., 1989a, p. 17). Figure 3-5 illustrates the organization of a common alternate practice model of case management.

Some case management models focus on a division of nursing work based on the assessment of client needs by a qualified (often more experienced) nurse (i.e., the nursing case manager) (Tonges, 1989, p. 34). Plans are devised to direct the nursing work group in providing care to ensure that it meets specified standards of quality. Depending on the context of care, the nursing staff may include varying ratios

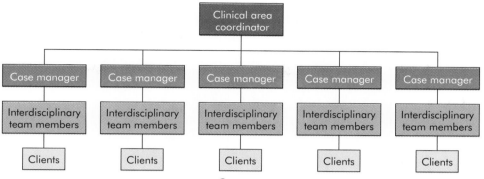

FIGURE 3-5 Case management.

of RNs, LPNs, nursing assistants (NAs), and unlicensed assistive personnel (Goodwin, 1994, pp. 29–31) or health-care technicians. The health-care technicians perform specific tasks involved in implementing plans developed by the nursing case manager when the client is on a complex acute care unit; whereas RNs, LPNs, and NAs provide care corresponding to the plan when the client is on a convalescent or general nursing unit.

Other common case management models of nursing service delivery differentiate nursing practice on the basis of the nurse's educational preparation. The organizational structure is designed so that nurses prepared at the BSN level are nursing case managers. Nurses with diploma or ADN preparation are associate nurses expected to implement plans of care developed by case managers. LPNs and NAs are assigned as needed to meet client needs. In this way, some believe that the case management method makes judicious use of scarce nursing resources.

As the role of case managers evolves, they will coordinate and lead multidisciplinary staff in the use of care maps and critical pathways. They will work closely with client care managers and other direct service multidisciplinary work group members from the management level of health-care organizations. Figure 3-6 depicts a service organization (Schneider and Bowen, 1995, p. 7) and describes the case manager's typical location on the organizational chart; the typical location of the client care manager on the organizational chart is also described in Figure 3-6 for comparison.

In case management patterns of nursing service delivery, the health-care organization focuses on varying the use of resources on a case (client)-by-case basis to address requirements imposed on it by government and private insurance financing limitations (Goodwin, 1994, pp. 32–34; Olivas et al., 1989b, pp. 13–16). Models of case management used to deliver nursing services are, and will be, studied thoroughly and researched qualitatively and quantitatively. The survival of the case management method is related closely to its effectiveness in satisfying client needs and allocating scarce resources (i.e., cost-effectiveness).

The major advantage of the case management method of service delivery is its focus on the complexity of client needs and multidisciplinary strategies to satisfy

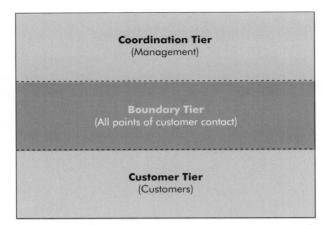

FIGURE 3-6 Case manager's position in a three-tiered organization. The case manager is located in the coordination tier, which is made up of interdisciplinary management. The client care manager is located in the boundary tier, or direct service level. The customer tier is made up of health-care clients. (From Schneider B, Bowen D: *Winning the service game*, Boston, MA, 1995, The Harvard Business School Press, p. 7.)

them, cost-effectiveness, and efficiency in promoting timely discharge plans and continuity of care. In addition, it selectively uses scarce nursing resources.

The major disadvantage of the case management system is its reliance on adequate numbers of highly skilled professional nurses and organizational systems that promote professional autonomy, accountability, and collaboration with the client and family and the multidisciplinary work groups, all of which are costly scarce human resources. As nursing service departments change into shared governance systems promoting professional practice, case management models of service delivery are expected to increase in their popularity (Parkman and Loveridge, 1994, p. 68). Entry-level staff nurses probably will assist case managers as associates, implementing care plans or pathways emphasizing client outcomes.

In a similar manner, the role and functions of nursing work group leaders, team leaders, and nurse managers probably will evolve into clinical care coordinators and operations managers. Frequently, nursing work group leaders or nursing team leaders coordinate staffing and clinical care for a group of clients for a specified time (e.g., work shift or 8- to 12-hour day, depending on the nature of the settings). An inpatient acute care unit might be organized around an 8-hour shift, whereas an ambulatory clinic might operate for 10 hours daily during a 4-day week. These nursing work group leaders often strive to obtain adequate staffing to provide care for a specific number of clients, assign client care to available staff, and coordinate nursing efforts with other departments and nursing shifts. They also collaborate with multidisciplinary work group members in a timely fashion to resolve conflicts and make adjustments in the client's treatment schedules on the basis of client responses and evolving priorities of care. Typically the nursing work group leader focuses on a specified time.

With the evolving professional practice delivery models, nursing work group leaders probably will coordinate clinical services to maximize client benefits efficiently and effectively in an effort to provide seamless care over the continuum. They will expend considerable effort toward coordinating care, often in accordance with care paths designed by the multidisciplinary team, using the nursing process to identify individual client needs throughout the client's entire length of stay or service episode, including follow-up. They will contribute to nursing staff development, CQI, and collaboration with multidisciplinary work groups. The focus will be on the desired client outcomes, minimizing costly complications, continuity of care, and cost-effective discharge preparations. In addition, they are likely to receive assistance from unit managers with day-to-day operations (i.e., adequate staffing, supplies, equipment, and technical support).

Because health-care organizations are managed as business enterprises, considerable effort will continue to be expended to improve the operational performance of acute care agencies. With the intensity of demands resulting from the increased pace of change, careful review of the processes of health care will be required and determination made as to how best to divide work of providing quality health care (Vestal and Massey, 1994, p. 9). That is, restructuring will be needed to address continued cost constraints, needs for safety, and results-oriented seamless (as perceived by customers) care. The increasing shortage of highly skilled licensed nurses is a growing concern. Lyne and Williams (1995, pp. 57–58) reported that planned packages (e.g., reimbursement on basis of DRG) devised to provide seamless care have been inadequate and propose a "care frame" model. This model is designed to address the inadequacies of previous models and is described as a combination of episodes of care, each described within a specific type of care context. As a client's status changes, the care frame provided is changed to correspond to the services and expertise required to provide the necessary care. Figure 3-7 illustrates a care frame model.

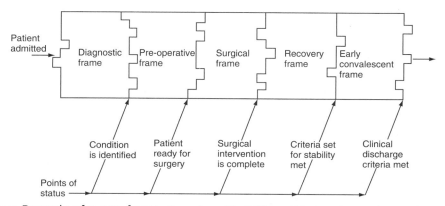

FIGURE 3-7 **Example of a care frame.** (From Lyne PA, Williams SM: Care frames: interactive units of health-care delivery, *Journal of Management in Medicine 9*[4]:58, 1995.)

## JOB DESCRIPTIONS

The entry-level nurse is expected to understand the philosophy of the nursing department and the organizational pattern or patterns of delivering care within the health-care setting. As mentioned previously, the nursing department's philosophy of nursing or mission should be consistent with the purpose of the health-care agency. The nursing philosophy usually reflects attitudes held by practicing nurses, including their attitudes toward practice, education, and research. Consequently, these values and beliefs reflect the organization of the nursing department and its division of the work involved in meeting client needs. The nursing department's organizational chart visually depicts the relationship of nursing staff to client care. Position or job descriptions include a list of the duties and responsibilities of nursing staff. Position descriptions also indicate the qualifications for each category of nursing staff and to whom each nursing staff member is expected to turn for supervision and guidance.

## Entry-Level Staff Nurse

The **position description** for the entry-level staff nurse describes the level of organizational decision making expected. It typically indicates to whom the entry-level nurse turns for help with organizational management matters and clinical decisions affecting client well-being. Box 3-3 is an example of a typical position description for an entry-level nurse in an acute care setting. Box 3-4 is an example of a typical position description of a nursing unit manager, who often supervises and guides staff nurses. This position description describes the nursing unit manager's involvement in preparing budgets. This level employee is in a position to carry out strategic plans at the nursing unit level as well as to develop resources needed to coordinate nursing services with other departments. Staff nurses often are acutely aware of the organization's gaps and overlaps as they affect client care and possible solutions. They sometimes are asked for input into budget planning, but typically are not expected to prepare a budget for a nursing unit. The staff nurses benefit from being aware of the process of budget processing so that timely and meaningful input is provided when opportunities arise.

The type of facility, its primary purpose, the types of clients it serves, and the patterns of nursing service delivery determine the functions of the staff nurse. The pattern of nursing service delivery reflects the organization's expectations of the nurse, influencing how the nurse relates to others in the nursing and multidisciplinary work groups.

Current position descriptions for entry-level staff nurses employed in many long-term care facilities outline expectations of modified team nursing, in which elements of team nursing and primary nursing are combined. In many acute care facilities, position descriptions for entry-level staff nurses incorporate expectations of an associate nurse in which modified primary nursing and case management methods of nursing service delivery are used. All entry-level staff nurses are responsible for reviewing the descriptions of the nursing position for which they are employed. This review helps ensure that the nurse understands his or her responsibilities toward clients, nursing staff, and multidisciplinary work groups.

BOX 3-3

## Typical Position Description of Entry-Level Registered Nurse

**Lakeside Community Medical Center**
**458 Lincoln Avenue**
**Centerville, WI**

**Qualifications**

Is a graduate of an NLN accredited program for RNs and currently licensed to practice as an RN.

**Functions**

The entry-level staff nurse at Lakeside Community Medical Center provides direct care to clients, including teaching them and their support systems in self-care strategies; manages resources effectively; and adheres to ethical codes of conduct, "Patient Bill of Rights," standards of care, and standards of nursing practice.

**Core competencies**

1. Systematically uses the nursing process to identify client needs, sets mutually acceptable goals with clients and families/support systems, formulates plans of care, and assists in implementation and evaluation of plans in a timely manner.
2. Manages resources, including staffing, equipment, supplies, and time, effectively in providing care for assigned groups of clients, including using the classification system to identify staffing needs and working cooperatively with other nursing department staff to ensure adequate staffing.
3. Communicates nursing concerns verbally, in writing, and electronically to clients, their families, and nursing and other multidisciplinary group members in a timely and courteous manner, documenting responses to services provided.
4. Adheres to agency standards, policies, and procedures and sets a positive example for staff under supervision.
5. Actively participates in CQI activities on his or her assigned nursing unit, including completion of required continuing education programs for safety, infection control, and human resource management.
6. Reviews pertinent literature and shares relevant findings with coworkers.
7. Seeks agency support to resolve conflicts and ethical dilemmas encountered in providing client care and staff supervision.
8. Seeks learning experiences to maintain core competencies and unit-specific competencies.

**Reports to**

Designated case manager or nursing unit manager.

**Performance review**

At the satisfactory completion of the first 6 months and annually thereafter. The entry-level staff nurse accepts a 1-year temporary position, which converts into a permanent position after 1 year of successful employment.

**BOX 3-4**

## Typical Position Description of Nursing Unit Manager

**Lakeside Community Medical Center**
**458 Lincoln Avenue**
**Centerville, WI**

**Qualifications**

Is a graduate of an NLN accredited program for RNs and is currently licensed to practice as an RN. In addition, has a minimum of a Bachelor's Degree in Nursing and 4 years of nursing experience as a staff nurse. Preferably has a Master's Degree in Nursing.

**Functions**

The Nursing Unit Manager at Lakeside Community Medical Center oversees the work of nursing staff providing direct care to clients. He or she directs and guides staff in the fulfillment of their duties and responsibilities. He or she sets an example for complying with ethical codes of conduct and "Patient Bill of Rights" and provides organizational support for providing standards of care and nursing practice, including budgetary planning. He or she manages organizational resources that interface nursing with other departments.

**Core competencies**

1. Systematically uses the nursing process to solve clinical problems, set mutual goals, and evaluate progress with staff in meeting the nursing unit's needs.
2. Develops a staffing plan and corresponding schedules to provide for anticipated client needs using an established classification system.
3. Procures resources, including staffing, equipment, supplies, and consultation needed by direct staff to provide established standards of care. Maintains a positive work culture and safe environment for clients and staff.
4. Communicates nursing concerns verbally, in writing, and electronically to direct service staff, Vice-President for Nursing, and other departments in a timely and courteous manner.
5. Adheres to agency standards, policies, and procedures and sets a positive example to influence nursing staff under her or his supervision by empowering direct service staff to participate in shared governance activities and contribute to organizational development.
6. Promotes nursing staff development through participation in CQI programs on assigned unit, including completion of required continuing education programs for safety, infection control, and human resource management.
7. Collaborates with peers to provide administrative coverage.
8. Applies relevant research findings toward the improvement of quality of care and cost-effectiveness.
9. Requests agency support to resolve conflicts and ethical dilemmas encountered by direct service staff in the provision of care.

BOX 3-4

## Typical Position Description of Nursing Unit Manager— cont'd

10. Writes performance reviews of every nursing staff member under supervision.
11. Seeks professional development needed to maintain clinical core competencies and unit-specific competencies.
12. Contributes to the evolution of nursing as a profession, through scientific community programs or creative approaches to interdisciplinary team building.

**Reports to**
Vice-President for Nursing

**Performance review**
After the satisfactory completion of the first 6 months of employment in the position and every 2 years thereafter. The nursing unit manager accepts a 2-year temporary position, which converts to a permanent position after 2 years of successful employment.

To understand the scope of nursing practice expected, the entry-level staff nurse needs to pay close attention to several aspects of the position description (i.e., the expected use of the nursing process and responsibilities for assessing client responses, analyzing client data to formulate nursing diagnoses, establishing written care plans or use of care maps, and revising care plans or adding variances to care maps on the basis of client outcomes and responses to treatment). It is crucial that nurses understand the extent of their responsibilities to communicate client needs to multidisciplinary staff and to provide the necessary feedback about client responses. In addition, the nurse needs to comprehend the extent of expected involvement in teaching clients about routine and complex self-care regimens. The nurse needs to know the scope of practice expected of the entry-level staff in the nursing department to avoid gaps in care or duplication of efforts and to coordinate multidisciplinary and interdepartmental efforts.

## CLASSIFICATION SYSTEMS

With the increasing complexity and costs of care, the need for accurate, reliable information about client care from staff nurses also has increased. Entry-level staff nurses employed by health-care agencies providing institutionally based services are expected to participate in collecting such information and regularly monitoring the reliability and validity of the classification system in use.

## Purposes and Uses

A **classification system** is a method of regularly collecting information about the nursing needs of clients to provide adequate staffing for a specific time period. This system may be referred to as *acuity levels* at some acute care agencies. Information from the classification system often is used to plan for adequate staffing, budgeting, billing for services, and CQI processes. To satisfy these varied purposes, it is crucial that the data collected be consistently accurate. Staff nurses generally are expected to use information about their assigned clients to provide the data needed for the classification system and to record these data permanently in client records. Staff nurses need a basic understanding of the elements of classification systems to enable them to produce the needed data and document it accurately.

## Essential Components

Accurate and dependable classification systems have six basic parts (De Groot, 1989a, p. 30). These six basic parts are: (1) critical indicators (concepts used to describe essential features of quality care) that accurately describe all of the important parts of nursing care; (2) a way to measure critical indicators so that the data accurately reflect the amount and type of care each client needs on each shift on every nursing unit; (3) a way to judge the adequacy of staffing ratios; (4) a way to monitor the accuracy of data obtained by the system; (5) a way to compute staffing requirements; and (6) a way to check the suitability of the critical indicators over time.

Critical indicators are the foundation of a classification system, and they must reflect accurately the many dimensions of client care. The critical indicators of nursing care reflect the nursing department's philosophy. When complete, these descriptive concepts measure all components of nursing care provided to all the types of clients served by the health-care agency. These measuring tools quantify by categorizing and rating all varieties of client needs and the degree of nursing expertise required to address them, rather than merely listing specific activities and tasks done by nursing staff.

To quantify client needs accurately and consistently, these needs are defined according to the perceptions of agency staff. The definitions must have the same meaning for all staff nurses who rate client needs and related nursing expertise. In addition, for purposes of consistency, each staff nurse needs to rate critical indicators in the same way. To gain a common understanding of these measuring tools, it is helpful if nurses understand how the agency's classification system was developed. This background information helps nurses understand critical distinctions in the categories of client needs and the nursing skills needed to address them.

To promote consistency in quantifying client needs, each staff nurse needs to categorize and rate nursing care as it is provided on the unit (practice environment or context). This quantification often requires staff nurses to distinguish between the routine and nonroutine care provided by various members of the nursing staff on different shifts. The staff nurse should understand that the classification system is used by all nursing units to enable the nursing department to calculate overall requirements for nursing staff. Understanding the relationship of the needs of clients on the unit to the context of the total nursing department helps the nurse rate client needs more accurately.

A reliable classification system produces data that accurately measure client needs. Repeated monitoring of the accuracy of data obtained from staff nurses on each unit with varied types of clients is necessary. Staff benefit from feedback about their accuracy and from in-service programs that keep them informed of system modifications.

In acute care settings, the data produced by staff nurses are converted into staffing requirements on a shift-to-shift basis. Usually staffing requirements are calculated by computers programmed according to the specifications of the agency's classification system. Calculated staffing requirements guide the distribution of nursing resources, which include the number of staff and their levels of nursing skills and qualifications. In this way, the quantity and the quality of nursing expertise are matched with client needs.

As a nursing management tool, a classification system is only as good as the data provided by staff nurses. It is crucial that all levels of nursing staff be committed to maintaining the classification system (De Groot, 1989b, p. 26). Regular efforts are necessary to ensure that staff nurses receive adequate orientation to the system. Changes in client needs must be addressed accurately by the definitions used to measure the critical indicators. From time to time, client records might be reviewed to check on the accuracy of the classification of client needs. This monitoring is particularly important if persistent shortages of nursing staff occur.

This facet of the client care manager role is so critical to an agency's success that it frequently is included in the entry-level staff nurse's position description. The data provided by the staff nurse's use of the agency's classification system also frequently are incorporated into quality assurance processes. Indirectly, using the agency's classification system may contribute to monitoring the quality of care.

As nursing organizational structures change in an effort to promote professional nursing practice, classification systems are likely to evolve into data information systems (Simpson, 1995, pp. 16–17). These nursing data sets will be used to evaluate the cost-effectiveness and impact of nursing input on client outcomes. Consequently, nursing may be reimbursed more readily for its impact on client health and treatment programs (Zbylot et al., 1995, p. 54).

## SUMMARY

The entry-level staff nurse is expected to understand how all departments within the health-care organization work together to enable the agency to achieve its objectives. The nurse uses this information to communicate with the multidisciplinary work group and coordinate organizational resources on clients' behalf. To foster effective working relationships within the health-care team, the nurse follows communication protocols including electronic transmission methods and practices telephone etiquette.

The staff nurse may contribute to establishing and maintaining nursing policies and procedures by involvement in liaison activities between administrative and direct service staff and participation in CQI programs. When CQI strategies are consistently unsuccessful, external agencies and the public will work to establish more effective methods of maintaining safety and protecting clients. To support the internal organization, the staff nurse must focus on meeting client needs as first priority. He or she also must serve as a client advocate when conflicts arise concerning policies, procedures, care paths, or agency interests.

The nurse needs to understand common patterns of nursing service delivery to determine the scope of practice intended by position descriptions for various categories of nursing staff. Background information about the classification system used at the specific agency helps the nurse accurately rate client needs so that nursing resources can be used effectively and efficiently to meet client needs. As nursing organizations evolve to support professional nursing practice, classification systems may be used to finance nursing resources consumed to meet client needs.

## APPLICATION EXERCISES

1. Describe how your agency's organizational chart reflects how its departments work together to achieve its purposes. How would you change it to increase its accuracy and clarity? Is it conducive to providing seamless care consistently?
2. Discuss the pros and cons of using computerized interdepartmental and interpersonal communications to satisfy the need for current, accurate information between various parties. How are written protocols (i.e., care pathways) used to increase communication effectiveness between departments and disciplines?
3. Give three examples of explicit and tacit knowledge that you used to manage your assigned clients' care. What were the sources for each of the examples of the different types of knowledge?
4. Identify the predominant pattern of nursing service delivery used on the unit to which you have been assigned. Is it consistent or in conflict with the agency's formal organization? Does it promote professional nursing practice? Give reasons for your answer.
5. Review the position description for the entry-level nurse on your assigned unit at your agency. Does it explicitly describe components of the nurse's role as a client care manager?
6. Classify an assigned client, using your agency's classification system. Did your rating agree with the staff nurse's rating? How is the consistency and accuracy of this classification system monitored? By whom?

## CRITICAL THINKING SCENARIO

Picture yourself employed in a subacute care setting that says it provides "seamless" care between admissions. You are assigned to a multidisciplinary work group. Within that group, you also are assigned a specific group of clients receiving nursing care on a 24-hour basis. Your nursing work group leader has requested that you provide coverage for another staff nurse today. You do not have the time to assess personally the other nurse's clients' needs and need to rely on current care paths and clinical records for up-to-date information. The

**CRITICAL THINKING SCENARIO—cont'd**

multidisciplinary work group meets within half an hour and expects you to contribute to discharge planning discussions for the clients assigned to the other nurse as well as for those to whom you have been assigned.

1. What would you do to acquaint yourself with the nursing needs of the clients in preparation for a multidisciplinary discussion about discharge plans?
2. Who or what supplementary resources would you bring to the discussion?
3. What would you change, if anything, to help you manage similar situations in the future? Explain.

## REFERENCES

American Nurses' Association: *Facts about nursing 84–85,* Kansas City, MO, 1985, American Nurses' Association.

American Nurses' Association: *Standards of clinical nursing practice,* Washington, DC, 1991, American Nurses Publishing.

Becher EC, Chassin MR: Improving the quality of health care: who will lead? *Health Affairs 20*(5): 164–179, 2001.

Brailer DJ: Management of knowledge in the modern health care delivery system, *The Joint Commission Journal on Quality Improvement 25*(1):6–19, 1999.

Cook JE: Professional practice committee: right on target, *Nurs Manage 21*(2): 54, 1990.

De Groot HA: Patient classification system evaluation, part I: essential system elements, *J Nurs Admin 19*(6):30–55, 1989a.

De Groot HA: Patient classification system evaluation, part II: system selection and implementation, *J Nurs Admin 19*(7):24–30, 1989b.

Donahue MP: *Nursing, the finest art: an illustrated history,* St. Louis, MO, 1985, Mosby.

Evans B: Customer service vs. profits, *Information Week,* November 26, 2001, p. 96.

Freeman BA, Coronado JR: A supportive clinical practice model, *Nurs Clin North Am 25*(3):551–560, 1990.

Goodwin DR: Nursing case management activities: how they differ between employment settings, *J Nurs Admin 24*(2):29–34, 1994.

Grinstead N, Timoney R: Seamless service, research and action, *Health Manpower Management 20*(2):4–7, 1994.

Hannan MT, Freeman J: *Organizational ecology,* Cambridge, MA, 1989, Harvard University Press.

Hunter KM: Electronic health records. In Englebardt SP, Nelson R (editors): *Health care informatics,* St Louis, MO, 2002, Mosby.

Institute of Medicine: *To err is human: building a safer health care system,* Washington, DC, 1999, Academy Press.

Jacobson E: Three new ways to deliver care, *Am J Nurs 90*(7):24–26, 1990.

Klingman-Brundage J, George WR, Bowen DE: "Service logic": achieving service system integration, *International Journal of Service Industry Management* 6(4):20–39, 1995.

Kramer M: Trends to watch at the magnet hospitals, *Nurs 90* 20(6):67–74, 1990.

Lang JC: Managerial concerns in knowledge management, *Journal of Knowledge Management* 5(1):43–57, 2001a.

Lang JC: Managing in knowledge-based competition, *Journal of Organizational Change Management* 14(6):539–553, 2001b.

Lyne PA, Williams SM: Care frames: interactive units of health-care delivery, *Journal of Management in Medicine* 9(4):53–62, 1995.

Marram GD, Schlegel MW, Bevis EO: *Primary nursing: a model for individualized care,* St Louis, MO, 1974, Mosby.

Olivas GS, Del Togno-Armanasco V, Erickson JR, et al: Case management: a bottom-line care delivery model: Part I. the concept, *J Nurs Admin* 19(11):16–20, 1989a.

Olivas GS, Del Togno Armanasco V, Erickson JR: Case management: a bottom-line care delivery model: Part II. adaptation of the model, *J Nurs Admin* 19(12):12–17, 1989b.

Parkman CA, Loveridge C: From nursing service to professional practice, *Nurs Manage* 25(3):63–68, 1994.

Porter-O'Grady T: *Implementing shared governance: creating a professional organization,* St Louis, MO, 1992, Mosby.

Schneider B, Bowen DE: *Winning the service game,* Boston, MA, 1995, Harvard Business School Press.

Simpson RL: Ammunition in the boardroom: the clinical nursing data set, *Nurs Manage* 26(6):16–17, 1995.

Tonges MC: Designing hospital nursing practice: the professionally advanced care team (ProACT) model, part 1, *J Nurs Admin* 19(7):31–38, 1989.

Vestal K, Massey R: Work transformation in health care, *Health Manpower Management* 20(3):9–13, 1994.

Wechsler J: Medication errors draw congressional scrutiny, *BioPharm,* March, 2000, p. 22.

Young S, Duncan B: From primary to modular nursing, *Nurs Manage* 21(5):97, 1990.

Zbylot S, Job C, McCormick E, et al: A case-mix classification system for long-term care facilities, *Nurs Manage* 26(4):49–50, 52, 54, 1995.

# Managing Time Purposefully

*When you complete this chapter, you should be able to:*

1. Explain the differences between effectiveness and efficiency.
2. Describe four categories of client care priorities.
3. Describe principles of priority setting that staff nurses use when managing care for a group of clients.
4. Rank the nursing priorities of a group of clients for a specified time period.
5. Describe the principles of work organization.
6. Compare the client care manager's role in disaster preparedness with that of disaster management.

effectiveness
efficiency
categories of priority nursing needs
  of individual clients
  first-order priority
  second-order priority
  third-order priority
  fourth-order priority
ranking priority needs
  urgency
  timeliness

plan for meeting priority needs of
  a group of clients
  flexibility
  creativity
principles of work organization
disaster preparedness
disaster management

## TIME: A VERY PRECIOUS RESOURCE

Managing time purposefully begins with the nurse's attitude, or how the nurse values time. As discussed in previous chapters, it is a new age of health care. The uniqueness of nursing as a critical profession in society provides its members an opportunity to transform health care in such a way that it changes people's lives for the better. Nurses' time is being leveraged by health-care organization, and considerable effort is being expended to maximize benefits of nursing knowledge and skills to benefit clients (Gerke, 2002, p. 23; Porter-O'Grady, 1999, p. 5). Witness the increased use of electronic devices to "free up" nursing time to improve quality of care for clients (Donnelly, 2000, pp. 28–29; Enger and Segal-Isaacson, 2001, pp. 60–62; McConnell, 1999, p. 43; McConnell, 2000, pp. 37–40; McConnell, 2001, p. 45; Parker, 2001, p. 46; Platt, 2001, pp. 40–43; Rosenthal, 2002, pp. 47–48). To manage time competently would enable the nurse to maintain effectiveness over time. To become proficient in managing time purposefully requires critical thinking throughout one's lifetime. If available, a mentor, preferably a nurse who perceives herself or himself as a good time manager (Francis-Smythe and Robertson, 1999, pp. 333–347), can be a wonderful resource for assisting the beginning nurse to develop this competency as quickly as feasible (Herrin, 2001, p. 16). When done conscientiously, learning to manage time is well worth the effort. The process increases focus on results and reflection for improved assessments and analyses. Many of the principles used by client care managers can be applied in the nurse's personal life, too (Servan-Schreiber, 2000).

The client care manager's time is a precious resource. Time is money. To waste time is to waste money. Each nurse is expected to manage time purposefully every day on every shift. This chapter addresses the many different principles that client care managers apply to ensure that they spend their time effectively and efficiently. It also describes principles of disaster preparedness and disaster management.

## DIFFERENCE BETWEEN EFFECTIVENESS AND EFFICIENCY

Effective use of time entails doing the right things. **Effectiveness** depends on the nurse's assessment and analysis of client needs. Efficient use of time entails doing things right. It depends on the nurse's work organization and ability to complete nursing activities smoothly without using excessive effort, time, or resources. Purposeful time management requires that each nurse select the appropriate activities and complete them correctly without waste.

Beginning and intermediate nursing courses provide opportunities for nursing students to practice using the nursing process. Students assess the client's health status, diagnose the client's health problems, and formulate plans to carry out nursing interventions. Research evidence indicates that nursing assessments are not recorded; these findings focus attention on the need for nursing assessments before establishing priorities (Ehrenberg and Ehnfors, 1999, pp. 65–76). When the nurse's assessments, diagnoses, and plans are appropriate, the nurse is likely to be effective. That is, the nurse is likely to do the right things to assist the client.

**Efficiency** refers to the smoothness with which the care is performed, without compromising effectiveness. Efficient care conserves effort and minimizes interruptions. With practice, the beginning nurse usually becomes more efficient in performing nursing procedures. The nurse is not managing time purposefully if inappropriate nursing care is performed efficiently or if appropriate nursing activities are performed but take excessive time, resources, or effort.

To be effective and efficient, the client care manager assesses each client's needs at the beginning of the shift, ranking needs in order of priority and setting out to meet them accordingly. As a nurse gathers information about each client, he or she ranks the priority of nursing needs immediately, often while receiving change-of-shift report, and makes a mental note of the ranking to set priorities for an assigned group of clients. After completing the initial assessments of individual clients, the client care manager is in a position to prioritize needs for the total group. With practice, the entry-level staff nurse becomes more effective and efficient in assessing client needs and ranking their priority. The discussion that follows focuses on addressing client needs, although the author is aware that other work requirements requested by one's supervisor also might be incorporated into a client care manager's work assignment. The nature of the client care manager's work has social and temporal (monitored and limited time) contexts that might be helpful or detrimental to successful time management (Perlow, 1999, pp. 57–81). The social context of the work setting is discussed further in Chapter Ten.

## PRIORITY NURSING NEEDS OF INDIVIDUAL CLIENTS

A priority client need relates to its importance to the client. Staff nurses are expected to judge the urgency of common client situations and to respond automatically in a timely manner to ensure that each client's needs are met. Staff nurses judge common situations in terms of their urgency or the amount of time available to provide the needed care without putting the client at undue risk. The major **categories of priority nursing needs of individual clients** used to rank their urgency are presented in Box 4-1. Another framework might be a four-category classification: *A*, needs to be done immediately; *B*, needs to be done soon; *C*, can be done later; and *D*, does not need to be done (Puetz and Thomas, 2001, p. 23). Setting priorities requires consideration of time expectation or temporal context.

## First-Order Priority Needs

**First-order priority** nursing needs are threats to a client's immediate survival or safety and demand immediate nursing intervention. A client with an obstructed airway has a first-priority need. The airway obstruction threatens the client's immediate survival. A client who is about to fall faces a threat to immediate safety and urgently needs nursing intervention to prevent injury. If this need is unmet, the fall may cause additional first-priority needs. Staff nurses are expected to apply nursing knowledge (e.g., use the nursing process) when identifying priority needs (Riegel and Dracup, 1986, pp. 307–309).

BOX 4-1

### Priority Ranking of Individual Needs

**First-order priority need**
An immediate threat to client's survival or safety

**Second-order priority need**
Actual problems for which the client or family have requested immediate help

**Third-order priority need**
Actual or potential problems that the client or family does not recognize

**Fourth-order priority need**
Anticipated actual or potential problems with which the client or family will need help in the future

## Second-Order Priority Needs

**Second-order priority** needs are problems for which the client or family has asked for immediate help. These problems frequently relate to comfort. Relief of pain, nausea, or full bladder or bowel often requires urgent nursing responses to prevent the client's problems from becoming worse. Minimizing the urgency of these needs may put the client at risk physiologically, psychologically, and emotionally. If the nurse does not respond promptly, the client's confidence in the nurse is likely to be threatened, and the health of their working relationship may suffer. The nurse is expected to respond to second-order priority nursing needs as soon as possible. Zeollner-Hunter (1999, p. 12) reported an effective response to changing the work routines and available equipment that helped client care managers respond to second-order needs in a more timely manner. By making more keys available, clients waited less for oral narcotics, which resulted in increased satisfaction with care received. This example is included to show that systematic study of a repetitious client care situation often results in improved service.

## Third-Order Priority Needs

**Third-order priority** needs concern actual or potential problems that the client or family does not recognize. They are characterized by relative urgency. The nursing staff must monitor closely and manage these needs because they can rely on neither the client nor the family for help in managing them. A client who is not aware of the side effects of drugs is usually at greater risk than a client who is aware of the side effects. An example of a third-order priority nursing need is a client who is experiencing cognitive dysfunction resulting from sedation. Other common situations involve interventions that prevent potential complications of diseases or treatments. Satisfying third-order priority needs often involves teaching the client and family about the condition in an attempt to reduce the urgency of the need for the nurse's watchfulness. It can involve teaching the client and the client's family to provide self-care to reduce the need for nursing care.

## Fourth-Order Priority Needs

**Fourth-order priority** needs involve actual or potential problems with which the client or family may need help in the future. These concerns often relate to the client's need for continuity of care within the facility or in preparation for discharge. The nurse may help the client learn about self-care and treatment procedures long before leaving the health-care facility. These needs often include teaching plans for managing anticipated discomforts, nutrition, skin integrity, or elimination problems. Teaching plans often are limited by the learner's readiness and ability to use new knowledge and skills within the time available during the length of stay. Written instructions often are used to help the client and family recall essential facts and related instructions. To the extent possible, the nurse assists clients and families to perform care to assess their capabilities, instead of asking them to describe the care verbally. The nurse also tries to enable the client to make alternative plans for anticipated continued care should anything unexpected occur.

## Ranking Priority Needs

In **ranking priority needs,** the nurse assesses the client's condition and responses to health problems and their treatment. This ranking is performed by taking into consideration the anticipated length of stay and requirements for continued care. Care maps or critical pathways often identify critical tasks, drugs, and instructional plans that have a high priority in the client's treatment and are helpful in prioritizing client needs. The priority ranking often relates to predictable consequences of not meeting the client's needs, the perceived **urgency** of preventing such risks, and the client's and family's resources to provide the indicated care. Importance and **timeliness** are of the essence when responding to priority nursing needs. The nurse typically has less time to address more urgent needs and more time to plan to meet nursing needs that are less urgent. If plans for meeting less urgent priority needs are not carried out, less urgent needs become urgent, and the work life patterns become a cycle of crises (i.e., repeated days of "putting out fires"). When daily routines become a repeated pattern of managing crises, it is important to analyze the social context of care to identify factors that reward the work group in this cycle and what might be done to change it.

## PRIORITY NEEDS OF A GROUP OF CLIENTS

Staff nurses use several principles in planning to meet priority nursing needs for a group of clients. These principles commonly are understood and treated as basic assumptions by experienced nurses. With practice, entry-level staff nurses can learn to apply these principles while providing care efficiently without compromising effectiveness.

## Know Needs and Priorities of Each Client

To **plan for meeting the priority needs of a group of clients,** the nurse needs to know both the needs and priorities of each client and those of the assigned group of clients. This is not to imply that the nurse does not respond to client needs until all individual client needs are assessed. Rather, the nurse completes assessments as soon as possible while addressing first-priority and second-priority needs in a timely manner. Every nurse develops a unique pattern of sequencing nursing activities to ensure that each client's condition is assessed and priorities are identified early in the shift. To identify which clients need assessment first, the nurse uses information from the change-of-shift report and the agency's classification system to help identify the client's acuity level (need for nursing resources). When initial nursing assessments are completed, the nurse spontaneously ranks individual client needs in terms of priority or urgency.

## Factors to Consider When Determining Priorities of Care

To determine the priorities of care needed by a group of clients during a specified time or shift, the nurse considers many factors. First, to help promote appropriate use of resources, the nurse thinks about the amount of time and skills required to do the nursing activities. Clients who need complex dressing changes, protective isolation, or encouragement to increase self-sufficiency in completing personal hygiene measures often require more nursing time and skill than clients who do not. The nurse also tries to match client needs with available resources and the number and qualifications of staff. The number and type of available staff frequently are related to the agency's classification system and the acuity and predictability of clients' needs. In addition to educational credentials, some nursing staff have unique skills and talents that, when matched with client needs, bring out the best in both client and nurse.

Depending on the purpose of the agency, the nurse also may consider the need to make provisions for each client's continued care or discharge preparations. If the client's needs are simple (predictable), as determined by the client's diseases, treatments, and responses, the nurse matches them with less complex nursing services. The needs of these clients are likely to be addressed satisfactorily with care provided by licensed practical nurses and nursing assistants. These needs also frequently are addressed by nursing routines, policies, and procedures. Typically, repeated nursing assessments and related interventions by a registered nurse are needed less frequently when the client's acuity level is low or the client is physiologically stable.

When the client's needs are more complex, often because the client's physiologic status is less predictable, the nurse often plans to provide the care. This approach ensures that more frequent assessments and corresponding interventions are made. If the client's care depends on various diagnostic study results and requires considerable interdisciplinary collaboration, the staff nurse frequently provides the needed nursing attention. For example, if clinical laboratory study results will be used to identify a client's likelihood of continued internal bleeding and to determine the need for further diagnostic workup, the staff nurse might care for the client to reinforce the diagnostic plan and to lessen the client's anxiety. This plan enables the nurse to teach the client to adhere to various interdisciplinary requirements and to help complete the diagnostic process and follow-up, which might, in this example, include blood transfusions.

By evaluating each client's needs and matching them with corresponding resources, the nurse addresses the priorities of the group of assigned clients. While matching client needs with available nursing staff, the nurse considers (i.e., tries to anticipate) what the staff needs to do, the amount of time required to complete the tasks, and the amount of monitoring needed. The nurse also considers and tries to anticipate the equipment, routines, policies, and procedures involved in each individual's care during the shift.

## Flexibility

When possible, the nurse is expected to be flexible in response to priority client needs. Client and staff preferences are incorporated in nursing responses. To provide for unpredicted first-order and second-order priority client needs, the nurse allocates nursing resources so that nursing staff capable of making complex assessments of client needs are continuously available. To provide such flexibility, registered nurses must be available to meet client needs throughout the shift, including during staff rest and meal breaks.

**Flexibility** in responding to priority needs requires that the nurse remember each client's primary goals. The goals often are described in terms of the client's symptoms, responses to treatment, or preparation for continued care in another

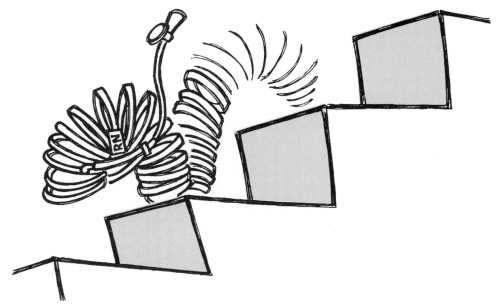

Flexibility in responding to priority needs requires that the nurse remember each client's primary goals.

setting. Keeping these goals clearly in mind, the nurse determines which policies, procedures, and routines best meet the client's needs. The nurse also helps the client understand the available options. The nurse assesses the effectiveness of approaches being used to alleviate postoperative pain, including the client's use of patient-controlled analgesia. If the client is not obtaining adequate relief, the nurse looks for other causes of discomfort, such as anxiety, atypical response to the analgesic, errors in medication administration or use of equipment, or evidence of postoperative complications. On the basis of repeated assessments, the nurse provides other comfort measures to reduce anxiety, teaches the client about anticipated progress, and collaborates with other disciplines to manage potential complications. The focus is on the desired goals and problem solving to achieve them.

The entry-level staff nurse is expected to understand how various routines promote continuity of care. Various client responses to postoperative routines often are described in the change-of-shift report. The client's responses to treatment also are described. The nurse is expected to modify routines if they do not help the client meet specific goals. For example, postoperative coughing and deep-breathing exercises need to be modified if the client is unable to perform them due to discomfort. The timing of these exercises might be scheduled to coincide with the client's response to analgesia. By focusing on the client's responses and progress, routines can be used flexibly to enable clients to reach their goals. As clients progress, different routines can be emphasized to reinforce attention to priority needs.

## Creativity

In addition to incorporating flexibility, the beginning staff nurse is expected to use **creativity** in responding to the priority needs of assigned clients. Clients usually have limited abilities to complete the activities of daily living. These limitations often are emphasized to the detriment of the client's abilities. The nurse strives to emphasize clients' abilities and strengths without ignoring disabilities or vulnerabilities (i.e., strengths are emphasized to encourage clients to continue their chosen lifestyles). To preserve client autonomy and independence, the nurse creatively encourages each client to use remaining abilities and skills rather than to focus on disabilities. Often the nurse must help the client alternate periods of activity with periods of rest to promote self-care and to control symptoms. Or the nurse might offer the client choices in various aspects of self-care, such as the sequencing of self-care activities or methods of performing treatments, when possible. These approaches are used to maximize client control and decision making when real choices are available. Nurses collaborate with other members of the health-care team to incorporate individual client choices in treatment programs. In this way, nurses act as client advocates.

The nurse also encourages client and family participation in care. Client and family involvement helps motivate clients to learn about the changes needed to facilitate their adjustment to their circumstances. This helps avoid compromising the client's autonomy or independence any more than absolutely necessary. Some client choices require the nurse to collaborate with other members of the health-care team to coordinate the client's treatment program.

A client's cultural background may increase his or her vulnerability for having priority needs overlooked. Effective nursing care requires application of knowledge of cultural differences. Cultural and ethnic dimensions of nursing care require the nurse to apply knowledge of the individual client's beliefs and values about health, illness, family dynamics, and healing practices (Kagawa-Singer, 1987, p. 59; Varricchio, 1987, p. 57). Frequently, additional knowledge and assessment skills are needed to care for clients with cultural backgrounds different from one's own (Stewart, 1991, p. 192). When adequately assessed, cultural differences require flexibility when they are addressed in corresponding plans of care. Sensitivity to cultural backgrounds of individual clients enables the nurse to prioritize their needs effectively.

With practice, priority setting for a group of clients enables the nurse to rate spontaneously the urgency of nursing attention needed to meet individual needs. This information is used to allocate available nursing resources. Through continued effort, the nurse learns to modify nursing routines, interpret policies, and perform procedures to address priority needs in a timely manner. The complexity of client needs also guides the nurse's response so that appropriate skills are consistently available to address first-priority and second-priority needs.

## PRINCIPLES OF WORK ORGANIZATION

The acuity levels of many clients needing nursing care in acute care and long-term care settings can be overwhelming if nurses do not have an effective method for organizing their work. Using **principles of work organization** may prevent the nurse from feeling overwhelmed and promote feelings of success. Box 4-2 lists principles of work organization. Entry-level staff nurses are expected to use these principles to manage time effectively and efficiently. This section discusses how these common principles are used in the nursing practice context.

---

### BOX 4-2

### Principles of Work Organization

---

Determine the short-term and long-term goals of assigned clients.
Make a "things to do" list and rank each activity.
Estimate how much time is needed to complete various activities.
Set limits by saying no to unreasonable assignments.
Eliminate unnecessary steps or work.
Reserve time to respond to unexpected demands. Plan to "free up" time of a more skilled staff member to provide for unexpected demands placed on the work group.

## Determine Short-Term and Long-Term Goals of Assigned Clients

To reach a destination, you need to know where it is. Then the journey can be made in single steps. In a similar manner, staff nurses need to know the short-term and long-term goals for each of their assigned clients. Short-term goals are desired client outcomes to be met within specified time periods, such as a shift, day, or week. Sometimes short-term goals refer to a particular phase of hospitalization, such as the immediate postoperative period or the first week of residence at a long-term care facility. All short-term goals rarely are identified on a nursing care plan or pathway, although many frequently are described in terms of quality assurance standards of care. For example, nursing assessments are done to detect potential postoperative complications; their frequency depends on individual client responses. Standards of care typically address interventions needed to prevent complications.

Long-term goals might be the desired outcome of a client's hospitalization or of a 3-month stay in a long-term care facility. These goals relate to the client's priority needs; when they are satisfactorily met, the client's response reflects desired progress. When the nurse knows the client's short-term and long-term goals, it is possible to identify priorities and evaluate the client's progress. Typically, when priorities are identified, the nurse performs more focused assessments as a method of diagnostic reasoning to collect information useful in establishing the interventions needed to achieve the client's goals successfully.

## Make a "Things To Do" List

With an overview of the work to be done, the nurse should jot down the essential tasks facing the work group (Zyry and Neumann, 1999, p. 262). When the nurse cares for one client, it is easier to remember the various activities that need to be done to complete the care. When the nurse is assigned several clients, however, it is more difficult to remember all the activities that need to be done throughout the entire shift. Consequently, to complete a work assignment, the nurse makes a "things to do" list at the beginning of the shift. Activities may be added to this list throughout the shift as they occur. Depending on the number of these items, they may need to be grouped in categories (e.g., telephone calls, e-mails, intravenous lines, medications) or by the times certain activities need to be done. This list enables the nurse to recall activities efficiently to meet client needs and personal goals that need to be accomplished in a timely manner. Sometimes nurses use a nursing worksheet to help organize their activities. Figure 4-1 illustrates a nursing assignment worksheet that might be used as a "things to do" list.

## Rank Activities

The nurse ranks each item on the "things to do" list in accordance with its importance or the order in which activities are to be done. Ranking these items takes only a short time, but the gains from spending concentrated thought early in the shift are invaluable later, especially since nursing practice entails multiple distractions

| Client | Room | VS/Time | Meds | Rx | Special needs/Observations |
|---|---|---|---|---|---|
| TD | 107 A | TDR @ 8-12 | 730 800 1130 1300 | Incentive Spirometry I & O | Assess breath sounds; reinforce activity restrictions |
| CM | 108 B | BP, TRR @ 800 | 800 1200 | I + O I + @ 1100 1500 | Encourage fluids; Reinforce teaching plan in prep for D/C |
| LR | 109 A | BP, TPR @ 800 1200 | 800 1300 | Drug I+O Change in AM | Assess breath sounds; Monitor adherence to fluid restrictions |
| AP | 109 B | TPR @ 800 | 900 | PT @ 1000 1400 | Monitor use of crutches, safety of transfers |

FIGURE 4-1 Nursing assignment.

and interruptions (Shaffer, 2000, pp. 24D-24F). With practice, the nurse can design a unique "things to do" list, rank the importance of each nursing activity spontaneously, and fit the activity into a unique pattern of activities. Until work organizational skills are well developed, however, the nurse needs to take time early in each shift to rate the desired sequence of completing activities on the list. Four suggestions may help in the sequencing of a "things to do" list.

First, consider items that have specific time limits in terms of addressing client needs. For example, the nurse cannot prepare a client for discharge from the health-care facility if the client has already gone. When clients gain more benefit from physical therapy if they receive analgesia beforehand, these clients need to receive analgesia sufficiently in advance of their treatment.

Second, compile the client care worksheet or "things to do" list at the beginning of the day, while or immediately after receiving the change-of-shift report. Developing it at this time helps the nurse recall details and specific tasks that promote doing the right thing when it needs to be done. This approach to immediate recall of details is likely to increase effectiveness and efficiency.

Third, analyze the "things to do" list to identify activities that are scheduled due to agency policies or routines developed for the sake of all involved (Bernhard and Walsh, 1995, p. 96). Note which activities need to be done "on time" to enable health-care team members to maintain efficiency. Identify the activities that can be done at the nurse's own discretion. Then plan to "work around" the scheduled activities (e.g., administering intravenous antibiotics as scheduled), and identify what else might be done while with the client. This approach often helps decrease fragmentation of client care as well as footwork. It also should help the nurse make efficient use of the time consumed by scheduled activities. For example, by gathering equipment and supplies needed for an individual client after you have done your initial assessment rather than before, you might avoid bringing what you do not need and interrupting your care to get what is needed but not available.

Fourth, try to estimate how much time is needed to complete the various activities in the assignment. Include longer amounts of time for activities with which the nurse will need help from another staff member. These activities often take more time because the nurse must plan and coordinate her or his efforts with the schedule and efforts of one or more persons.

Many of the assigned activities involved in care require the nurse to work with one or more of the nursing work group, especially in the beginning of the nurse's career, when the nurse needs more frequent supervision (Holcomb, 2001, pp. 38–39; Mastrian, 2001, pp. 36–37). It is crucial that the nurse plan time to do everything that she or he believes is important; the nurse needs to rank it accordingly with her or his ranking of importance and urgency (Brink, 2000, pp. 383–384). Learning time management skills in a specific practice context requires the nurse to gain considerable tacit knowledge. When the initial "things to do" list is developed with others on the nursing work group and with clients, the nurse can begin to plan when to do what. This planning helps to gain the cooperation of others and to identify any "impossible" plans early so that they can be changed to make them feasible.

As you proceed throughout the shift, check off completed activities to reinforce your success and progress. Refer to the list at regular intervals. Check it to see what else you had planned to accomplish that you did not include in your plan, and try to avoid similar omissions in the future (Dawes, 1999, pp. 374–377). Add activities that have high priority but that you had not anticipated earlier. Use of a current "things to do" list helps you feel successful in managing time purposefully.

Developing time management skills is a continuous process. Practice estimating how much time you need to complete various assigned client care activities. Research findings indicate this is difficult but can be learned with practice (Francis-Smythe and Robertson, 1999, pp. 333–347). Notice what types of activities consume more time than you expected and what types of interruptions delay your completion of various nursing tasks. You may find that you frequently attend to several clients' needs concurrently and efficiently. The smoothness with which you complete your assignment will increase as you learn to monitor your assigned clients regularly throughout your shift. The beginning nurse will gain confidence as she or he identifies client needs that respond to preventive nursing measures. The beginning nurse also will learn how much time is needed to respond to unanticipated activities that require attention.

As the client care manager continues to develop time management skills, she or he also will learn to multitask (i.e., work at more than one task of the total assignment at any one point in time) (Grensing-Pophal, 1999, pp. 55–56). Concurrently, it will become apparent that small amounts of time can be used to work on more or less complex tasks. Usually, it is better to work on more complex or time-consuming work early in the shift so that it is accomplished, given the potential for multiple interruptions throughout a workday.

## Set Limits by Saying No to Unreasonable Assignments

Keeping a time log for several consecutive days may help the nurse distinguish between reasonable and unreasonable assignments. Unreasonable assignments are those that cannot be done with the available resources and time (Cushing, 1988, pp. 1635–1637). Figure 4-2 is a form that might be used at two or more intervals to help the nurse identify patterns of time management throughout a workday. Data are compared at intervals to help distinguish assignments that merely need an improved method of delivery from assignments that are unreasonable. Patterns of response to reasonable client care assignments are analyzed to determine which aspects of each assignment required more time or resources than the nurse had anticipated. If the nurse is unable to monitor and respond to clients' needs adequately, the nurse's clients are in danger. By continuously looking for improvements in time management, the nurse will develop a clear understanding of which assignments are reasonable, given the available staffing, and which are unsafe for clients and staff. Consultation with a trusted mentor could prove valuable in providing insight given the specific characteristics of the practice context.

No amount of education, good will, or practice enables the nurse to complete unreasonable client care assignments. Unreasonable assignments often reflect inadequate staffing, which can occur for many reasons and place impossible demands on the nurse. With the persistent shortage of qualified nurses, some entry-level staff nurses may be given unreasonable assignments. If, after careful analysis of the assignment, the nurse thinks that the assignment reflects understaffing, he or she has an immediate obligation to inform the supervisor on behalf of the assigned clients (Fiesta, 1990, pp. 22–23).

You need to explain in detail to your supervisor the reasons you believe you are understaffed (Mallison, 1987, p. 151) and why you think the assignment is unreasonable (Cushing, 1988, pp. 1635–1637). Saying, "I won't have enough time to do all the care my clients need" is not as helpful as describing what the client needs are; for example, "I have three clients who need continuous careful monitoring of vital signs, three others receiving blood transfusions who need careful watching, and another client is expected to be admitted within the hour."

You also have a responsibility to inform your supervisor if you think your assignment exceeds the limits of your educational preparation and clinical expertise. Take time to discuss the situation with your supervisor to identify alternative options. If adequate staffing is unavailable and you believe you have the necessary skills to provide the needed care but not enough time to do so, you must proceed with your assignment to the best of your ability (Nurse's Reference Library, 1984, pp. 124–129). If the situation is not remedied, you need to decide your next course of action and whether to continue your employment. Make your concerns known throughout every level of the organization. Keep a written log of actions you have taken to find solutions to inadequate staffing.

The nurse needs to determine how he or she will say no to unreasonable assignments (Knippen and Green, 1990, pp. 6–7). To not recognize unreasonable assignments due to inadequate staffing is to accept compromised standards of sound nursing practice and to jeopardize clients' safety and well-being.

TIME LOG

Date:_____

| Time | Activities | Comments |
|------|-----------|----------|
| 6:30 | | |
| 6:45 | | |
| 7:00 | | |
| 7:15 | | |
| 7:30 | | |
| 7:45 | | |
| 8:00 | | |
| 8:15 | | |
| 8:30 | | |
| 8:45 | | |
| 9:00 | | |
| 9:15 | | |
| 9:30 | | |
| 9:45 | | |
| 10:00 | | |
| 10:15 | | |
| 10:30 | | |
| 10:45 | | |
| 11:00 | | |
| 11:15 | | |
| 11:30 | | |
| 11:45 | | |
| 12:00 | | |
| 12:15 | | |
| 12:30 | | |
| 12:45 | | |
| 1:00 | | |
| 1:15 | | |
| 1:30 | | |
| 1:45 | | |
| 2:00 | | |
| 2:15 | | |
| 2:30 | | |
| 2:45 | | |
| 3:00 | | |
| 3:15 | | |
| 3:30 | | |
| 3:45 | | |
| 4:00 | | |
| 4:15 | | |
| 4:30 | | |

Totals:  Direct client care activities:_____
   Planning activities:_____
   Staff conferences:_____
   Documentation activities:_____
   Telephone communications:_____
   Socialization:_____
   Breaks and lunch:_____

FIGURE 4-2 Time log: analysis of time management patterns.

The nursing shortage is expected to continue in the foreseeable future. It will continue to be important that professional nurses direct nursing care while collaborating with others when indicated (Hendrickson and Doddato, 1989, pp. 281–283). Identifying what nursing actions need to be taken is a crucial function of staff nurses if care is to be safe and effective. Assignment of nursing tasks to promote efficiency may contribute to cost-effectiveness if done wisely (e.g., if it focuses on individual client needs and is consistent with the organization's primary purpose).

## Eliminate Unnecessary Steps or Work

As the nurse strives to improve time management skills, it is necessary to eliminate unnecessary steps or nursing activities. It is crucial that efforts to increase efficiency not compromise effectiveness. To reduce footwork, assemble needed equipment and supplies before entering client care areas to do specific nursing procedures. It takes a short time to review a procedure mentally and identify needed equipment and supplies when you are in the client's room completing your initial assessment. Noting your findings can help you assemble needed equipment, avoid contaminating unneeded supplies, and avoid interruptions in procedures due to lack of supplies or equipment.

Another method of promoting efficiency is to reduce fragmentation of a client's care by grouping similar activities done at the bedside. A nurse can gather needed information, monitor symptoms and client responses, administer treatment, and assist with personal hygiene activities during one contact with a client. Grouping procedures means fewer interruptions for the client, allowing him or her to rest. If the client's care is expected to take considerable time, the nurse might block off time in the work plan and make provisions to ensure that other clients' needs are addressed during that time. This approach may require planning with peers or coworkers to provide the necessary coverage, but it benefits clients and helps the nurse to manage time.

To manage time well, it is best to complete the nursing tasks for one client's care before starting with another client. Usually clients appreciate the reduced fragmentation and prompt assistance. It is usually easier to recall detailed observations of a client's assessment if it is documented immediately, rather than waiting until the end of the shift.

Collaboration with coworkers avoids or reduces duplication of staff efforts. It ensures that everyone involved in the client's care knows exactly what is expected in terms of the nursing assignment. Clients who must repeat requests for help or reiterate information for assessments several times bear the burden of duplication or gaps in staff efforts. Client confidence in such staff efforts cannot be sustained if duplicated efforts or gaps occur repeatedly.

To the greatest extent possible, involve support staff in performing tasks (nonclinical activities) for which they are prepared and employed to do (Hendrickson et al., 1990, p. 35). Use computers or electronic communication methods to relay common requests when feasible (e.g., for requisitioning supplies or equipment, transcribing orders [Hendrickson et al., 1990, p. 36]). This method of information relay is rapid and can be accessed by others without untimely interruptions or long waiting periods.

To judge the success of time management efforts, evaluate the extent to which plans and use of nursing routines met the clients' needs. By listening to what clients and their significant others say or questions they ask, a nurse can identify needs for modification of nursing routines and ways to eliminate duplicated efforts and unnecessary steps. It also is helpful to ask coworkers for feedback about the plans used to provide the needed care. This information often provides helpful insight into the interrelationships important in effective and efficient use of resources.

## Plan for Unexpected Demands

Because many unpredicted client needs arise during a shift, it is necessary to plan to provide for them. Initially the nurse may need to allow more time to deal with unpredicted situations. Later, as the nurse becomes more experienced with the agency's routines and variations in clients' needs, there should be fewer unpredicted needs. To manage these needs, whenever possible, plan to "free up" a more skilled team member, preferably a registered nurse, to respond to unexpected demands placed on the work group. A more skilled worker can be expected to respond more flexibly and creatively to a greater variety of client needs than a less skilled one. This flexibility enables more members of the work group to carry out their plans to complete their work assignments. Although this method or strategy may seem to be preferential treatment, this approach actually promotes increased satisfaction and positive feelings about staff work assignments.

The principles of work organization assist the entry-level staff nurse to manage time purposefully. To manage time effectively with the assigned group of clients, the client care manager also must rely on an accurate assessment of the clients' conditions, analyses of needs, and formulation of nursing plans, including short-term and long-term goals.

Purposeful time management also requires the nurse to allocate nursing resources to match assessed client needs. Consistent delegation of client care according to nursing staff skills and qualifications within the context of the agency's position descriptions promotes efficiency. Principles of proper delegation are discussed further in Chapter Twelve. With the shortage of qualified nurses, it is important to maximize the effectiveness and efficiency of available staff members.

By repeated use of a time log, the entry-level staff nurse can gain insight into realistic work assignments and expectations for accomplishing them. Frequently, nurses omit rest or lunch breaks to complete various aspects of client care. Although this behavior is well intentioned, such patterns of time management often reduce the nurse's effectiveness. Nurses are aware that to prevent fatigue and excessive physiologic stress, they must include breaks in their work schedule and stick to them. Ultimately, such an approach preserves the nurse's resources and decreases potential for burnout.

Time management skills are learned approaches, not inherited characteristics. Work organization skills develop from careful attention to determining what needs to be done in a specified time and how it can best be accomplished with the available resources: staff, equipment, supplies, and time. Clients and nurses benefit from continuous efforts to improve.

## DISASTER PREPAREDNESS AND MANAGEMENT

With the increased widespread fear of terrorism, the need for disaster preparedness and management increases. Terrorism attacks are a category of disaster causes. The other common type of disaster is a natural disaster (e.g., flood, tornado, fire, earthquake). One could compare disaster management strategies in categories similar to the types of broad categories within the health-care continuum (Table 4-1).

Just as in the provision of health care throughout the continuum, disaster management involves preventive, early detection and treatment programs. As with disease management, predictably the circumstances and approaches differ for each of the various types of disasters (Dawes, 2002, pp. 730–732). Similarly, although established disaster programs are reviewed and practiced, every actual disaster is unexpected; effective disaster management relies on the faith that enough information will be retained so that planned organized staff responses occur to provide effective care. Responding to a disaster is anything but routine. Actual disaster management is highly dependent on disaster preparedness and regular review and revision.

**TABLE 4-1**

## Disaster Management

| Category | Health Care | Disaster Management |
|---|---|---|
| Primary prevention | Immunizations | Recognize and respond to vulnerabilities and increasing risks, such as increasing poverty or oppression and changing physical structure of the environment due to urban development, deforestation, and decreased waste management; may involve immunization programs |
| Secondary prevention | Early detection | Recognize unusual case presentations, expected symptoms of anticipated diseases or health problems, increased incidence of disease presentations or screening for evidence of infectious agents, and appropriate reporting and follow-up treatment |
| Tertiary prevention | Disease treatment and prevention of complications | Provide urgent disease treatment to prevent complications of disease, biologic or chemical exposure, floods, tornadoes, fires, or bomb threat |

Consequently, every disaster practice or drill needs to be reviewed carefully and evaluated to make the plan focused and comprehensive; these reviews depend on the input of client care managers as to what worked and what did not and what else should be considered.

## Disaster Preparedness

There is growing evidence that increased vulnerability associated with poverty and poor coordination of public safety measures and communication increases risk and potential for disaster (Horwich, 2000, pp. 521–542; Ozerdem, 2000, pp. 425–439; Perez-Lugo, 2001, pp. 55–73). The first priority of **disaster preparedness** is to prevent the disaster by identifying risks and decreasing vulnerabilities and losses (Gerber and Feldman, 2002, pp. 61–64). Most commonly in the United States, considerable effort is expended to provide safety in transportation and workplaces in addition to monitoring weather conditions for risks of tornadoes, floods, and severe weather. The media are involved in broadcasting preventive measures and impending weather conditions. Despite these efforts, most disasters are unexpected by their victims.

Consequently, it becomes crucial that work groups of well-informed and experienced persons be involved in public education programs that address the types of disasters that should be anticipated, given the local resources and environmental characteristics (e.g., vulnerability for floods, tornadoes, fires, or earthquakes) (Howard, 2001, pp. 527–528). In addition, this team, interdisciplinary in nature, establishes a risk management plan, defining evacuation routes and plans, alternative sites for care, and vertical and horizontal communication patterns so that everyone will know what needs to be done, who to report to, and how to preserve valuable records and documentation.

It is essential that the client care manager understand the disaster (risk management) plan in sufficient detail so that it makes sense. It is not enough to read the plan; the client care manager needs to know whom to report to, where to find needed information quickly and understand evacuation plans in effect. At regular intervals, it is necessary to review the disaster plan because it is likely to change as the health-care organization gains experience and vulnerabilities change. The purpose of the plan and implementation practice is to enable employees to know and follow the plan in an autocratic way. Time is of the essence until officials directing the plan notify employees otherwise.

## Disaster Management

When a disaster occurs (it is likely to be unexpected), the client care manager needs to implement the established plan as directed to the extent possible; when it is not feasible, the circumstances need to be communicated to the supervising staff for review and response. The **disaster management** approach will involve many different departments and specialists, corresponding to the cause and magnitude of the disaster. If the disaster relates to chemical weapons, environmental specialists will be involved, whereas a disaster caused by an infectious biologic weapon would involve the Centers for Disease Control and prevention staff. Not only victims but also members of the community, family members, and employees need to be safe and adequately protected or decontaminated. It is also important that feedback about the effectiveness of the plan be given when requested because the experience will be valuable for developing awareness of vulnerability and improving the plan.

When a disaster occurs, it becomes priority one. Client care managers can best participate in effective disaster management by concentrated effort on carrying out the plan based on one's understanding the health-care agency's plan and knowing where more detailed information is readily accessible and the communication methods and codes that will be used to follow through. Consideration needs to be given to providing care to disaster victims and clients already assigned to the nurse's care. After the disaster plan is implemented, the client care manager needs to provide feedback about the plan in an effort to improve it based on experience.

## SUMMARY

The client care manager's time is a precious resource. Client care managers are expected to manage their time purposefully when providing care to an assigned group of clients. Time management requires commitment to effectiveness and efficiency; staff nurses are expected to do the right things for clients and perform them without excessive use of time, energy, equipment, or supplies.

Priority client needs require urgent nursing attention. The priority needs of individual clients can be ranked in several categories: (1) threats to immediate survival or safety, (2) actual or potential problems for which the client or family have asked for immediate help, (3) actual or potential problems unrecognized by the client or family, (4) actual or potential problems for which the client or family needs help in the future, and (5) problems that do not need intervention. Timeliness is of the essence when the client care manager responds to priority nursing needs. The more urgent the client need, the less time the nurse has to respond. More urgent needs rank as higher priorities.

Staff nurses follow several principles when planning to meet the priority needs of a group of clients. The nurse must focus on the primary goals of clients to provide flexible and creative responses. In addition, client strengths and abilities should be emphasized without neglecting disabilities or vulnerabilities. The effective nurse promotes client and family participation in decisions that affect them. Nurses collaborate with multidisciplinary work groups to incorporate client choices in treatment programs.

Staff nurses apply a variety of principles of work organization to address assigned client needs. After determining short-term and long-term goals, effective nurses compile a "things to do" list early in the workday and refer to it often to ensure that priority client needs are met. They try to estimate time needed to complete various client care activities, plan with others, and avoid interruptions and delays. If inadequate staffing jeopardizes client well-being, staff nurses report unreasonable assignments to supervisors to obtain the needed help. To promote efficiency, client care managers strive to eliminate unnecessary steps and work by planning activities on the basis of nursing assessments, clustering activities with one client before beginning care of others, and collaborating with others. By repeated analyses of a time log, nurses can gain insight into patterns of time management that reduce their effectiveness. Although it is sometimes difficult, development of purposeful time management skills is a necessity in modern health care as well as a continuous process. Clients and nurses benefit from the use of these skills.

Disaster management involves preparedness and implementation of established plans. Disasters, similar to diseases, can be prevented or decreased through public education and increased awareness of vulnerabilities. Preparedness is key to effective responses to disasters. The client care manager needs to understand the agency's disaster plan and where to find additional information if needed and to whom implementation problems need to be reported. Disaster management principles correspond to the type, specific causes, and magnitude of the disaster. Autocratic leadership is used, and experience is maximized through the use of feedback to improve existing plans.

## APPLICATION EXERCISES

1. Observe a staff nurse's activities during the first hour of a shift. List six sources of information the nurse used to complete nursing assessments to increase effectiveness.
2. Observe a staff nurse's activities during the last hour of a shift. List six techniques the nurse used to increase efficiency in completing nursing assignments.
3. Review previous client care assignments that you completed within the last month. Give an example of each category of nursing priority as described in this chapter. Be prepared to give reasons for your selections.
4. Describe three examples of creativity involved in adapting nursing routines to increase the quality of client care.
5. Application of principles of work organization is an individualized activity. Describe at least one principle of work organization that you use or know of that is not described in this chapter.
6. State where the written disaster plan is located in your work environment. Are there additional databases that you will use if the disaster is of a biologic or chemical nature?
7. Describe how the disaster plan is likely to meet the emotional and psychological needs of a victim of a disaster caused by fire, by flood, and by bomb threat.

## CRITICAL THINKING SCENARIO

Picture yourself practicing your profession at a community-based home care agency. You are expected to provide services for clients who already have been assessed initially by a lead community health nurse who functions as their primary nurse. You also are expected to document your visits and communicate with the lead community health nurse if any client's condition or needs change, necessitating revision in the frequency or amount of services provided

**CRITICAL THINKING SCENARIO—cont'd**

each visit. You typically make four to six visits per day, depending on the quantity and complexity of services needed and travel time required. It is a busy holiday weekend. In addition to "taking call" (requests for unscheduled visits), you have been asked to make eight visits today: some to provide scheduled infusion therapy for pain management and others for local wound care. It is not feasible to complete this assignment without altering the scheduled times established with the clients and extending your day beyond 10 hours.

1. After you take four slow deep breaths, what would you do?
2. Who would you contact to establish a workable visit schedule for today?
3. Would you plan to change anything about your typical visit pattern to accommodate all of your assigned clients? Explain.

## REFERENCES

Bernhard LA, Walsh M: *Leadership: the key to the professionalization of nursing*, ed 3, St Louis, MO, 1995, Mosby.

Brink PJ: I'm too busy, *West J Nurs Res* 22(4):383–384, 2000.

Cushing M: Refusing an unreasonable assignment: Part 2. strategies for problem solving, *Am J Nurs* 88(12):1635–1637, 1988.

Dawes BSG: Perspectives on priorities, time management, and patient care, *AORN J* 70(3):374–377, 1999.

Dawes BSG: Disaster management requires planning, improvising, and evaluating, *AORN J* 75(4):730–732, 2002.

Donnelly J: Integrated communication cascade: better information, faster response, *Nurs Manage* 31(3):28–29, 2000.

Ehrenberg A, Ehnfors M: Patient problems, needs, and nursing diagnosis in Swedish nursing home records, *Nurs Diagnosis* 19(2):65–76, 1999.

Enger JC, Segal-Isaacson AE: 2002 guide to new technology—PDAs: the ABCs of PDAs, *Nurs Manage* 32(12):60–62, 2001.

Fiesta J: The nursing shortage: whose liability problem? Part II, *Nurs Manage* 21(2):22–23, 1990.

Francis-Smythe JA, Robertson IT: On the relationship between time management and time estimation, *Br J Psychol* 90(3):333–347, 1999.

Gerber JA, Feldman ER: Is your business prepared for the worst? *Journal of Accountancy* 193(4):61–64, 2002.

Gerke ML: Find nursing's essence, *Nurs Manage* 33(4):23, 2002.

Grensing-Pophal L: Round the clock: multitasking made easy, *Nursing* 29(2):55–56. 1999.

Hendrickson G, Doddato TM: Setting priorities during the shortage, *Nurs Outlook* 37(6):280–284, 1989.

Hendrickson G, Doddato TM, Kovner CT: How do nurses use their time? *J Nurs Admin* 20(3):31–37, 1990.

Herrin DM: Time for a leadership tune-up? *Nurs Manage* 32(12):16, 2001.

Holcomb S: Homegrown: CC interns take root, *Nurs Manage 32*(5):38–39, 2001.

Horwich G: Economic lessons of the Kobe earthquake, *Economic Development and Cultural Change 48*(3):521–542, 2000.

Howard E, Wiseman K: Emergency and disaster planning: patient education and preparation, *Nephrol Nurs J 28*(5):527–528, 2001.

Kagawa-Singer M: Ethnic perspectives of cancer nursing: Hispanics and Japanese-Americans, *Oncol Nurs Forum 14*(3):59–65, 1987.

Knippen JT, Green TB: Knowing how and when to accept responsibility, *Supervis Manage 35*(10):6–7, 1990.

Mallison MB: Protesting your assignment, *Am J Nurs 87*(2):151, 1987.

Mastrian KG: An advantageous alliance, *Nurs Manage 32*(8):36–37, 2001.

McConnell EA: Get the buzz on nurse call systems, *Nurs Manage 30*(7):43, 1999.

McConnell EA: Get the right information to the right people at the right time, *Nurs Manage 31*(12):37–40, 2000.

McConnell EA: Open the lines of communication, *Nurs Manage 32*(3):45, 2001.

Nurse's Reference Library: *Practices*, Springhouse, PA, 1984, Springhouse.

Ozerdem A: After the Marmara earthquake: lessons for avoiding short cuts to disasters, *Third World Quarterly 21*(3):425–439, 2000.

Parker P: Subacute monitoring systems: vital advantages for vital signs, *Nurs Manage 32*(2):46, 2001.

Perez-Lugo M: The mass media and disaster awareness in Puerto Rico: a case study of the floods in Barrio Tortugo, *Organization and Environment 14*(1):55–73, 2001.

Perlow LA: The time famine: toward a sociology of work time, *Administrative Science Quarterly 44*(1):57–81, 1999.

Platt A: Meet the pain standards with new technology: documentation takes a leap-into the palm of your hand, *Nurs Manage 32*(3):40–43, 2001.

Porter-O'Grady T: Nurses dance to a different tune, *Nurs Manage 30*(7):5, 1999.

Puetz B, Thomas DO: Here's how to manage your time more efficiently, *RN 64*(2):23, 2001.

Riegel BJ, Dracup K: Teaching nurses priority setting for patients with pain of acute myocardial infarction, *West J Nurs Res 8*(3):306–320, 1986.

Rosenthal K: Monitoring vital signs in vital times, *Nurs Manage 33*(3):47–48, 2002.

Servan-Schreiber JL: The art of time: gain new mastery over your life and the power to live your time instead of simply spending it, New York, NY, 2000, Marlowe & Company.

Shaffer DP: Do not interrupt, *Nurs Manage 31*(4):24D–24F, 2000.

Stewart B: A staff development workshop on cultural diversity, *J Nurs Staff Dev 7*(4):190–194, 1991.

Varricchio C: Cultural and ethnic dimensions of cancer nursing care, *Oncol Nurs Forum 14*(3):57–58, 1987.

Zeollner-Hunter J: End long waits for pain relief, *Nurs Manage 30*(7):12, 1999.

Zyry P, Neumann M: Time management networking session, *ANNA J 26*(2):262, 1999.

# MANAGING CLIENT CARE

# 5

# *Managing Resources Cost-Effectively*

OBJECTIVES

*When you complete this chapter, you should be able to:*

1. Conserve resources when providing client care.
2. Describe rationale for fairness in allocation of resources.
3. Use critical thinking to develop strategies for allocating scarce resources.
4. Describe expectations of staff nurse participation in planning for financial management.
5. Contribute to research efforts for cost-effective care.
6. Allocate resources judiciously to meet specific client needs.
7. Describe the intent of the HIPAA Privacy Rule.

KEY CONCEPTS

retrospective financing mechanisms
prospective financing mechanisms
primary care
tertiary care
fairness
allocation of resources
justice
rationing
managing
resources
costs
  direct

indirect
fixed
variable
total
cost-effectiveness
care maps
Health Insurance Portability and
  Accountability Act (HIPAA)
budgets
master staffing plan
full-time equivalents

## GAINING A NURSING PERSPECTIVE ON CONSERVING SCARCE RESOURCES

This chapter is intended to help the learner gain and maintain perspective. As discussed in earlier chapters, many trends are affecting the health-care industry. The steadily increasing cost of health care is shaping the nature of nursing services delivered. Nurses witness the consequences of scarce health-care resources on a daily basis while total health-care costs continue to escalate. Public discussions about health-care rationing are common. Health-care reform continues to be a complex political issue: Private citizens support major changes, but elected officials have not mobilized political support effectively for changes without the approval of representatives of vested interests (Jacobs et al., 1999, pp. 161–180). As discussed in previous chapters, competition associated with a global economy has stimulated public awareness of the increasing costs of health care within the context of overall economic productivity. Subsequent chapters will expand on skills needed by staff nurses to increase their cost-effectiveness as health-care providers.

## Payment Mechanisms and Types of Care

The growth of health maintenance organizations (HMOs) and corresponding insurance mechanisms, including the transition from retrospective (fee for service) to prospective (premiums paid in advance for a range of health and illness services) payment financing mechanisms, have reinforced the need to reconsider health-care costs and benefits over the long-term. In the past, **retrospective financing mechanisms** were commonly used (i.e., illness care was financed largely by insurance mechanisms). The emphasis was on meeting the immediate needs of a person's illness. In the early 1980s, diagnosis-related groups (DRGs) heralded efforts reflecting the interests of providers and insurers to restrain costs by using prospective financing mechanisms to pay for costly health care. **Prospective financing mechanisms** reflect the emphasis of future health-care payments, if needed, and are provided to individuals over a specified time or prepaid premium period (e.g., 1 or 3 months). Individuals insured by an HMO receive not only acute care, which tends to be the most expensive, but also a broad range of health services, including primary prevention, diagnostic, and treatment services in a variety of settings. Since the advent of DRGs and increased prospective payment mechanisms, health maintenance and promotion strategies have gained stature. Consequently, these strategies have generated increased support for primary care. **Primary care** involves providing disease prevention (e.g., immunizations, health teaching) and disease detection services (e.g., screening for age-related health conditions, annual check-ups) as well as episodic care needed to treat illnesses. The emphasis on primary care is beginning to address accessibility for a "decent minimum of health care" (Beauchamp and Childress, 1994, p. 387). Much of the care provided for persons with chronic illnesses has shifted from acute care hospitals to subacute or long-term care facilities (Shah et al., 2001, pp. 86–100). Concurrently, outpatient and community-based services have gained in popularity as an alternative method of reducing health-care costs by trying to reduce need for costly inpatient care. Consequently, providing **tertiary care** (treatment of acute and chronic illnesses and their complications) is being deemphasized.

## Ethics of Resource Allocation

The basic ethical dilemma inherent in the cost-effective allocation of scarce health resources involves meeting individual health needs in a manner that is acceptable, available, and affordable within social standards (i.e., what is a fair or just standard of care for the individual within socially acceptable guidelines for providing the greatest good [optimal health care] for the greatest number of people).

Societal perceptions of health-care priorities are changing. Health-care organizations are shifting emphasis from illness-oriented to health maintenance–oriented care. Individuals continue to pay more for health care. Health insurance plans have required individuals to pay increased premiums and deductibles for clinic, outpatient, and inpatient services. Whenever feasible, outpatient and community-based settings are used instead of inpatient stays to reduce health-care costs. These strategies devised by insurers and providers have not always been accepted readily by recipients of health care; the strategies do not receive much political support. The recipients of care who are paying more are articulating expectations more actively through their evaluations of services received (Cardello, 2001, pp. 36–38; Curran, 1998, p. 169). The evolving publicly funded insurance programs (Medicare Parts A and B) parallel these predominant trends. Frequently, explanations for unrelenting escalating health-care costs include the increased cost of technology used to provide health care, the scarcity of qualified health-care providers, and public expectations of minimally acceptable standards of care as being synonymous with optimal care accessible to everyone when it is needed (Moody, 1995, pp. 4–6).

Clients may be confronted by increased costs if they choose to maintain relationships with specific providers (e.g., physicians or other primary care providers). Insurance providers are gaining control over selection of other health-care provider options. Health insurance premiums have become so expensive that insurance is affordable only when it is funded partially by employers.

More people are realizing that health-care resources are finite and limited. Two issues—accessibility and affordability—are now in the spotlight. Large numbers of American citizens have no health insurance. Rising public concern about the accessibility of health care is leading many people to support politically universal health care (a national health service program, publicly funded and available to every citizen) as a remedial strategy for making a basic level of health care accessible (Beauchamp and Childress, 1994, pp. 351–361). Universal health care is promoted politically as a reasonable method for decreasing gaps in the insurance financing mechanisms.

Distributive justice, the ethical issue of equality of health care, involves the question of how to provide "fairness of opportunity" (i.e., equal access to health care versus equal right to health care), a moral commitment that carries a heavy economic burden (Beauchamp and Childress, 1994, pp. 351–361; Callaway and Hall, 2000, pp. 87–97; Emanuel, 2000, pp. 8–16). There is some evidence that there is significant political backlash associated with the managed care approach to health care (Hokanson, 1998, p. 1; Stone, 1999, pp. 1213–1218; Stone, 2000, pp. 16–18).

The concept of **fairness** (balance of equal justice) in the provision of health care is extraordinarily complex. Individual health-care needs vary widely because of genetic, physiologic, psychological, social, and cultural factors. Consequently, rising costs of health care are forcing ethical choices. Emphasis is being placed on providing equal opportunity (i.e., equal access to care) designed to manage risks to health (primary care) rather than on providing care for everyone corresponding to need. The evolving health-care system and its **allocation of resources** is often not questioned until individuals, believing they are insured, learn that they must rely on more of their personal resources and support systems to cope with and manage an illness episode. Approvals for inpatient admissions or emergency department, diagnostic tests, or specialty provided visits are required from insurance representatives, rather than being determined by the client and the primary provider of the care. Early discharges from inpatient settings in the interest of reducing costs of care frequently require the client to draw on personal resources, instead of relying on health insurance benefits as in the past. An eroding public sense of fairness inherent in the allocation of health-care resources is often a consequence of clients receiving less financial support for managing the costs of their health care.

Insurance programs were one type of response to the resolution of ethical issues of fairness and justice. Issues of **justice** in the allocation of health-care resources are stimulating further discussion of a coherent health (versus illness) system and ethical mechanisms for the allocation of costly scarce resources (Beauchamp and Childress, 1994, pp. 361–378; Hurley, 2001, pp. 234–239). Discussion of allocation of resources incorporating ethical criteria for **rationing** health-care services on the basis of limited resources and ethical priorities is likely to continue.

Changing health-care financing mechanisms and escalating health-care costs increase competition among providers (Viprakasit, 2000, pp. 67–70). To accommodate the increasing emphasis on primary care, traditional health-care organizations develop collaborative relationships with other agencies, employers, and insurance companies to contract for prospective payments in the form of HMO premiums as a source of income.

## Emergence of Managed Care

A consequence of competition among providers of health care is the emergence of managed care. The ultimate goal (i.e., reducing health-care costs) of this model of service delivery originated with health insurance financing mechanisms. As a model of service delivery that focuses on client outcomes, managed care uses a multidisciplinary approach and emphasizes cost. Providers of care are asked to develop and use specific multidisciplinary programs as foundations for their activities. That is, critical pathways or care maps guide services that clients receive for specific health conditions. These guides are integral parts of the clinical information systems and typically provide a framework for documentation by multidisciplinary staff. When individual clients deviate from specified plans, variances (changes in the established plans that may include more, different, or fewer services) are used to describe these changes so that information can be incorporated into the database used to evaluate services provided. Frequently, desired client outcomes that indirectly relate to costs are depicted in continuous quality improvement (CQI) processes (e.g., decreasing lengths of stay in acute care settings). Providers are expected to use CQI strategies to monitor complications or client situations that do not fit service programs specified in the managed care system.

It is critical that priorities of health-care professionals not be replaced by the priorities of those responsible for financing health care. Clients prefer being served as individuals with unique health needs to being managed as cases (Jacobson and Kanna, 2001, pp. 291–326). Health-care providers need to maintain commitment to providing quality care that focuses on these health needs. Allocating resources wisely is an integral part of such a commitment, but not its primary goal or first priority.

To maintain fiscal survival, health-care organizations articulate their specific missions, goals, and strategic plans to delineate their range of service programs. These defining characteristics help health-care providers understand their primary

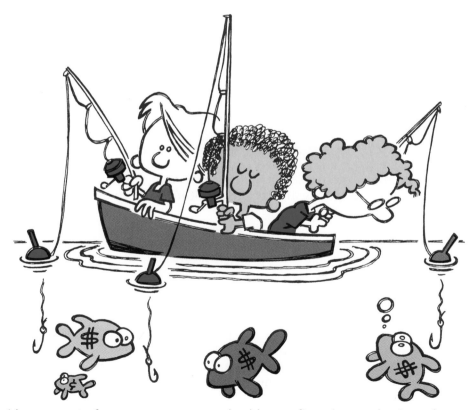

Providers compete for scarce resources as health-care financing mechanisms change and costs continue to escalate.

function, the related purposes of an organization, and its corresponding structuring of services. The processes of care focus on individual client needs along the health (instead of illness) continuum, available resources, and long-term cost-effectiveness.

## DEFINING FUNCTIONAL HEALTH-CARE RESOURCES

As Curran (1998, p. 169) has described, "many organizations are having a difficult time 'keeping the main thing the main thing'." With the evolving chaotic health-care scene, key components of the operating system need to be defined clearly and kept in focus.

## Managing

The concept of **managing** refers to the process of mobilizing or setting in motion various resources to accomplish desired outcomes. In the health-care setting, service begins with a request for a service and ends when client needs are met or transferred to others in a coordinated way. Managing is a dynamic interaction between the client and available resources, which translates into money. If more money is spent for resources than is received for services provided, the long-term survival of the organization becomes questionable. Expenses cannot exceed income from all sources over the long-term. Consequently, knowing exactly what resources are consumed in providing services is important for managers.

## Using Resources: Tangible and Intangible

**Resources** include things of value (i.e., anything that can be converted into money). The value of money corresponds to the purposes for which it is used. In a similar way, the value of health-care resources is defined by their use. *Tangible resources* are property or assets that can be identified or "touched" (e.g., tables, chairs, and computers). *Intangible resources* are assets that cannot be touched and are difficult to measure (e.g., goodwill or positive attitudes of employees).

### *Organization*

A health-care organization's mission, goals, and strategies for reaching them are intangible resources. Although intangible, they are organizational assets used to guide its members. By attending to these variables, health-care providers gain a sense of purpose, direction, and perspective. These organizational resources might be used as guides for reaching described health-care destinations via strategic plans. The organization's mission describes the nature of the work to be done, the values used to set priorities, and the manner in which the health-care providers expect to coordinate their efforts. By using these resources, effectiveness and efficiency are likely to increase, resulting in less costly provision of health-care services (Hirtzel-Trexler, 1994, pp. 23–29). By using the agency's mission statement as a resource to gain a sense of direction, nursing divisions or departments gain organizational support for mobilizing resources that are needed ultimately to address individual client needs in the short-term and long-term.

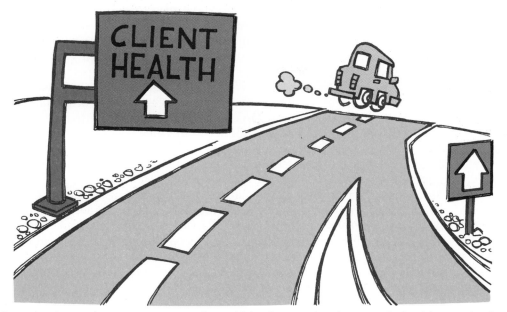

Organizations rely on resources as the vehicle that carries them to their ultimate destination—client health.

## Nursing Resources

Nursing departments are designed to mobilize nursing resources, which include structure, culture, quality and quantity of nursing staff, time, and personal attributes, as well as their methods of service delivery (Beyers et al., 1992, pp. 1–10; Curtin, 2000, pp. 7–13; Flannery and Grace, 1999, pp. 35–46; Schroeder et al., 2000, pp. 71–78). Client care managers need to recognize that the nursing organizational structures in place are designed to enhance their professional practice. Increasing numbers of organizational structures are being designed to promote nursing autonomy and accountability for clinical decision making. As these practice-oriented nursing structures (e.g., shared governance or self-governance) and processes evolve, nursing values, knowledge, strategies, and skills are strengthened (Garcia et al., 1993, pp. 73–74; Parkman and Loveridge, 1994, pp. 63–68). Nursing departments focus nursing resources on meeting client needs. Nursing values (attitudes), knowledge, and skills respond to client needs via delivery systems. The quality of nursing care provided reflects the types and amount of nursing resources consumed (Kramer, 1990, pp. 70, 73).

## Standards of Care and Practice

Evolving health-care organizations and nursing departments should be designed to "free up" nurses to practice nursing, with less emphasis on organizational relationships and more attention paid to the processes entailed in meeting client needs.

Changes being made in patterns of using traditional nursing resources should correspond with changes in nursing departments to reflect the emphases on primary care and less costly services. Client care managers need support to provide care according to critical pathways and care frames, rather than expecting to provide all care needed by the client during the entire inpatient stay or episode of care. Less emphasis should be placed on adherence to policies and procedures, with more emphasis being placed on standards of care and practice (Krueger and Mazuzan, 1993, pp. 467, 470). Standards of care and practice, developed with staff nurse input, are used to *guide* nursing activities. Practice guidelines are professional "yardsticks" used to evaluate quality of care provided over the long-term. In a similar way, standards are integrated into CQI efforts to revise care processes to increase desired outcomes.

This is not to imply that procedure manuals, equipment indexes, and other manuals are not nursing resources; they are. Standards of care and practice are being compiled to help staff nurses as client care managers make clinical decisions and guide processes of care involving clients, families/social support systems, and other members of the health-care team effectively and efficiently in a cost-effective manner. Deviations or variances to these processes may be necessary and legitimized by documented assessments, interventions, and evaluations.

### Knowledge, Skills, and Competencies

Other common nursing resources include the nursing knowledge, skills, and competencies embodied in the nursing work group. Although philosophically committed to holistic care, individual nurses vary in their nursing beliefs, knowledge, skills, competencies, and unique talents. To the extent that these individual nurse resources are identified and used, quality of client care is enhanced (Marks et al., 1999, pp. 44–46). By applying nursing knowledge and skill as the organizing principle for practice, education, and research (including quality improvement), nurses mobilize resources to meet client needs cost-effectively.

To the extent that nursing staff mixes (e.g., various combinations of registered nurses, licensed practical nurses, nursing assistants, and support staff) are combined to complement rather than substitute for professional nursing staff, effectiveness, efficiency, and cost-effectiveness are enhanced. For example, with more nursing work group members who possess more narrowly defined skills, staff nurses (registered nurses) are required to assess client needs and allocate nursing resources to meet them. Staffing mixes increase demand (i.e., time for communication, teaching, and supervision) for staff nurses, depending on the changing nature of client needs related to increased acuity, client education, and discharge planning. As these demands increase, staff nurse resources (effort and energy) available to provide and coordinate direct client care are diminished. The culture or work climate in which these functions are carried out affect whether the quality of care is enhanced or diminished. The attitudes, values, and mindsets of the nursing staff are crucial resources. Staff nurses who value themselves as vital members of the various health-care work groups are much more likely to maintain self-esteem and convey a deep sense of respect for their colleagues and profession (Droes et al., 1992, pp. 53–60). The skills needed to manage the varied nursing resources are discussed in greater detail in later chapters.

### Staff Time, Equipment, and Supplies

Traditional resources include nursing staff time, equipment, and supplies. As described in Chapter Four, nursing staff time is a health-care resource, and it needs to be allocated carefully. Equipment and supplies also cost money. To be used cost-effectively, they need to be used for the purposes for which they were designed and made available. To minimize risks and costs, in-service programs and team building are needed to reinforce staff in proper use of new or different supplies and equipment. Work group members are expected to monitor and assist each other. Videotaping information-sharing sessions (i.e., when presented by product representatives or staff) are often an inexpensive strategy for making the information available to staff at various times throughout the 24-hour day. In addition, compiling files for product information and vendor sources and equipment reference guides are other strategies that might be used to develop inexpensive additional resources to enhance appropriate usage by staff. These information resources might be used creatively to provide client instruction as well.

### Nursing Information Systems

Perhaps less traditional, but frequently used equipment and resources are nursing information systems. Nursing information systems typically are used as components of integrated health information systems. These information systems store data that can be accessed to communicate to interdisciplinary work group members and request specific services from other departments. As increased emphasis continues to be placed on cost-effectiveness, the North American Nursing Diagnosis Association (NANDA) taxonomy, Nursing Interventions Classification (NIC), and Nursing Outcomes Classification (NOC) are likely to become more integrated within clinical information systems. There is growing evidence that these taxonomies when computerized are used by nursing and multidisciplinary work group members to increase efficiency (Dienemann and Van de Castle, 2002, pp. 317–319).

Further development of nursing data sets and clinical decision support systems is expected. These electronic resources will consume valuable time and require nursing staff to develop computer literacy competencies. As integrated information system databases and equipment are developed to enable nursing staff to input data where it is collected, increased savings of nursing time and greater efficiency are projected (Turley, 1992, p. 181).

Other less complex resources in the form of electronic equipment frequently are provided to conserve nursing time and effort and promote timely communication of concerns among clients and involved staff. These resources include paging systems, monitoring systems, scanners, and software programs used to collect, document, and store data to make them readily accessible to other health-care providers.

## QUANTIFYING COSTS

To help quantify the value of their professional skills and their multidisciplinary work group efforts with other providers, equipment, and supplies, staff nurses need to understand how costs of care typically are quantified. Exact classifications vary from one health-care agency to another. **Costs** may be classified as direct, indirect, fixed, or variable.

**Direct costs** include activities (e.g., hands-on care provided directly to clients consisting of human labor, paid overtime), equipment (beds, monitors, suction machines), and supplies (catheters, disposables, dressings, drugs). All departments providing services directly to clients incur direct costs.

**Indirect costs** are paid expenses incurred to support the provision of direct care. Examples of indirect costs include clerical staff wages, supplies, equipment, and educational programs (staff time paid for preparation and attendance); paid holiday time; paid professional dues; and paid sick leave (Pelfrey, 1990, pp. 10–11).

**Fixed costs** are expenses incurred to provide care that remain the same over time. For example, the cost of heating a room, whether it is occupied or unoccupied, remains the same. Similarly, salaries of staff not providing direct care (not affected by volume of client care services needed) remain essentially the same over time. Fixed cost staff might include educators, unit secretaries, or unit managers (Keeling, 1999, pp. 16–18).

In contrast, **variable costs** increase or decrease with the frequency of use. For example, intravenous treatments and wound dressings are variable costs. Similarly, salaries or wages of staff providing direct care that are consumed on the basis of volume of client care services needed above those planned generate variable costs. Variable costs increase **total costs** when their frequency (use) increases. To "break even," billing fees for services rendered need to reflect total costs (i.e., all costs—direct, indirect, fixed, and variable), and income (reimbursement) needs to equal or exceed costs (expenses). How costs are classified varies from agency to agency. Costs are classified carefully and compiled to obtain maximum benefits for reimbursement or billing purposes. To the extent that expenses incurred (labor, equipment, and supplies) in providing care remain within limits of income, financial health is maintained. In planning and providing care, staff nurses need to consider direct and variable costs, so as to maximize cost-effectiveness.

**Cost-effectiveness** relates to the ratio of benefits to costs. This concept was first introduced by the U.S. Department of Defense and was used to describe a technique that "attempts to establish whether a specific expenditure or an alternate one would produce more benefits, or whether the same results could be obtained with less spending" (Terry, 1992, p. 331). A cost-effective health service provides benefits that are worth the costs of resources consumed. For example, in selecting a wound dressing (its therapeutic effects being equal), the cost of the intervention in terms of frequency, staff skill, effort, time, and supplies must be considered. Cost-effectiveness is considered *after* clinical decisions are made based on assessments and *after* needs and desired therapeutic effects, including potential risks associated with these benefits, are identified. Priority setting in determining cost-effectiveness evolves from determining client need before selecting the intervention based on cost/benefit analysis. To provide care on the basis of cost instead of assessed need is like putting the cart before the horse. It increases risk of complications and decreases the chances of obtaining therapeutic benefit. Staff nurses can increase cost-effectiveness by using current knowledge, experience, and data about the cost of equipment and supplies, amount of staff skill and time required, and the effectiveness of various interventions.

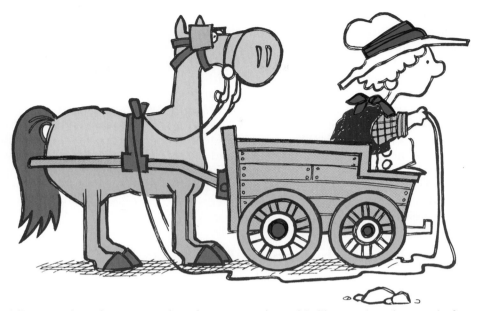

Providing care based on cost rather than assessed need is like putting the cart before the horse.

## USING EVOLVING NURSING MANAGEMENT MECHANISMS

As mentioned earlier, financing mechanisms for health-care costs are shaping nursing practice. As client care managers apply nursing knowledge related to their role, it is hoped that nursing practice will be less shaped by economic considerations and more reflective of the application of nursing knowledge, creativity, and flexibility. Each type of setting has specific purposes, with a corresponding range of services. Inpatient care is typically most expensive and consequently provided only when it cannot be provided at less cost in outpatient or ambulatory care settings. Traditionally, nurses have valued the client's active participation in care, involvement of ethical considerations, and extensive client education. With the increasing emphasis on outcomes, these components of care, sometimes neglected for varied reasons, need to be included to enable the client to manage his or her health-care needs in the short-term and long-term (Taunton and Otteman, 1986, pp. 33–34). Often less costly settings have less complex equipment and less multidisciplinary involvement and are less able to respond to client needs for constant or frequent monitoring. When clients' complex needs require frequent monitoring of physiologic and psychological functions, their care is likely to be more costly. Nurses, as knowledge workers, are needed to analyze the information gathered and determine whether further medical intervention is indicated.

## Responding to Trends Using an Outcome Orientation

In response to trends influencing insurers and health providers for the short-term and the long-term, **care maps** (client profile–driven) or critical pathways are created to promote cost-effectiveness. These care maps delineate desired outcomes and types of multidisciplinary input required within specified periods. Care maps are a type of nursing resource (i.e., they save nursing time and effort) that helps to communicate expectations, including client/family education, and coordinate interactions with the client, family/social support systems, and nursing and multidisciplinary work groups. Care maps are used to document care provided and client responses. In the past, nursing care plans and multidisciplinary plans of care were used in a similar manner. As the increased use of information technology makes clinical information accessible, less time is used to communicate data needed to make timely clinical decisions. Subsequently, effectiveness and efficiency are increased as components of cost-effectiveness.

## Using Available Technology

Although electronic care paths (e.g., electronic medication administration records and clinical records as current nursing care references) may be costly to establish, the accessibility and timely communication of clinical information to nursing staff make them valuable nursing resources. When easily accessible, these resources save scarce nursing staff time and effort. Nurses who have learned to practice before the availability of these electronic resources know the frustration experienced when such records were inaccessible. These technologic resources aid client care managers in assessing priority nursing needs. This information can be integrated with communication tools used by nurses and the multidisciplinary work groups caring for clients and with classification systems used to determine nursing staffing needed. In a similar manner, technology can be used to track client outcomes and "cost out" nursing services provided. Nurses need to continue to develop data sets using nursing terminology (versus medical terminology, e.g., DRGs) as a foundation for nursing practice (Ozbolt and Graves, 1993, pp. 408–411). When nursing develops data sets responsive to needs of professional nursing practice that can be used to evaluate client outcomes and bill for services, nursing will establish its professional and income-generating accountability. (It is hoped this day will come.) These data sets would help nursing to determine staffing mixes needed for cost-effective use of labor based on measures of nursing resource consumption and outcomes (Phillips et al., 1992, pp. 47–52). More attention would be given to hourly nursing resource consumption rather than an estimate encompassing a 24-hour period. In addition, achievement of outcomes will continue to be a crucial part of analyzing the effectiveness of care provided.

## Mobilizing Nursing Staff

With the evolving emphases on primary care, electronic information management (clinical and administrative databases), and nursing department restructuring (promoting professional autonomy and accountability), nursing practice patterns are changing. Basically the sources of these changes are health-care system and agency organization redesign/restructuring and nursing work/practice redesign/restructuring (Dienemann and Gessner, 1992, p. 253). Amidst all this change, to ensure that nursing services are analyzed appropriately for efficiency and effectiveness, it is crucial that nursing interventions be documented accurately (Schroeder et al, 2000, p. 77). Not to do so threatens the nursing profession's credibility in the cost-conscious health-care industry.

The health-care system is changing to include more primary care, health maintenance, and outpatient services made possible by evolving technology. This trend has influenced the changing structure/formal organization of health-care facilities to include more outpatient care and community support for health maintenance. This range of services involves multidisciplinary work groups differently and requires increased coordination of effort (e.g., meeting time to collaborate with nursing and multidisciplinary work group members, taken from total time available for providing direct care).

The changing sources of income for health organizations require that consumer satisfaction be integrated throughout their programs and services. Cost-effectiveness studies and quality assurance efforts are likely to focus on consumer satisfaction. Data collection needed for analyzing program effectiveness requires input from various departments, depending on the nature of the consumer concerns and the processes of service delivery involved. Frequently, refining the processes of care by developing more effective structured communications results in cost savings. For example, consumers required to wait for needed services report increased frustration and decreased satisfaction. By improving communication networks for requisitioning, tracking, and billing for equipment and supplies, system redesign saves staff time and increases client satisfaction. Staff nurses involved in system redesign frequently are asked to provide input into how an activity might be done differently to decrease steps and effort and increase convenience and accuracy of communication among all departments involved. Staff nurses are likely to have less time available to provide direct care because valuable staff time is used to confer with others. System changes focus on cost-effective use of multidisciplinary work group resources. Making system changes often results in increased meeting time, however, to coordinate effort designed to reduce gaps and overlaps.

Associated nursing department changes revolve around the agency's needs for nursing and the intense need for cost-effective use of scarce nursing resources. As nursing departments develop sources of revenue by billing for nursing care provided (corresponding to nursing resources consumed), nursing is expected to increase its professional influence on multidisciplinary work group decisions in establishing client care priorities (Stepura and Miller, 1989, pp. 19–20).

Another major change is the redesign of nursing practice and care delivery patterns. As in the past, nursing practice is and will continue to be shaped by the availability of quality nursing staff. Application of nursing knowledge and skill is needed to identify client needs, select strategies to meet them, allocate available resources, and evaluate client responses within the context of specified outcomes. This change would require client care managers to view the practice of their profession differently, instead of trying to do more with less. Evolving case management delivery models vary, depending on the context of client characteristics and available nursing resources (Faherty, 1990, p. 20; Tahan, 1993, p. 60); client needs as delineated in care maps reflect services to be provided by various disciplines, including client and family education.

Coordination of care usually done by nurses is crucial to ensure seamless care (continuity of services) within the continuum of health agencies. Coordination activities also involve supervision of technical staff, documentation of services provided, and systematic review of effectiveness. Beginning with the need for comprehensive assessments, selection of appropriate plans by a multidisciplinary work group and coordinating their implementation requires a client-needs focus. Staff nurses are expected to coordinate and manage direct care provided. These functions require clinical decisions based on specific knowledge of client health problems. In addition to allocating available nursing resources, staff nurses oversee non-nursing staff who assist clients with non-nursing activities (e.g., safe transport of clients from one location to another within the facility). The types of support staff and their assigned duties vary from agency to agency. For purposes of cost-effectiveness (however misguided), staff nurses often are expected to provide guidance to support staff whose involvement affects the quality of the client's care. By collaborating with non-nursing staff to perform their assigned duties safely, two major cost-effective goals are met: satisfying client needs and saving time and effort of scarce nursing staff.

As the need for coordination increases, so does the need to communicate with various staff. Combine the need to communicate in a timely manner with the use of electronic equipment and the potential for breaks in confidentiality become obvious. The Federal Government's response to expressed public concerns about maintaining privacy, the **Health Insurance Portability and Accountability Act (HIPAA)** was passed and was enacted in full in April 2003 (Health Privacy Project, 2002; Michael and Pritchett, 2001, pp. 524–528). This legislation was designed to preserve security and privacy of individually identifiable health information, including all oral, paper, and electronic communications. The HIPAA established standards for communicating health information from one provider to another after the individual client's permission to do so has been obtained. The HIPAA may be modified after 1 year if deemed necessary.

Health services will continue to be in demand, whereas the supply of human resources needed to provide them is predicted to be less than adequate. Health-care costs will continue to be a major public concern. Individuals will be required to assume personal responsibility for health by adopting lifestyles that maintain or promote well-being. Consequently, without regard for specific financing mechanisms, cost-effectiveness will remain a high priority. All health-care providers will be expected to maintain or increase productivity through cost-effectiveness while providing quality care. As the amount of care provided in outpatient and community-based settings increases, the need for cost-effectiveness will increase in these settings, as has occurred in inpatient settings.

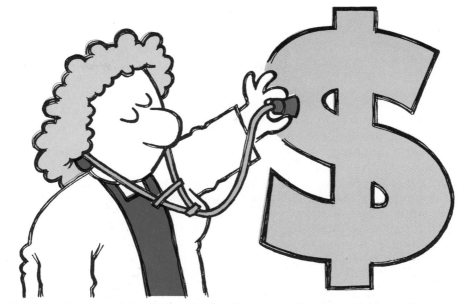

Providers must focus on delivering cost-effective care as the demand for health-care services continues to rise.

## Collecting Data Systematically

With the restructuring of health-care organizations and nursing departments, staff nurses will be expected to gather data needed to evaluate the cost-effectiveness of services they provide. Because services involve fixed and variable costs, staff nurses will continue to be asked to provide input for designing programs and processes of care. It is crucial that staff nurses clearly understand the benefits of nursing values, knowledge, and skills so that nursing time and efforts are included appropriately in evaluations of cost-effectiveness. Nursing practice, as well as the costs of supplies and equipment, needs to be converted into itemized costs (versus being included in room rates).

Staff nurses need to seek and act on opportunities to provide input into strategic plans and participate in decision making for implementing them. These activities are likely to involve interdisciplinary team building. Multidisciplinary work groups will be asked to provide "seamless" (continuous, unfragmented), cost-effective care throughout the integrated delivery system (Rovinsky, 1999, pp. 31–34). These work groups will design care maps integrating essential components of services and select data collection methods to help the group and each discipline to monitor cost-effectiveness.

The process of care delineated in the critical path or care map outlines the types of services and the disciplines expected to provide them. When the client's care deviates from the path because of special client needs or characteristics, variances or modifications are documented. These documented circumstances are a source of data related to increased or decreased costs (e.g., delays in discharge due to complications or unusual client characteristics, unavailability of less costly settings/services, or equipment). Documenting clinical responses to special client circumstances provides clues to possible solutions. Data collected during the process of care provide information about possible needs for program revisions. The work group's response to these situations has an immediate and direct effect on cost-effectiveness.

To monitor overall effectiveness, a multidisciplinary work group usually collects data about outcomes achieved. Frequently, this data collection involves classifying client characteristics on discharge (e.g., functional status; type and amount of services needed after discharge; or through retrospective clinical record reviews, interviews, or surveys). Key outcomes typically relate to (1) decreasing length of stay or service episodes, (2) decreasing complications and mortality, (3) increasing client satisfaction or quality of life indicators, (4) decreasing need for costly care over the long-term, and (5) decreasing use of scarce resources. These data often are extracted from clinical records or indirectly from clients and family by surveys or interviews. Frequently, statistical comparisons of outcomes achieved by providers in other facilities are made to evaluate cost-effectiveness (Angelelli et al., 2000, pp. 646–653; Chen et al., 2001, pp. 359–375).

## Using Research Methodology

Two types of research can be done to evaluate the effectiveness of clinical services provided (Webb and Mackenzie, 1993, pp. 132–133). The term *organizational research* refers to the use of systematic data collected to evaluate cost-effectiveness. Frequently, CQI programs use such data to redesign specific processes involved in providing services (e.g., timely distribution of medications from the time of prescription to delivery to the client). Usually, CQI programs involve ad hoc teams whose membership has a vested interest in its findings. Given nursing's broad functions and role in coordinating client care, nursing staff input is needed on many CQI teams. This input includes helping to diagram processes of care, what and how data are collected, and how the data are interpreted; it also is used to revise these processes. This information is useful to other staff nurses not directly involved in a specific CQI team; findings need to be communicated in a timely manner. Sharing of CQI findings encourages collaboration, helping health teams learn from experiences (by reflecting on successes and mistakes), and usually results in revision of policies, procedures, or care maps. This type of systematic study is embedded in the practice environment and usually has less generalizability (Beyea and Nicoll, 2000, pp. 228–231).

Another type of research involves clinical nursing practice. Clinical nursing research focuses on developing nursing practice (i.e., nursing theory, knowledge, and interventions) (Lindemann, 1988, pp. 5–6; Parker et al., 1992, p. 58). The methods of sampling and data collection depend on the purpose of the clinical study. Findings may be used to change nursing practice, depending on their generalizability and applicability. The staff nurse role in research varies with the nature of the practice setting, clinical study, and one's position description (Sidani, 1998, pp. 621–635).

Given the shortage of nurses, it comes as no surprise that more research is needed to determine nursing's contribution to client outcomes (Lee et al., 1999, pp. 1011–1032). The nature of the staff nurse's activities puts her or him in a key position for contributing to nursing research. Nursing practice (i.e., providing direct client care) is a rich source of ideas, questions affecting clinical decisions, and care map content. On a daily basis, nurses consider special characteristics and needs of clients, including cultural backgrounds and lifestyles, teaching and health maintenance strategies, and the effectiveness of long-term follow-up of treatment as it relates to quality of life and use of family resources. Clinical documentation describes nursing responses to these variables and differences in client responses to nursing interventions. Depending on the nursing department's philosophy and purposes, staff nurses may be invited, or strongly encouraged, to provide input into nursing research methodology, including sampling and data collection using a wide variety of research instruments and information technology. In addition, staff nurses may assist in the dissemination of findings, compiling reports and presenting new nursing knowledge to other interested people. Generally, nursing departments have resources (i.e., expertise [staff, consultants], supplies, and equipment) to support clinical research (Price, 2001, pp. 24–28).

In addition to active participation in research processes, staff nurses are expected to use research findings in practice. They are expected to read pertinent research reports and attend conferences at which research findings are disseminated to maintain a current nursing knowledge base. Subsequently, if findings are pertinent, staff nurses are expected to use the nursing department structure and resources to apply them in efforts to improve nursing practice.

## DEVELOPING PERSPECTIVE BY USING COST-EFFECTIVE STRATEGIES

As mentioned earlier, using resources in a cost-effective manner benefits clients directly and nurses indirectly by increasing productivity. Given the trend in decentralizing clinical decision making and restructuring organizations to promote nursing autonomy and accountability, staff nurses are expected to act on their values to be cost-effective without compromising quality care. After identifying client needs and aligning priorities, staff nurses use nursing knowledge about costs and benefits to select cost-effective interventions (Lessner et al., 1994, p. 458).

While providing direct client care, staff nurses use strategies to enhance cost-effectiveness of nursing services at the department and agency levels. Some key strategies for decreasing direct costs include consideration of (1) purposeful use of nursing staff time to set priorities of client care and act on them as described in Chapter Four; (2) amount of time it takes to complete treatments using different equipment and supplies to achieve the same therapeutic benefit; (3) all nursing tasks involved in each client's care as a foundation for assigning and delegating them; (4) care maps used to guide the process of care; and (5) the layout of the physical plant to reduce nursing "footwork" and untimely interruptions in caregiving.

Another strategy for increasing nursing cost-effectiveness involves attention to the indirect costs of care. A major indirect cost of care involves staffing methodologies.

Patient classification systems need to focus on the nursing resources required to provide quality care to specific clients (Phillips et al., 1992, p. 46). If staff nurses providing direct care need to spend time obtaining staffing on a shift-by-shift or daily basis, these efforts subtract from the nursing resources immediately available to provide direct client care. Nursing unit managers need to help staff nurses set priorities when less staff are available than the number calculated as necessary by the classification system for each shift that fewer staff are available. Staff nurses may be asked to do workload analyses by completing activity logs to determine how workloads can be managed without compromising quality of care or nursing practice (Kirk, 1990, pp. 22–29).

**Budgets** are plans for allocating anticipated income to pay anticipated expenses. Staff nurses often are invited by administrative staff to provide input for budgetary purposes. Special needs associated with strategic plans influence budgets. In addition to staff maintenance and supplemental staffing needed to implement strategic plans, costs of equipment and supplies corresponding to anticipated client needs are incorporated in budgets.

Administrative staff accept responsibility for developing budgets and monitoring their implementation. Staff nurses often contribute data and information to evolve staffing methodologies (i.e., data from time studies are used by administrative staff to develop a master staffing plan for budgetary purposes). A **master staffing plan** specifies core nurse staffing on a daily or shift-by-shift basis, corresponding to anticipated client needs, often in terms of full-time equivalents. **Full-time equivalents** represent the number of staff nurses needed, according to the agency's definition of full-time status and staff nurse benefits (e.g., holiday, vacation, and in-service benefits [indirect costs]) provided by the agency. The master staffing plan must address staffing mix to meet the increasing acuity of client needs and to obtain maximum benefit from available nursing staff (e.g., "ensure that registered nurses do only those tasks that require a registered nurse" [skills, knowledge, and beliefs about nursing]) (Davis, 1994, p. 78). Licensed practical nurses, nursing assistants, and support staff are assigned to perform tasks for which they are adequately credentialed and prepared. Staff nurses are aware of components of care that must be completed within specific periods (e.g., monitoring, treatments, and services needed on a daily basis, such as personal hygiene, or as a component of an episode of care, such as discharge planning or client/family education). Staff nurses can provide valuable insight into cyclic or seasonal variations in specific client populations so that corresponding changes in staffing can be budgeted for accordingly. Frequently, staff nurses can readily define unit-based staffing needs and identify factors that require supplemental staffing that affect overall staffing budgets and are required to meet standards of care. Staff nurses also can provide insights regarding methods of maximizing use of "float pool" or traveling nurse staff when supplementary staffing is needed. Ultimately, staff nurses share responsibility with administrative staff for adequate staffing.

Staff nurses are expected to provide direct care, manage care of groups of clients whose direct care is provided by others, and strive toward increasing cost-effectiveness without compromising standards of practice or quality of care provided. To do so, application of nursing knowledge is needed to assess client needs. Critical thinking is required to identify cost-effective alternative interventions. To meet the client needs cost-effectively, the nurse may need to integrate clinical problem-solving skills with information about the client, nursing department, other agency resources, community-based alternatives, and existing clinical options. A positive attitude toward conserving scarce resources and open-mindedness (creativity and flexibility) toward setting priorities as a foundation for selecting and providing cost-effective nursing interventions are priceless, invaluable assets.

## SUMMARY

Rising health-care costs are shaping the nature of nursing practice. Financing mechanisms are providing for health promotion and maintenance with an evolving emphasis on primary care. Issues of justice and fairness must be considered in the allocation of health-care resources. As individuals are required to pay for more of the costs of their health care, "fairness of opportunity" (i.e., equal access versus equal care) is becoming the accepted standard. Cost-effectiveness in managing resources is a popular topic in today's health-care management scene.

Managing health-care resources involves selecting options with the best benefit-to-cost ratio or expending resources on alternatives that produce the most benefits in the short-term and the long-term. Nurses, as client care managers, need to integrate the agency's mission, strategic plans, and values, as well as those of nursing, in developing structures and processes supportive of quality client care and nursing practice. Nurses need to value their professional resources as clients value them, including traditional resources (e.g., equipment and supplies) and resources that are less traditional (e.g., nursing's holistic perspective, information systems).

Total costs of health care need to be quantified to bill for them properly. Classifications of costs include direct, indirect, fixed, and variable. Quantifying these costs enables providers to use budgets to manage income and expenses.

Cost-effective management of health-care resources requires heavy reliance on electronic information systems. Clinical and financial information needs to be integrated to assist nurses to provide cost-effective care. Often these systems involve care maps used by multidisciplinary work groups to guide provision of services and documentation. Individual client deviations from these guides and solutions developed to address them provide clues as to possible revisions to increase cost-effectiveness. HIPAA legislation has established standards for preserving privacy of identifiable health information and will need to be integrated in the systems used to provide integrated health care.

Nursing staff are mobilized by the nature of the health-care facility's organization, strategic plans, and nursing department structure and function. These components are evolving to support nursing practice and cost-effective deployment of available staff. Patterns of service delivery vary with the characteristics of the client population and agency resources. Nursing staff typically contribute to multidisciplinary work group planning and coordination of care.

Much work needs to be done to develop systems for evaluating cost-effectiveness of nursing care. Data incorporating nursing beliefs and nursing interventions used must be collected systematically. These data need to be incorporated in the development of standards of practice and care as a foundation for analyzing cost-effectiveness. The multidisciplinary work group needs to evaluate data about client outcomes to evaluate progress in providing cost-effective programs. Consequently, nurses need to become involved in organizational and clinical research.

Using cost-effective strategies to provide care benefits clients and nurses. These strategies include consideration of all costs but especially direct and variable costs. Master staffing plans specify needs for adequate staffing based on anticipated client needs. Calculation of full-time equivalents helps to include direct and indirect costs of nursing staff as employees. Staff nurses often complete workload analyses and evolve classification systems that quantify nursing activities completed to meet specific needs of groups of clients. Staff nurses share responsibility with administrative staff for obtaining resources needed to provide cost-effective quality care. Nurses are valued health-care resources. They need to value themselves and maintain a positive attitude and open mind about increasing their cost-effectiveness.

## APPLICATION EXERCISES

1. As a group, interview one of the clinical area coordinators of a nursing unit to which you are currently assigned. Delineate how the agency's strategic plan is changing the characteristics of the client population served and how the agency recovers the costs of the services provided.

2. Interview two staff nurses with whom you practice on a nursing unit about the admission and discharge planning policies. Identify criteria used to determine who is eligible for care on this unit, criteria used to set discharge dates, and resources used to provide seamless care after the client is discharged.

3. Quantify the cost of care you provided to an assigned client as if you were an entry-level staff nurse on your unit, including your time, time of others who directly supervised your practice, equipment, and supplies. If you were following a care map, would you have deviated from it on the basis of the client's needs? How? Explain.

4. Observe a staff nurse's activities for the first 3 hours of a shift or work period. List the types of data entered into the clinical information system used to evaluate client care, care maps, availability of equipment and supplies, adequacy of nurse staffing, nursing network communications, and organizational effectiveness (e.g., client satisfaction, quality of life).

5. Write a letter to yourself, describing yourself as a nursing resource and how you plan to allocate your assets to provide a "decent minimum of health care" to your clients. Compare your statement with statements written by two colleagues.

## CRITICAL THINKING SCENARIO

Imagine yourself as a staff nurse employed in a busy extended care setting specializing in care of neurologically impaired middle-aged and older adults. The agency's primary mission is to provide rehabilitation services that enable clients to manage satisfying lifestyles in private residences. It also provides clinical experiences for students of dietetics, exercise physiology, physical medicine and rehabilitation, nursing, occupational therapy, physical therapy, speech therapy, and social work. The strategic plan (to be implemented within the next 2 years) indicates a need for shorter lengths of stay and more use of outpatient care. This agency is installing an integrated health information system.

1. What types of computerized information would you, as a client care manager, need to provide nursing care?
2. Make a list of information system characteristics that would increase cost-effectiveness of the nursing and multidisciplinary work groups.
3. What suggestions would you make to redesign the current system, making cost-effective use of resources and promoting timely communication while minimizing service interruptions?
4. Who would you designate to guide and coordinate care programs of individual clients? Explain.

## REFERENCES

Angelelli JJ, Wilber KH, Myrtle R: A comparison of skilled nursing facility rehabilitation treatment and outcomes under Medicare managed care and Medicare fee-for-service reimbursement, *Gerontologist 40*(6):646–653, 2000.

Beauchamp TL, Childress, JF: *Principles of biomedical ethics*, ed 4, New York, NY, 1994, Oxford University Press.

Beyea SC, Nicoll LH: Evaluating patient care programs, *AORN J 71*(1):228–231, 2000.

Beyers M, Hill B, McClelland MR, et al: New-wave nursing: back to the basics? *Nurs Clin North Am 27*(1): 1–10, 1992.

Callaway ME, Hall J: Distributive justice in the Medicaid capitation: the evidence from Colorado, *J Behav Health Serv Res 27*(1):87–97, 2000.

Cardello DM: Improve patient satisfaction with a bit of mystery, *Nurs Manage 32*(1):36–38, 2001.

Chen Q, Kane RL, Finch MD: The cost effectiveness of post-acute care for elderly Medicare beneficiaries, *Inquiry 37*:359–375, 2001.

Christmyer CS, Catanzariti PM, Langford AM, et al: Bridging the gap: theory to practice: Part I. clinical applications, *Nurs Manage 19*(8):42–50, 1988.

Curran C: On measuring and managing . . ., *Nurs Econ 16*(4):169, 1998.

Curtin LL: The first ten principles for the ethical administration of nursing services, *Nurs Admin Q 25*(1):7–13, 2000.

Davis B: Effective utilization of a scarce resource: RNs, *Nurs Manage 25*(2):78–80, 1994.

Dienemann J, Gessner T: Restructuring nursing care delivery systems, *Nurs Econ* *10*(4):253–258, 1992.

Dienemann J, Van de Castle B: The impact of health care informatics on the organization. In Englebardt SP, Nelson R (editors): *Health care informatics: an interdisciplinary approach*, St Louis, MO: Mosby, 2002, pp. 303–320.

Droes N, Kramer M, Halton D: How much are nurses worth? Nurses evaluate themselves, *Nurs Manage 23*(6):5353–5355, 5358–5360, 1992.

Emanuel EJ: Justice and managed care: four principles for the just allocation of health care resources, *Hastings Rep*, May-June 2000, pp. 8–16.

Faherty B: Case management—the latest buzzword: what it is and what it isn't, *Caring 9*(7):20–21, 1990.

Flannery TP, Grace JL: Managing nursing assets: a primer on maximizing investment in people, *Nurs Admin Q 23*(4):35–46, 1999.

Garcia MA, Bruce D, Niemeyer J, et al: Collaborative practice: a shared success, *Nurs Manage 24*(5):72–74, 78, 1993.

Health Privacy Project: *Myths and facts about the new Federal privacy regulations and overview of HIPAA privacy regulation*, Institute for Healthcare Research and Policy, Georgetown University, Washington, DC. Available at http://www.healthprivacy.org. Accessed June 10, 2002.

Hirtzel-Trexler BJ: Permeation of organization-level strategic planning into nursing division-level planning, *J Nurs Admin 24*(11):23–29, 1994.

Hokanson MO: Nobel Prize winner decries market medicine, *Nurs Matters 9*(2):1,6, 10, 1998.

Hurley J: Ethics, economics, and public financing of health care, *J Med Ethics 27*:234–239, 2001.

Jacobs L, Marmor T, Oberlander J: Report from the field—the Oregon Health Plan and the political paradox of rationing: what advocates and critics have claimed and what Oregon did, *J Health Politics and Law 24*(1):161–180, 1999.

Jacobson PD, Kanna ML: Cost-effectiveness analysis in the courts: recent trends and future prospects, *J Health Politics, Policy and Law 26*(2):291–326, 2001.

Keeling B: How to allocate the right staff mix across shifts, part 2, *Nurs Manage 39*(10):16–18, 1999.

Kirk R: Using workload analysis and acuity systems to facilitate quality and productivity, *J Nurs Admin 20*(3):21–30, 1990.

Kramer M: Trends to watch at the magnet hospitals, *Nursing 20*(6):67–68, 70, 73–74, 1990.

Krueger NE, Mazuzan JE: A collaborative approach to standards, practices, *AORN J 57*(2):467, 470–474, 478, 1993.

Lee JL, Chang BL, Pearson ML, Kahn KL, Rubenstein LV: Does what nurses do affect clinical outcomes for hospitalized patients? A review of the literature, *Health Serv Res 34*(5):1011–1032, 1999.

Lessner MW, Organek NS, Shah HS, et al: Orienting nursing students to cost effective clinical practice, *Nurs Health Care 15*(9):458–462, 1994.

Lindemann CA: Research in practice: the role of the staff nurse, *Appl Nurs Res 1*(1):5–7, 1988.

Marks L, Dennis RS, Borozny H, Ferrone K: The "new team" triad, *Nurs Manage* 30(2):44–46, 1999.

Michael P, Pritchett E: The impact of HIPAA electronic transmissions and health information privacy standards, *J Am Diet Assoc* 101(5):524–528, 2001.

Moody J: Health care reform: the shape of the debate to come, *Bioethics Bull* 8(1):4–6, 1995.

Ozbolt JG, Graves JR: Clinical nursing informatics—developing tools for knowledge workers, *Nurs Clin North Am* 28(2):407–432, 1993.

Parker ME, Gordon SC, Brannon PT: Involving nursing staff in research: a nontraditional approach, *J Nurs Admin* 22(4):58–63, 1992.

Parkman CA, Loveridge C: From nursing service to professional practice, *Nurs Manage* 25(3):63–68, 1994.

Pelfrey S: Cost categories, behavior patterns, and break-even analysis, *J Nurs Admin* 20(12):10–14, 1990.

Phillips CY, Castorr A, Prescott PA, et al: Nursing intensity: going beyond patient classification, *J Nurs Admin* 22(4):46–52, 1992.

Price A: Commissioning nurse "in-house" consultancy projects, *Nurs Econ* 19(1):24–28, 2001.

Rovinsky M: Provisions of the Balanced Budget Act challenge IDS care coordination patterns, *Healthcare Financial Management*, August 1999, pp. 31–34.

Schroeder CA, Trehearne B, Ward D: Expanded role of nursing in ambulatory managed care: Part II. impact on outcomes of costs, quality, provider and patient satisfaction, *Nurs Econ* 18(2):71–78, 2000.

Shah A, Fennell M, Mor V: Hospital diversification into long-term care, *Health Care Manage Rev*, Summer 2001, pp. 86–100.

Sidani S: Measuring the intervention in effectiveness research, *West J Nurs Res* 20(5):621–635, 1998.

Stepura BA, Miller K: Converting nursing care costs to revenue, *J Nurs Admin* 19(5):18–22, 1989.

Stone D: Managed care and the second great transformation, *J Health Politics, Policy and Law* 24(5):1213–1218, 1999.

Stone D: Rationing compassion—a fable for our time, *The American Prospect*, May 22, 2000, pp. 16–18.

Tahan H: The nurse case manager in acute care settings: job description and function, *J Nurs Admin* 23(10):53–61, 1993.

Taunton RL, Otteman D: The multiple dimensions of staff nurse role conception, *J Nurs Admin* 16(10):31–37, 1986.

Terry JF: *International management handbook*, Fayetteville, AR, 1992, The University of Arkansas Press.

Turley JP: A framework for the transition from nursing records to a nursing information system, *Nurs Outlook* 40(4):177–181, 1992.

Viprakasit DP: Balancing their budget: the potential ethical decision facing skilled nursing facilities, *Top Stroke Rehabil* 7(3):67–70, 2000.

Webb C, Mackenzie J: Where are we now? Research mindedness in the 1900s, *J Clin Nurs* 2(3):129–133, 1993.

*When you complete this chapter, you should be able to:*

1. Describe basic nursing competencies required to develop the client care management skills expected of entry-level staff nurses.
2. Describe the relationship of other core nursing roles to the client care manager role.
3. Compare the nursing process with the management process.
4. Describe how client care managers use the nursing process.
5. Describe a client care manager's typical day.
6. Describe how client care manager routines may vary with organizational patterns of nursing service delivery, during evening or night shifts, and with the personal strengths of individual nurses.
7. Describe strategies being used to address common resource utilization issues related to the continuing transformation of health care.

## KEY CONCEPTS

core nursing competencies
core nursing roles
  provider of care
  member within the discipline of
    nursing
  manager of care

nursing process
management process
typical client care management
  routines
variations in client care management
  routines

## BUILDING ON BASIC NURSING ROLES

Key elements of the client care manager role were introduced in Chapter One. The relationship of basic nursing competencies to the client care manager role is described in this chapter.

**Core nursing competencies** are required of all entry-level nurses. These competencies are the learned skills and attitudes that are integral to practicing nursing safely. The basic or core nursing competencies described in this chapter initially were delineated by groups of entry-level staff nurses and supervisors of such nurses (Wywialowski, 1987, pp. 145–164). As the transformation of the health-care industry continues, the key elements of the core competencies are changing in response to evolving trends in financing health care and the increased emphasis on the "bottom line" (minimal overall requirement of avoiding losses) (Apker, 2001, pp. 117–136; Ray et al., 2002, pp. 1–14; and Turkel, 2001, pp. 67–82). These competencies are described within the parameters of the **core nursing roles** common to all entry-level nurses, as described by the National League for Nursing (Council of Associate Degree Programs, 1990, pp. 3–12). The specific core competency tasks expected of the entry-level staff nurse depend on the employing agency's mission and purpose, client characteristics, the governance and structure of the nursing department, and patterns of nursing care delivery. Competence is context specific (i.e., skills needed to practice nursing competently vary among acute, long-term, and ambulatory care settings).

A role describes a set of expectations or characteristic forms of behavior imposed on a person because of status within a group. A role includes the essential components of the person's function or tasks to be done by the employee in an organization (Terry, 1992, p. 483). Within health-care organizations, core roles expected of entry-level staff nurses include **provider of care, member within the discipline of nursing,** and **manager of care**. Nurses prepared at the baccalaureate level may take on additional nursing roles, such as communicator, client teacher, and investigator. In accordance with their broader liberal education, they are prepared to "evaluate research findings for applicability to nursing practice" and participate in community health programs "to meet the emerging health needs of the general public in a changing society" (Council of Baccalaureate and Higher Degree Programs, 1987, p. 2).

As health-care organizations have become increasingly complex, the need for clear communications from administrative staff also has increased to help staff nurses "make sense" of expectations placed on them for meeting increased managerial and clinical responsibilities (Apker, 2001, p. 118). Apker (2001, pp. 123–131) described an example of how staff nurses needed to change their roles on the basis of information gleaned from other organizational members (e.g., physicians, nurse managers, pharmacists), while they were providing care needed by their assigned clients. Apker (2001, p. 132) reported that nurses were expected "to do it all," although they were not provided with adequate support (e.g., supplies and equipment); consequently, nurses responded to these expectations with increased stress, burnout, and turnover. Apker (2001, p. 132) suggested that nurses can enact evolving roles but would benefit from instructional programs, support groups, and recognition programs for their expended efforts.

## Providing Client Care

### Develop a Knowledge Base

As a provider of care, the entry-level staff nurse is expected to develop a knowledge base pertinent to nursing practice. The nurse uses the nursing process to apply this knowledge as a basic strategy for clinical decision making. In addition, as a provider of care, the entry-level nurse performs various nursing procedures to meet client care requirements. The entry-level nurse's knowledge base includes information about:

1. Normal anatomy and physiology and its relationship to diseases and dysfunction.
2. Psychology, sociology, and spirituality as they relate to human needs.
3. Pharmacology as it relates to responsible administration of medicines; this includes drug actions, side effects, and indicators of toxicity.
4. Aging processes related to changes in self-concept and physiology.
5. Behavioral manifestations of diseases.
6. Nursing implications of normal nutrition and diet therapy.
7. Hydration.
8. Oxygenation.
9. Common normal and abnormal laboratory values and related symptoms.

The entry-level staff nurse must be able to locate information about laboratory values and disease processes with which he or she is unfamiliar and to use the client record and other general resources of information available on nursing units. In addition, the nurse, as a member of the profession, integrates a code of conduct into practice committing the nurse to provide care corresponding to assessed client needs. When circumstances do not allow the nurse to provide care while communicating within a caring relationship, the nurse experiences moral distress. Turkel (2001, p. 81) identified the conflicting messages that caring is valued but the emphasis is on survival, reducing costs, and making a profit. She indicated that administrators need to restructure the practice environment (especially acute care organizations because they are typically the most expensive type of care) to maximize and focus nursing time on nurse-client interactions in an effort to preserve or increase the quality of care. Although challenging, nurses need to remember that they are the essence of quality care as clients perceive it. To bill clients for care not provided would not lead to organizational survival based on the "bottom line." The crises of cost control in health care can be managed so that financial and clinical performance are integrated rather than presented as competing forces (Meliones et al., 2001, pp. 21–29). Surviving organizations need to work toward achieving desired financial and clinical quality outcomes.

### Use the Nursing Process

Entry-level nurses are expected to use the nursing process to make clinical decisions that they can defend. The nursing process consists of five phases: assessment, analysis, planning, implementation, and evaluation.

Entry-level staff nurses also are expected to view the client holistically (i.e., as a unique person with varied physical, psychological, spiritual, and social needs). Each nursing assessment includes a health history, data about subjective and objective symptoms, data about current health status and functional abilities, and information about the client's participation in self-care. Adequate analysis of assessment data by entry-level staff nurses includes:

1. Identifying health problems and formulating nursing diagnoses.
2. Identifying multidisciplinary approaches needed to address client needs.
3. Listing the client's health problems.
4. Ranking the client's needs in order of priority and acuteness.

The nurse is expected to analyze the nature of the client's responses and distinguish between dependent and independent nursing functions as collaborative problems or nursing diagnoses arise. In addition, the entry-level nurse is expected to use information from the agency's system of classification or level of care to estimate the client's acuity level and the complexity of nursing needs.

Entry-level staff nurses are expected to plan client care. The nurse helps the client set realistic goals and develop discharge plans within the context of the multidisciplinary approaches and available agency and community resources. The nurse helps the client understand her or his own health needs, identify realistic short-term and long-term goals, and plan to use available resources to meet them. As a conclusion to these activities, the nurse writes a nursing care plan to communicate with other members of the nursing and health-care team. As pressure increases to conserve scarce resources, staff nurses will be required to use assertiveness and collaboration to advocate for clients in an effort to meet complex client needs in a timely manner, often in collaboration with a nursing case manager (Gardner and Cary, 1999, pp. 64–77).

As a provider of care, the beginning staff nurse carries out the client's plan of interventions. While performing various nursing procedures, the nurse is expected to apply principles of restorative nursing and encourage clients to participate in the rehabilitation process. Based on the treatment plan, the nurse is expected to monitor the client's responses and to propose alternative approaches. Depending on the nature of the health-care agency and the client's health needs, the nurse performs various procedures to help the client meet basic human needs. For example, the nurse uses methods of infection control to administer parenteral therapy, oxygen therapy, and skin and wound care. To meet long-term goals, the nurse is expected to involve family members in the client's care.

With the evolving nursing service delivery patterns associated with the escalating costs of health care and the increasing acuity levels of clients, entry-level staff nurses are likely to be expected to adhere to standards of practice and care (Dienemann and Gessner, 1992, p. 254). Nursing departments are likely to expect the entry-level staff nurse, as a provider of care, to select cost-effective interventions, as discussed in Chapter Five.

Finally, as a provider of care, the nurse must evaluate the client's responses. Evaluation efforts involve comparing the client's responses with quality assurance criteria and desired client outcomes. The nurse's evaluation is expected to result in a clinical decision to continue or revise the plan of care on the basis of current nursing data. The client's progress is measured and judged in terms of indicators (measures) of client progress.

### Use Communication Skills

Entry-level staff nurses are expected to use communication skills when providing direct client care. They communicate with clients, families, nursing staff, and the multidisciplinary work group. Nurses are expected to modify their communication for clients with sensory deficits, language barriers, and speech deficits. In addition, they should use terminology that enables clients and families to comprehend information about health needs and treatment.

Nurses also are expected to communicate in a manner that enables all members of the nursing and interdisciplinary work groups to comprehend the terminology used. At the same time, they need to comprehend the terminology used by others. These skills include written and verbal techniques used to communicate oral, printed, or electronic messages.

## Fulfilling Role Obligations as a Member Within the Discipline of Nursing

### Exhibit a Sense of Professionalism

Another core nursing role is that of a member within the discipline of nursing. Entry-level staff nurses are expected to exhibit a sense of professionalism. They should accept responsibility for adhering to ethical codes of conduct, which includes maintaining confidentiality and accepting points of view that differ from their own. In addition, ethical conduct mandates that entry-level nurses provide required nursing care and that cost cutting is an unacceptable explanation for not doing so. They should show self-respect and respect for others. These attitudes enable nurses to provide quality care and maintain the client's dignity, regardless of the type of payment the client uses to finance health care. Entry-level nurses should expect continued pressure to provide cost-effective care and prepare to adapt within reasonable limits. They should be receptive to constructive criticism and suggestions for improvement. Entry-level nurses serve as role models to other members of the nursing work group.

### Interpret Health-Care Legal Issues

Entry-level staff nurses need to be able to interpret legal issues involved in health care. They are expected to practice within the parameters of state licensure laws and nurse practice acts, American Nurses Association standards of practice, and institutional quality assurance standards. They are expected to comply with their employing agency's policies and procedures and implement standards of practice and care. In addition, they should adhere to "patient rights" guidelines and comply with state laws requiring informed consent and reporting of child or elder abuse or neglect.

### Demonstrate Accountability for Nursing Actions

Entry-level staff nurses are expected to show accountability for their nursing actions and the actions of their subordinates. With the increased financial pressures to use less expensive alternate care providers, staff nurses need to supervise and direct others in an effort to provide coordinated care. It is incumbent on nurses to understand the roles of each member of the nursing work group (Cosolo, 2002, pp. 34–42). This function is discussed in greater depth in Chapters Thirteen and Fourteen.

To remain competent, entry-level staff nurses need to participate in lifelong learning programs to enable them to remain competent as the practice environment changes. This includes continuing and in-service education programs and other activities that promote personal growth. At times, these activities enable entry-level staff nurses to identify evolving ethical issues (e.g., advanced directives) and available alternatives that could be used to resolve them.

## Managing Client Care

As described in Chapter One, the manager of care role requires that nurses coordinate the services received by a group of clients during a specific period, often an 8-hour workday. It is generally more complex than and builds on the other two core nursing roles. With emphasis on escalating costs in the evolving health-care system, the staff nurse's client care manager role explicitly includes aspects of cost-effective use of resources (e.g., managerial and financial tasks) (Meliones et al., 2001, pp. 21–29; Seaman, 1990, pp. 177–180; Tahan, 1993, pp. 54–60; Turkel, 2001, pp. 67–82).

### RELATIONSHIP OF MANAGER ROLE TO OTHER CORE ROLES

Every entry-level staff nurse is expected to show competency in all three core nursing roles. As described in Chapter One, client care management skills are essential for success as a beginning staff nurse.

In reality, the three core nursing roles are interrelated. Depending on the nature of the practice setting and client needs, the nurse enacts varying degrees of the interrelated roles concurrently, rather than separately from each other. While the nurse provides client care, he or she also enacts varying degrees of the manager-of-client-care and member-within-the-discipline-of-nursing roles in any setting. Generally the nature of the client's needs and the context of practice guide which nursing actions are taken. For example, entry-level staff nurses employed to provide care for critically ill clients emphasize the provider-of-care role, whereas nurses employed in long-term care settings caring for less acutely ill clients often use client care manager skills more extensively.

Because the core nursing roles are interrelated, students develop varying degrees of the skill inherent in each role as they gain practical experience. Refining the skills needed for competency in each of the core roles is a continuous process. Typically, students learn to practice nursing by developing less complex skills and proceeding to more complex skills. Accordingly, as students' nursing skills develop, they practice managing care in increasingly complex situations. To manage client care successfully in common nursing situations, the entry-level staff nurse builds on the less complex skills needed to provide client care and to fulfill obligations as a member within the discipline of nursing.

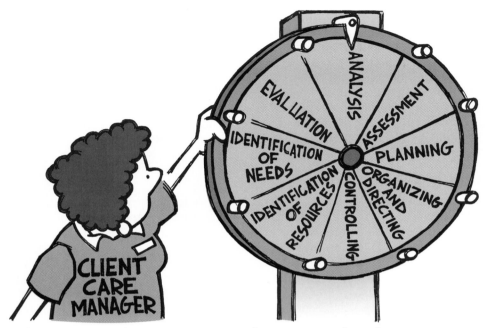

The client care manager performs many nursing roles.

## COMPARISON OF NURSING AND MANAGEMENT PROCESSES

### Nursing Process

The nursing student builds on previous nursing skills to develop more complex client management skills. As described previously, nursing students learn to use the five phases of the **nursing process** (i.e., assessing, analyzing, planning, implementing, and evaluating) to apply knowledge needed to provide care. Although these phases typically are listed in this order, in actual practice the nurse might engage in any of these activities at any time, depending on the circumstances. For example, the nurse admitting the client to a nursing unit spends considerable effort assessing client needs. The nurse assisting the client with personal hygiene activities might be involved in implementing, evaluating, and planning activities to correspond to the client's response to treatment.

### Management Process

Basically the **management process** is used to meet client needs in an efficient and effective manner with available resources (i.e., to allocate resources cost-effectively). The management process consists of five phases: (1) identification of needs, (2) identification of resources, (3) planning, (4) organizing and directing, and (5) controlling. Box 6-1 compares the phases of the nursing process with the phases of the management process.

## Identification of Needs

For the client care manager to address client needs, the needs must be identified clearly. Often they can be prioritized on the basis of the purposes and objectives of the health-care agency. That is, the client care manager determines specifically what nursing services each assigned client needs during the workday and identifies group priorities. Without determining what the group of assigned clients need, the client care manager cannot establish what resources are required.

## Identification of Resources

The assessment of the nursing service needs of an assigned group of clients is related closely to the client care manager's need to identify available resources. Usually entry-level staff nurses obtain information about community and agency resources from orientation, in-service, and continuing education programs and from internal communications from various departments within the agency. In addition, a staff nurse assigned the care of a group of clients is informed about the number and type of nursing staff available during the shift. The nurse obtains preliminary information about client needs and available resources when receiving the change-of-shift report.

## Planning

The planning phase of client care management should begin immediately after client needs and available resources have been identified. Additional planning may be needed throughout the shift, depending on the success of the initial plan, the changing needs of the assigned group of clients, and the availability of resources. The priorities of clients' needs might change, or the client care manager might be requested to "share" staff with other managers or nursing units as overall agency needs change. When establishing a plan for matching agency resources with client

---

**BOX 6-1**

### Phases of the Nursing Process and the Management Process

| Nursing Process | Management Process |
|---|---|
| Assessment | Identification of needs |
| Analysis | Identification of resources |
| Planning | Planning |
| Implementation | Organization and direction |
| Evaluation | Control |

needs, the client care manager attends to specific time constraints of scheduled activities, routines, and required treatments. Realistic plans reflect the client care manager's awareness that staff cannot be in more than one place at a time. The client care manager does not plan simultaneously to administer complex treatments for one client in one room while preparing another client for a diagnostic procedure in another room. When discussing the plan for caring for the group of clients, the client care manager might teach time management skills by the specific instructions given within the individual staff assignments.

### Organization and Direction

The entry-level staff nurse is expected to organize and direct the use of available resources in the best interest of assigned clients. On the basis of assessed client needs, the client care manager attempts to provide staff with an overview of client priorities and plans to meet them. The client care manager seeks input from other staff when planning activities that affect them. In addition, the client care manager assigns care and directs staff to ensure that specific needs are addressed in a timely manner (i.e., within the established time constraints of scheduled diagnostic tests, procedures, and operating room schedules). While providing direction, the client care manager might offer specific instructions to approach individual client needs or adhere to agency protocols for providing safe, effective care. A client care manager might request that a coworker adjust a plan of care to incorporate special family needs in preparation for discharge or adhere to a specific procedure to ensure control of infections while clients are transported between departments. The client care manager uses complex communication and teaching skills when organizing and directing activities. The skills needed to manage others are addressed in more detail in Unit Three.

### Control

As a provider of care, the staff nurse evaluates the extent to which desired client outcomes are met during the shift. At intervals throughout the shift, the client care manager seeks feedback from coworkers regarding their success in completing care plans for clients. Careful attention is given to the feedback received to determine whether care plans must be revised or adjusted to make more effective use of available resources. In this way, the client care manager monitors the progress of the client and of the work group in addressing priorities in a timely manner. Depending on the conclusions drawn, the client care manager revises the plan or redirects the use of resources to meet identified priorities.

Another facet of controlling the process of client care involves evaluating the overall management plan for the shift. Client care managers must provide positive feedback to coworkers about their efforts to implement the management plan. It is also important to provide accurate information about client needs and outcomes that need continued attention. The client care manager communicates progress in meeting desired client outcomes when giving a change-of-shift report. This information is used to help client care managers on the following shift identify the current needs of an assigned group of clients. More information about change-of-shift reports is provided in Chapter Eight.

## Combining Skills

As discussed earlier, the phases of the management process might occur in any order. The phase of the management process that is emphasized depends on the context and needs of the assigned group of clients. If clients' needs are less predictable due to physiologic instability, more emphasis might be placed on planning allocation of highly skilled staff. If the assigned clients are physiologically stable, more emphasis might be placed on evaluating the extent to which clients are achieving desired outcomes (e.g., adequacy in performing new skills in accordance with established standards of care).

Client care managers combine the skills needed as a care provider with those needed to mobilize agency resources to care for a group of clients. The client care management process also requires that the entry-level nurse use more complex skills: setting priorities for a group of clients on the basis of assessed need, communicating with and teaching clients and coworkers in a timely manner, planning the use of available resources within the constraints of established schedules and routines and changing client needs, and evaluating the work group's success in meeting desired client outcomes.

### CLIENT CARE MANAGER ROUTINES

During a typical workday, a client care manager follows a series of routines that promote effectiveness and efficiency. As mentioned previously, the client care manager's approach to caring for a group of assigned clients incorporates nursing skills inherent in each of the three interrelated core nursing roles. **Typical client care management routines** for an 8-hour day shift are listed in Box 6-2. Client care management routines commonly include the following sequence of activities.

## Typical Workday

At the beginning of the workday (7:00 to 7:30 A.M.), the client care manager receives a change-of-shift report for assigned clients. On the basis of this report, the client care manager completes a preliminary assessment of these clients' needs (7:30 to 8:00 A.M.). These activities might include reviewing available clinical information and conferring with coworkers. Finishing these tasks permits the client care manager to complete assigning client care activities to appropriate coworkers. During the same period, scheduled drugs and treatments are administered as prescribed (i.e., before meals or with meals).

After clients have received meals (8:00 to 9:30 A.M.), the client care manager typically administers drugs to be given after meals and per agency schedules. In addition, the nurse uses this time to complete detailed assessments of acutely ill or unstable clients and provides comfort and personal hygiene measures. Often changes in medical plans are noted during this time, as are changes made by the multidisciplinary work group needed to complete diagnostic and treatment programs.

At midmorning (9:30 to 10:00 A.M.), the client care manager often administers scheduled drugs and completes a detailed assessment of stable clients. These

BOX 6-2

## Typical Client Care Management Routines

7:00-7:30 A.M.: Receive change-of-shift report.

7:30-8:00 A.M.: Complete preliminary assessment of assigned client needs; complete assigning client care to coworkers; administer scheduled drugs and treatments before meals or with meals.

8:00-9:30 A.M.: Administer drugs to be given after meals and per agency schedules; complete detailed assessments of acutely ill clients and provide comfort and personal hygiene measures; note changes in medical plans and other interdisciplinary diagnostic or treatment programs.

9:30-10:00 A.M.: Administer scheduled drugs and detailed assessment of stable clients; provide comfort and personal hygiene measures; implement exercise treatments.

10:00-11:30 A.M.: Obtain feedback from coworkers regarding progress and special needs; provide assistance to coworkers, and plan to receive assistance from others for complex procedures; administer drugs before meals; involve clients in routine health education programs.

11:30 A.M.-1:00 P.M.: Take lunch break and cover for coworkers while they are on break; monitor unstable clients; assist clients with meals; administer scheduled drugs and those to be given with meals.

1:00-2:00 P.M.: Monitor client progress; provide comfort measures; promote client rest periods; administer drugs to be taken after meals and as scheduled.

2:00-2:45 P.M.: Monitor unstable clients; seek feedback from coworkers; complete care plan revisions and documentation not completed earlier; organize data for change-of-shift report; involve clients in health education programs.

2:45-3:30 P.M.: Give change-of-shift report.

activities often are done while the nurse is with these clients to provide comfort and personal hygiene measures. Sometimes the client care manager implements exercise treatments at this time.

If the client care manager shares responsibility with coworkers for some of the assigned clients, the manager obtains feedback about their progress and special needs (10:00 to 11:30 A.M.). Conferring with coworkers enables the nurse to assist them and to plan to receive help from others for complex procedures. The nurse also administers drugs before meals. In addition, the nurse might involve clients in routine health education programs.

During the lunch hour (11:30 A.M. to 1:00 P.M.), the client care manager takes a lunch break and covers for coworkers while they are on break. Specific efforts are made to monitor unstable clients, assist clients as needed with meals, and administer scheduled drugs, including those to be given with meals.

After meals (1:00 to 2:00 P.M.), the client care manager continues to monitor client progress. While visiting clients, the nurse provides comfort measures and promotes client rest periods. The nurse typically administers drugs to be taken after meals and as scheduled.

Before the change of shift (2:00 to 2:45 P.M.), the client care manager monitors the conditions of unstable clients. The manager also seeks feedback from coworkers to update the care plans. During this time, the nurse completes documentation not completed earlier. These activities help the nurse organize data for giving the change-of-shift report. This time also might be used to involve clients in health education programs.

At the end of the workday (2:45 to 3:30 P.M.), the client care manager gives the change-of-shift report to oncoming staff assigned to his or her clients. To the extent possible, the client care manager uses data gathered during the shift to relay information about client needs. These routines are similar to those used on other shifts.

## VARIATIONS IN CLIENT CARE MANAGEMENT ROUTINES

**Variations in client care management routines** occur frequently throughout each workday due to different organizational patterns of nursing service delivery and staffing, changes in client care routines associated with evening and night shifts, and changes in client needs and associated goals. In addition, client care managers adjust their typical routines to correspond to individual personal strengths, patterns of work organization, and use of time management skills.

## Pattern of Nursing Service Delivery

As mentioned earlier, the pattern of nursing service delivery used relates to the nature of client needs, available staff, and agency purposes and goals. Nurses using the primary nursing method of service delivery (often used in critical care units) might spend more time communicating with peers than directly supervising staff. This is because the clients' needs might require more skilled attention due to the increased acuity levels. In comparison, staff nurses using team nursing often spend more time communicating with subordinates. These clients may be less acutely ill but require consistent detailed attention to implement established individual client care plans. Nurses involved in functional nursing methods of service delivery might spend more time earlier in the workday ensuring that each task is assigned to available staff. They are more likely to emphasize providing the bare necessities of care and to pay less attention to identified individual client outcomes.

## Daily Activities of Clients and Departments (Day, Evening, and Night Shifts)

Client care management routines also vary according to the daily activities of clients and of other departments. Compared with day-shift client care managers, evening-shift managers spend less time feeding clients and performing related mealtime routines. Evening-shift workers may devote more time to communicating with families and to teaching programs. Nurses working during the evening shifts often communicate less with representatives of other disciplines or spend more time preparing clients for diagnostic procedures to be done the next day. They might use more time to communicate concerns to others through change-of-shift reports, in written form, or by interdepartmental methods.

In contrast, nurses working during the night shift often focus on monitoring client responses and promoting comfort in ways that do not interfere unnecessarily with sleep. As appropriate, nurses avoid unnecessary contact with clients. Their contact with representatives of other disciplines is often minimal. Staffing mix and routines may change to reflect these client needs and priorities. Fewer multidisciplinary work group members are available on other than an emergency basis, and almost nobody appreciates being awakened to discuss nonurgent concerns. Some clients benefit a great deal from a skilled caring listener when distressed and unable to sleep. Less time is likely to be spent on the routine administration of medicines. Many health-care facilities establish drug administration schedules to minimize involvement of night staff and disruption of typical sleeping hours. Interdepartmental communications for routine revision of care plans are rare. Nurses who work the night shift must provide feedback to and seek feedback from nursing staff and the multidisciplinary work group about client care to ensure that priority needs are addressed. This feedback promotes follow-through of individual treatment plans.

These common patterns of night-shift communication can place greater demands on staff working this shift to be assertive and extremely well organized. Often night-shift nurses are expected to complete all of the special diagnostic procedures and treatments in a timely manner to avoid interrupting the client's sleep. Nurses working during the night shift often tend to read the chart to ensure that all points of view are synthesized into the care plan. In addition, they are required to communicate current information about client needs to other departments in the early morning hours. Often less time is available to complete routine documentation before giving the change-of-shift report.

## Client Needs and Associated Goals

The staff nurse is expected to apply nursing process skills throughout each shift. Routines corresponding to the basic human needs of clients (e.g., nutrition, rest, and interaction with others) influence priorities and clinical decision making, however. Opportunities for communicating with clients, families, and multidisciplinary work group members affect how the nurse responds to evolving needs.

The entry-level nurse is expected to respond to client needs in a timely manner on any shift. Each nurse has a combination of unique strengths that influence her or his effectiveness as a client care manager in different contexts, however. Some nurses are more effective as primary nurses, providing care to acutely ill clients who need close monitoring. Others thrive on the social interactions involved in supervising subordinates caring for more physiologically stable clients. Some nurses have analytic skills that make them effective planners. Others are especially good at formulating detailed assessments to guide their work organization and use of available resources. Ultimately a client care manager's effectiveness in enabling clients to meet desired outcomes in a timely manner is the important factor.

## SUMMARY

Core nursing competencies basic to entry-level nursing practice are used to fulfill the obligations of three core nursing roles. These core roles, which are common to all entry-level staff nurses, are provider of care, member within the discipline of nursing, and client care manager. In practice, these roles are interrelated. The nurse emphasizes a specific role depending on the client's priority needs within a specific organizational context (e.g., practice setting). With the increasing emphasis on cost-effectiveness (i.e., the "bottom line"), nurses are pressured to provide quality of care with decreased or scarce resources. Staff nurses should remember, however, that their caring is the essence of quality of care. Consequently, staff nurses need to continue to focus (amidst considerable chaos) on meeting client needs. Client care managers should expect to participate in work force development efforts that promote the organization's mission in a measurable way.

Typically, client care managers develop their skills by building on skills used as providers of care and members within the discipline of nursing. In addition, they combine application of the nursing process with the process common to management. Consequently, client care managers mobilize and allocate resources of the nursing and interdisciplinary health work groups to meet the health needs of an assigned group of clients during a specified time.

Just as the nurse may use any phase of the nursing process at any point in time, he or she also might be involved in any phase of the management process. Consequently the client care manager's typical routines incorporate the allocation of agency resources to address established clients' needs and evaluation of the effectiveness of the group's efforts. A client care manager's typical day requires a plan that focuses on client needs and sensitivity to needs of coworkers. Typical routines vary with evolving priorities of client needs, with different patterns of nursing service delivery within organizational contexts, with the changes in emphasis of different shifts and the personal strengths of entry-level staff nurses.

## APPLICATION EXERCISES

1. Describe the differences between core nursing competencies and core nursing roles. List different expectations related to the client care manager role in an acute care inpatient versus a long-term care inpatient versus an ambulatory care setting.
2. Make a chronologic list of nursing courses you have completed. Indicate which client care management competencies you developed in each. Compare your findings with those of your peers.

*Continued*

## APPLICATION EXERCISES—cont'd

3. Make another chronologic list of nursing courses you have completed. Indicate which core nursing roles were emphasized in each. Compare your findings with those of your peers.
4. Keep a log of your use of time for two clinical days. Compare your findings with the typical routines of a client care manager described in this chapter. List three time management skills that you used each day to complete your assignment.
5. Observe a client care manager for a shift. Describe the typical routines for this nurse and how they increase effective and efficient use of available resources. Compare this client care manager's routines with those discussed in this chapter.
6. Describe any work force development activities that you became aware of while observing a client care manager on your assigned unit. What were the goals of these activities? What were the desired outcomes that made them worthwhile (i.e., a cost-effective use of scarce resources for the specific agency)?

## CRITICAL THINKING SCENARIO

You are an entry-level staff nurse employed in an acute care facility. Most of the clients you serve are admitted for orthopedic operative procedures, following care maps throughout the length of their stay. Some elderly clients with multi-system dysfunction struggle to accomplish all the goals in preparation for discharge. Your clients, with assistance from their families, need to use adaptive equipment and modify their patterns of activities of daily living due to self-care deficits. The staffing mix on your unit typically is 20% to 30% registered nurses, supplemented by 70% to 80% licensed practical nurses and nursing assistants. In addition to managing the nursing work group during the shifts you work, you attend multidisciplinary biweekly conferences. Often you struggle to complete tasks of care incorporated in the care maps. Frequently (every shift), assessments and discharge preparations by the assigned registered nurses are minimal due to other care management and coordination responsibilities.

1. What strategies would you use to prepare for the multidisciplinary work group conferences?
2. How would you mold your client care manager role so as not to compromise the quality of care (i.e., continue to provide skilled caring interactions with clients)?
3. What steps would you take to ensure that your clients' needs were assessed adequately in a timely manner?
4. How would you ensure that your clients were prepared adequately for discharge?

## REFERENCES

Apker J: Role development in the managed care era: a case of hospital based nursing, *Journal of Applied Communications Research 29*(2):117–136, 2001.

Cosolo N: Role-job functional mapping: a workforce design tool for 2000, *Nurs Admin Q 26*(2):34–42, 2002.

Council of Associate Degree Programs: *Educational outcomes of associate degree nursing programs: roles and competencies*, New York, NY, 1990, National League for Nursing.

Council of Baccalaureate and Higher Degree Programs: *Characteristics of baccalaureate education in nursing*, New York, NY, 1987, National League for Nursing.

Dienemann J, Gessner T: Restructuring nursing care delivery systems, *Nurs Econ 10*(4):253–258, 1992.

Gardner DB, Cary A: Collaboration, conflict and power: lessons for case managers, *Fam Community Health 22*(3):64–77, 1999.

Meliones JN, Ballard R, Liekweg R, Burton W: No mission—no margin: it's that simple, *J Health Care Finance 27*(3):21–29, 2001.

Ray MA, Turkel MC, Marino F: The transformative process for nursing in workforce development, *Nurs Admin Q 26*(2):1–14, 2002.

Seaman LH: Preparation: the key to nursing case management, *J Post Anesth Nurs 5*(3):177–181, 1990.

Tahan H: The nurse case manager in acute care settings, *J Nurs Admin 23*(10):53–61, 1993.

Terry JV: *International management handbook*, Fayetteville, AR, 1992, The University of Arkansas Press.

Turkel MC: Struggling to find a balance: the paradox between caring and economics, *Nurs Admin Q 26*(1):67–82, 2001.

Wywialowski E: *A study to determine skills expected of entry-level staff nurses using the DACUM methods: a MARP report presented to Nova University*, Fort Lauderdale, FL, 1987.

# 7

# *Identifying and Resolving Conflicts*

*When you complete this chapter, you should be able to:*

1. Differentiate between constructive and destructive conflict.
2. Identify symptoms of conflict.
3. Classify common types of conflict encountered by entry-level staff nurses.
4. Describe how personal beliefs, values, and biases might contribute to conflict.
5. Describe causes of conflict between nurses and clients.
6. Describe causes of conflict between members of the nursing work group.
7. Describe causes of conflict between nurses and other health care providers.
8. Describe techniques that staff nurses use to resolve destructive conflicts.

conflict  
  constructive  
  destructive  
  intrapersonal  
  interpersonal  

intergroup  
symptoms  
sources  
conflict resolution process

## IDENTIFYING CONFLICT

With the increasing importance of a global economy, conflict situations also are increasing (Gruen, 2001, p. 16; Jeong, 1999; McCaughan, 2001, p. 40). Not only are the costs of conflict a growing concern (Sandler, 2000, p. 723), but also the long-term consequences of unresolved conflict on public safety are drawing attention of private citizens and government officials. Conflict is so common that elementary schools are beginning to develop instructional programs designed to help children develop conflict resolution skills to prevent violence and aggressive behaviors (Parker Roerden, 2001, p. 24). Resolving conflicts is a competency needed by entry-level staff nurses that enables them to manage client care successfully.

A **conflict** exists when individuals, acting in their own best interests, participate in activities that generate tension. The participants in the conflict develop antagonisms (i.e., disagreements or an interactive relationship characterized by differences in their attitudes, values, interests, plans, or intentions) (Becker-Beck, 2001, p. 260). Tension results from significant disagreements or incompatible interests and activities (Gibson, 1986, p. 47). Important differences evolve and persist between the individuals involved and interfere with mobilizing resources to achieve common goals. A conflict can be caused by almost anything, result in disagreement, and produce stress.

The fast-paced and diverse work demands of common nursing practice settings provide fertile territory for conflict. The cultural diversity of staff and clients also frequently contributes to conflict. Entry-level staff nurses are expected to identify and resolve conflicts that interfere with client care. This chapter provides insight into sources of conflict and strategies that might be used to resolve them.

## Types of Conflict

Many nurses perceive all conflict as negative (Gibson, 1986, pp. 48–49; Jones, 1993, p. 68). Conflict itself is neither positive nor negative, but if conflict is not recognized and managed, opportunities for positive growth are missed (Brandt, 2001, p. 32). **Constructive** conflict (i.e., conflict that results in improved client care, work satisfaction, or communication among work group members) should be nurtured because it presents an opportunity to stimulate desired change that benefits the organization. When the participants begin to appreciate the opportunities being presented by a conflict and the appreciation that positive results are possible, the conflict is transformed into positive, constructive behaviors (Cloke and Goldsmith, 2000, pp. 5–6). In contrast, **destructive** conflict causes stress and interferes with the quality of client care provided, work satisfaction, and the effectiveness of communication between coworkers. Entry-level staff nurses are expected to identify destructive conflict and implement strategies to reduce or eliminate it. They also are expected to respond appropriately to constructive conflict.

Conflict can be intrapersonal, interpersonal, and intergroup (Douglass, 1992, p. 170). **Intrapersonal** conflict is conflict that occurs within the individual when he or she tries to engage in incompatible activities. Entry-level nurses often experience intrapersonal conflicts. A nurse might choose to work overtime to complete a work assignment and be unable to attend to scheduled commitments with family or friends. This type of conflict requires the nurse to use critical thinking and problem-solving skills to set personal priorities and goals.

**Interpersonal** conflict is conflict that occurs between individuals. Interpersonal conflicts occur when tension results from differences between two or more people, often people presumed to be working toward common goals. Common causes of interpersonal conflict include differences in cultural background, gender, race, ethnic diversity, and values (Caprioli and Boyer, 2001, p. 503; Davidson, 2001, p. 259; Easterly, 2001, p. 687; Morris and Fu, 2001, p. 324). Entry-level staff nurses frequently encounter interpersonal conflict as they supervise the work of licensed practical nurses or nursing assistants who hold different perceptions of client care needs and how they might be provided for. Entry-level staff nurses are expected to identify and try to resolve these conflicts by helping to clarify roles and functions (Beauchamp and Bray, 2001, p. 144). Conflict resolution techniques often include communication with the administrative staff to manage the conflict and work toward identifying problem solutions. These collaborative communications might lead to a systems change through a quality improvement process. The advocacy role of the staff nurse as a liaison between administration and the health-care team was described in Chapter Three.

Entry-level nurses experience **intergroup** conflict from time to time. Intergroup conflict often arises between groups with differing values, goals, and perspectives. It frequently involves more than one shift, work group, or combination of health-care work group members (e.g., between nursing groups working different shifts or between intradisciplinary or multidisciplinary staff assigned to provide care for a client with complex needs). Intergroup conflict often indicates potential systems problems (i.e., problems within the health-care organization). Frequently, members of work groups or interdisciplinary teams do not understand each other's roles and functions or are confronted with differing constraints of staffing, equipment, time, or supplies. These conflicts may be addressed by first-line (nursing unit) managers, "case managers," or higher levels of management rather than by client care managers. Administrative staff strive to manage intergroup conflicts in such a way that they nurture organizational development. Ultimately, leadership and direct care staff share accountability for using resources wisely to ensure safe care (Smith, 2002, p. 19).

## SYMPTOMS OF CONFLICT

**Symptoms** of conflict frequently include frustration, anger, missed or ineffective communication, or withdrawal from an interrelationship. Prolonged conflict frequently produces continued stress that is costly in terms of "wear and tear" on valuable human resources. In addition to the missed opportunities to provide quality of care, health problems such as hypertension, heart disease, muscular tension, and headaches frequently result from long-term conflict. Learning to differentiate between positive and negative stress and learning when to intervene is a fine art. The goals of conflict resolution include nurturing desired changes, while avoiding destructive conflict (i.e., conflict that interferes with providing quality care and erodes valuable human resources).

## SOURCES OF CONFLICT

**Sources** of conflict vary widely. Frequently, they originate in different personal beliefs, values, and biases of individual staff members, clients, or family members. When participants in the conflict listen carefully and empathically, additional sources of conflict may surface, such as differences in cultural backgrounds and expectations, gender, race, or ethnicity. When these covert (hidden) sources of conflict are combined with ineffective or missed communications, destructive conflict is likely. Destructive conflict can be transformed into an opportunity (i.e., constructive conflict).

### Recognizing Personal Beliefs, Values, and Biases

An entry-level staff nurse soon learns about the numerous sources of conflict by observing the behaviors of coworkers. Behavior reflects basic beliefs about human nature or motivation, and these beliefs vary widely from person to person. For example, individual perceptions about a person's capacities are often described in conversation. One person may say, "If you don't expect much, you avoid disappointment"; another will say, "I never cease to be amazed by what people can do, given half a chance." As a result of their differences in basic beliefs, these people might come into conflict when faced with demanding situations.

Personal values are reflected in individual attitudes. Attitudes influence how people perceive the demands of the workplace and often contribute to different perceptions and evolve into conflict. For example, individuals differ in how they

Sources of conflict vary widely

perceive their employment activities and the importance they place on making money. These perceptions affect the types of employment they accept and how they communicate with coworkers. Differences based on personal values may be a source of conflict in work settings that require flexibility and a focus on the needs of others. One employee may be concerned primarily with "making a living," whereas another is trying to provide the best possible care. Staff nurses are expected to recognize differences in perspective and work to accommodate them so that client needs are addressed satisfactorily.

Personal biases stemming from differences in socialization, gender, race, or ethnicity, when unrecognized or unchecked, also can contribute to conflict. They can contribute to negative feelings by communicating nonverbal messages that are perceived as devaluing the worth of others. For example, one coworker's lack of eye contact might convince another that he or she is being ignored or that the coworker is unfriendly, when the coworker merely may be trying to focus on the client's symptoms and needs. In another example, cultural or racial differences may result in more verbal responses to conflict instead of withdrawal that may be interpreted as aggressive behavior (Davidson, 2001, p. 259). To relate effectively with coworkers, entry-level staff nurses need to be aware of personal beliefs, values, cultural differences, and biases. This awareness helps avoid ineffective communication in stressful situations and behaviors that coworkers or clients might perceive as insensitive.

## Gaining Insight into Individual Client Differences

Clients have personal beliefs, values, and biases. Consequently, nurses need to confirm with the client their interpretations of client behavior to communicate effectively. For example, the nurse might interpret the client's facial expression as evidence of tension. By confirming this interpretation with the client, the nurse might learn that the client is feeling tense because of discomfort or frustration related to limitations of self-care or because he or she is bored because of the resulting limited involvement in diversional activities. As nurses confirm their interpretations of client behavior, they gain insights into the client's personal beliefs, values, and biases.

Conflicts may arise when individual client goals differ from those of the predominant culture of health-care providers. Differences between individual client goals and goals anticipated by the nurse often become apparent during the assessment and planning phases of care. A client might select health-care options on the basis of religious beliefs different from those held by the nurse. A client might place greater value on mystical powers than on a health-care professional's interventions to preserve human life, resulting in refusal to accept common medical procedures. If these conflicts are not recognized and managed constructively, they could lead to infringement of the client's right to refuse treatment.

Similarly, a client's ethnic or cultural background might result in responses that do not fit the nurse's expectations. Uncertainty or unfamiliarity often increases anxiety and ultimately results in conflict (Butrin, 1992, p. 249). Special attention is required in the initial assessment and continued evaluation efforts to ensure that differences in the spiritual and ethnic backgrounds of clients are recognized. For example, a client might not eat certain types of foods because he or she is unfamiliar with them. If not discussed with the client, this behavior might be interpreted incorrectly as a lack of appetite. If nurses are insensitive to a client's ethnic preferences, routines are often not adjusted to meet individual needs.

The family dynamics of clients with different religious and ethnic backgrounds can complicate communication processes. Members of some ethnic groups do not share the predominant American cultural norms and patterns of communication and decision making. For example, the "breadwinner" of a client's family might expect to make all major decisions about how money and family resources are used. Patterns of decision making among family members need to be recognized and incorporated in the strategies used to establish plans for continued care. Otherwise, implementation of discharge plans might be difficult or unworkable. Impoverished clients often may not hold the same value on follow-up care as do middle-class health-care providers; consequently, these clients do not commit scarce resources to follow-up care.

## Gaining Insight into Differences in the Personal and Professional Beliefs of Self and Coworkers

Consistent with American Nurses Association Standards of Nursing Practice, entry-level nurses are expected to provide care on the basis of assessed client need. This standard of practice does not allow nurses to provide the client care that they personally would prefer. Rather, nurses are expected to provide client care consistent with a plan mutually agreed on with the client.

Sometimes a nurse's professional experiences of caring for clients with various diseases and types of illnesses can color subsequent perceptions of the needs of clients experiencing similar illnesses. A nurse can be sensitized or emotionally affected by client situations, especially those involving intense pain or suffering. Experience also might influence a nurse's personal perceptions of death. These types of emotional response can influence the nurse's ability to remain objective in determining the client's best interest. The nurse must distinguish his or her personal perspectives about illness and death, however, from the professional perspective required to provide care to clients, who have their own varying perceptions of illness and death. The nurse is not in a position to choose for others what the clients want done on their behalf.

Similarly, nurses need to be sensitive to expressed personal perceptions of coworkers. Coworkers often have had similar experiences that affected each of them differently (Arnold et al., 1988, pp. 40–49). As client advocates, nurses are expected to help coworkers recognize when personal experiences and preferences conflict with those of clients. Particularly when situations involve intense emotions (e.g., following serious injury or death or during intense discomfort), special effort is needed to separate personal desires and professional responsibilities.

This is not to suggest that compassion be eliminated in the interest of objectivity. Compassion is an integral part of nursing care. Compassionate nursing effort focuses on client perceptions and needs instead of self-interests. Mutually satisfying and caring nursing actions minimize conflict. That is, when nurses are aware of how their own cultural values and behaviors stem from their unique cultural backgrounds, they are more likely to experience fewer conflicts and more satisfying relationships with clients having cultural backgrounds different from their own (Butrin, 1992, p. 249).

## Distinguishing Client and Family Expectations

Another source of conflict the entry-level nurse is expected to manage involves differences between the expectations of clients and their families. Although the client and family usually have similar spiritual beliefs and ethnic traditions, the process of adjustment to illness often differs among family members. In addition, the client's adjustment related to changing levels of dependency often changes the adjustments required of family members and consequently how the family uses its resources.

### Client Adjustment to Loss

Clients who live with a long-term health problem experience and adjust to varying degrees of loss. The duration and intensity of the adjustment experienced by each client varies. Stages of adjustment to loss of body function or health correspond to those described by Crate (1965, pp. 72–76) and by Kubler-Ross (1969, pp. 38–137). Box 7-1 compares the stages described by these two theories. An individual client's success in progressing from one stage to the next depends on the client's physiologic status and the availability of psychological, social, and spiritual resources. Because family members are usually the primary caregivers, clients usually expect to adjust their dependencies to match family resources. The client is expected to adjust to changing family resources as well as to lost or decreased body function.

### Family Adjustment

While the client strives to adapt to long-term loss of health and ability to meet the demands of daily living independently, family members cope with a realignment of priorities, use of time, and resources. Hasselkus (1988, pp. 60–70) described the various stages of family adjustment to a member of the family with a long-term health problem. Box 7-2 lists stages of family caregiver adjustment. Each family member, depending on the extent of support or care he or she provides to the client, adjusts at his or her own rate. As Hasselkus described, client and family attempt to adjust to demands placed on them by health-care providers. When the health-care provider's perspective differs from that of the client or family, conflicting expectations often arise. The client and the family usually try to cope with these conflicting expectations as they adapt to long-term health problems.

### Client and Family Progress and Use of Resources

As client care manager, the nurse is expected to assess the client's and the family's progress and to monitor how effectively they are using resources. Typically, clients expect the nurse to take the initiative in identifying and resolving conflicts. If conflicts arise that interfere with their progress, the nurse promotes communication processes that clarify perceptions, identify differences, and reduce misunderstandings. In addition, the nurse might initiate referrals and mobilize other agency resources to provide needed support. For example, in addition to regularly monitoring the client's progress, the nurse might refer the client and family to self-help

---

**BOX 7-1**

## Comparison of Crate's and Kubler-Ross's Models of the Adaptation Phases of Individuals to Illness

**Crate**
1. Disbelief
2. Developing awareness
3. Reorganization of relationships with others
4. Resolution of loss
5. Identity change

**Kubler-Ross**
1. Denial and isolation
2. Anger
3. Bargaining
4. Depression
5. Acceptance

---

groups and other social and pastoral services. The nurse may need to initiate support to assist the client and family to follow through. Constructive conflict resolution provides the nurse an opportunity to address client needs better.

## Ineffective Communication Processes

Many sources of conflict involve ineffective communication processes. Nurses can contribute to conflict by failing to recognize personal beliefs, values, and biases. The assumption that others hold the same beliefs, values, and biases leads to

---

**BOX 7-2**

## Stages of Family Caregiver Adjustment

**In-hospital**

They know best: Family caregivers believe the professionals know best.

Coming up with the reasons: Family caregivers search for causes of the client's illness.

**Discharge time**

Critiquing and modifying: Family caregivers try to do what they are "supposed to do" but change approaches to fit personal capabilities and perceptions.

Figuring it out together: Family caregivers work in parallel with professionals.

**On their own**

Teaching the professional: Family caregivers decide what the client needs and how to get it.

Sharing what works: Family caregivers develop their own special knowledge and seek to "teach the professionals" about what "works" for the client.

---

Adapted with permission from Hasselkus BR: Rehabilitation: the family caregiver's view, *Top Geriatr Rehabil 4*(1): 60–70, 1988 (© 1988, Aspen Publishers, Inc.)

communication errors in sending and receiving messages. Language barriers between people of different cultures or perspectives also contribute to misinterpretations of speech and behaviors (Tracy and Ashcraft, 2001, p. 297). Frequently, communication patterns involving language barriers are complicated by less interaction; when language barriers exist, more interactions usually are needed. In addition, differences in cultural patterns and family decision-making processes can complicate the nurse's efforts to provide for continued care. Clients and families do not adjust at the same rate. Conflicts may arise when client and family needs change frequently and they are expected to fit expected patterns of behavior.

In addition to retaining a client-centered focus, the entry-level nurse is expected to identify when destructive conflicts exist. The client care manager also should be familiar with specific approaches to resolve conflict to prevent such situations from interfering with the effectiveness of the client's care.

## Using Communication Techniques to Resolve Conflicts

As providers of care, nurses develop communication skills that enable them to assess client needs and evaluate responses to care provided. The nurse recognizes that lack of anticipated progress in meeting desired client outcomes could be an indication of conflict. If the client situation indicates potential for ineffective communications, several techniques can be used to determine if a conflict exists. Box 7-3 describes the **conflict resolution process**.

### Separate Facts from Opinion

Collect information about the facts of the client's situation or what actually happened. Listen to how the people involved describe their perceptions. Determine if the perceptions of the client and caregiver overlap or differ. Pay attention to the terminology used. Which concerns are difficult to discuss or are not discussed at all? Try to identify reasons for the opinions presented. Does the client understand his or her predominant health problem? Has the client received the information needed to participate in priority setting? Are you or other staff members aware of existing language barriers or misinterpretations of behavior? Were any inappropriate assumptions made?

---

BOX 7-3

## Conflict Resolution Process

1. Separate facts from opinion.
2. Identify the specific problem.
3. Seek suggestions and ideas from those involved.
4. Select the solutions that settle the disagreement.
5. Note the consequences of the solution.
6. Evaluate your success in resolving the conflict.

## Identify the Specific Problem

Describe the conflict in your own words. Try to locate the source of the conflict and how those involved have responded. It is likely that there are multiple sources for the evolving conflict. What is the underlying source of the disagreement? How have the participants contributed to ineffective communication processes?

## Seek Suggestions and Ideas from Those Involved

To the greatest extent possible, attempt to settle the conflict so that it results in a win-win situation for all involved. Various communication strategies might be used, depending on the nature of the entry-level staff nurse's relationship to the persons involved in the conflict. Collaboration typically results in win-win situations for those involved in the conflict, whereas avoidance, withdrawal, compromise, competition, and accommodation do not. Avoid blaming participants for the conflict. Rather, emphasize the problem-solving process, beginning with the positive value of their ideas and input about potential solutions. Because their perceptions have contributed to the conflict, discussing possible solutions can help you gain further insight into their beliefs, values, misinterpretations, and biases. If feasible, make a mental note of the words the participants use to describe their ideas. Think about the various possibilities and their acceptability to the involved persons.

## Select the Solutions That Settle the Disagreement

This step is not easy. Much of decision making, especially in situations in which participants feel threatened, is driven by emotion (Gordon and Arian, 2001, p. 197). Often the solution selected is not a suggestion from one of the participants, but rather a combination of ideas from participants on both sides of the disagreement. If the conflict is deeply rooted organizationally, you probably will be limited to a temporary solution. You should inform those involved of your intention to discuss the situation with your supervisor. Typically, you can expect your supervisor to support your efforts. Explain to the participants the expectations related to the solution. Request that the participants attempt to carry out the solution to the best of their abilities.

## Note the Consequences of the Solution

Observe the reactions of participants involved in the conflict. Note their attitudes and their behaviors. Do you believe each of the participants gained from the conflict resolution process, or did they perceive the solution as a lose-lose or win-lose situation? If you believe that some participants perceive the solution as a "lose" situation, the conflict may not be resolved completely. Positive individual self-concepts contribute to effective conflict management. If the solutions do not support individual self-esteem and dignity, more work needs to be done (Ting-Toomey et al., 2001, p. 197). Expect to spend more effort to maintain or improve communication and ultimately the relationship among the people involved.

## Evaluate Your Success in Resolving the Conflict

Recall that when you identified the conflict, you believed that the existing ineffective communication or disagreement was interfering with the client's care. Have your efforts increased the likelihood that the client will progress toward desired out-comes in a timely manner? Has communication improved among the participants involved in the conflict?

In general, efforts to improve communication when conflicts arise are well spent. Although client care managers frequently are under stress from multiple con-flicts in a fast-paced work environment, they are highly motivated to improve the quality of care provided. When conflicts are complicated by intergroup disagree-ments and organizational involvement is indicated, client care managers might rea-sonably "sink their heels in for a long haul." The more people perceive the solution to be an answer to an unselfish concern, the more they can focus on the greater good (Baron, 2001, p. 294). Conflict management leading to organizational change is often a lengthy process and may lead to filing a formal complaint (O'Connell, 2001, p. 761). As client care managers refine the communication skills used in con-flict resolution, their value to clients, employing agencies, and the nursing profes-sion increases as well.

As mentioned earlier, conflict can be perceived as an opportunity for positive change. Or it can be avoided, which increases the risk of its escalation. As members of complex organizations, entry-level staff nurses need to remain sensitive to con-flict and the potential for constructive change. Insight into the causes of conflicts that consume valuable scarce resources can be used to guide personal change. Changes in attitudes, behaviors, communication patterns, and styles of managing may be indicated (Barton, 1991, pp. 83–86; Collyer, 1989, pp. 77–80). Although these self-improvements are difficult to achieve, their benefits in effectiveness, effi-ciency, and satisfaction are likely to be well worth the effort (Mallory, 1985, p. 83).

## Unionization and Conflict Resolution

Historically, just as nurses too often have overlooked the value of constructive res-olution of conflict, they also have resisted identification with unionization (Wilson et al., 1990, p. 35). As the costs of health care continue to escalate in a labor-intensive industry, in which nursing salaries and wages account for more than half the expenses, unionization likely will be one possible alternative to resolving conflict. With increasing costs, threats to job security may lead to nurs-ing role changes to include more involvement in decision making affecting use of nursing resources.

The need for an intervention team (e.g., a union) is an indication that the inten-sity of conflict has escalated beyond the point at which the parties involved can resolve it. "When top hospital administrators and nursing administration become arbitrary and unfair with employees, union activity is bound to grow within the nursing profession" (Wilson et al., 1990, p. 39). Nurses need to understand the issues underlying the unresolvable conflicts that require "outside" intervention teams. They need to understand the crucial need for clear articulation of nursing concerns and needs and how these unmet needs affect client care. Ultimately, col-lective efforts are needed to resolve conflicts in the interest of providing cost-effec-tive quality client care. Whether or not unionization results may depend on the commitment of the parties involved to strive toward common goals.

## SUMMARY

Entry-level staff nurses are expected to identify and resolve interpersonal conflicts that interfere with client care. Conflict is stressful, but it can be helpful by providing an opportunity to work toward solving persistent or growing problems. Common symptoms of conflict include frustration, anger, missed or ineffective communication, and withdrawal. Prolonged conflict can result in health problems of individual participants.

Staff nurses are expected to distinguish between destructive and constructive conflict. Constructive conflict resolution often leads to organizational development. Destructive conflict decreases quality client care, work satisfaction, and the effectiveness of communication between workers.

To resolve conflicts that interfere with quality client care, nurses need to be sensitive to differences in personal beliefs, values, and biases of staff, clients, and families. Nurses also need to monitor the various phases of adjustment to health problems of clients and their families. Various illnesses involve intense pain or suffering and can influence the nurse's ability to remain objective in determining the client's best interest. Insensitivity to these issues can result in ineffective communication and potential destructive conflict. To comply with Codes of Conduct, nurses need to provide care consistent with assessed client needs, choices, and preferences.

To resolve conflict, six steps are suggested: (1) separate facts from opinion, (2) identify the specific problem, (3) seek suggested solutions from those involved, (4) select the solution that settles the disagreement, (5) note the consequences of the solution, and (6) evaluate success in resolving the conflict. Unresolved conflict is likely to escalate. If conflict involves large numbers of people at varying levels of the organization, collective efforts and an outside intervention team may become necessary. Ultimately, nurses are expected to acknowledge conflict actively and strive to achieve client care goals consistent with organizational purposes.

## APPLICATION EXERCISES

1. The assigned staff nurses on the day and evening shifts have expressed differing opinions about the intensity of a client's pain and its etiology. The client's family reported their concerns about the client's need to "wait" for 2 hours on the evening shift before receiving "something for pain." Identify the type of conflict involved in this situation, and its sources.
2. Describe the role of emotion in this conflict.
3. Describe likely consequences if facts are not separated from opinions when attempting to resolve this conflict.
4. Describe the likely consequences if the specific problem created by this conflict is not identified when attempting to resolve it.
5. Describe the difficulties likely to occur when the disagreeing parties are not involved in identifying possible solutions. Discuss the likely sequence of events in resolving this conflict if a win-lose situation is allowed to occur.
6. Resolution of this conflict may or may not occur. Describe how meeting desired client outcomes helps to evaluate success in conflict resolution.

## CRITICAL THINKING SCENARIO

Imagine yourself as an entry-level staff nurse, a graduate of a baccalaureate program, employed full-time on a busy surgical unit of an acute care facility, assigned to the evening tour of duty. Two of your colleagues are "new grads" of associate degree programs. The nursing staff is a homogeneous group of middle-class Hispanic and white Americans. The client population served are more heterogeneous, including African Americans, Hispanics, and Asians. Almost on a daily basis, family members or significant others stay later than regular visiting hours to complete client education programs and discharge planning discussions. Often these people have other family or employment commitments that do not allow them to come earlier in the day.

By agency policy, visiting hours end at 8:00 P.M. While completing your assignment, you overhear one of your colleagues requesting family visitors involved in client education programs to comply with the visiting hours policy. Later, as you are preparing to give change-of-shift report, a licensed practical nurse and nursing assistant on your nursing work group briskly inform you that "visitors need to be cleared out of here on time, so we can get our work done. They can learn earlier in the day, when there are more people on."

1. What would you do first? Would you delay your initiation of a conflict resolution strategy? Explain.
2. Are you in the best position organizationally to collaborate with the entire work group? Is this a problem that affects only your shift?
3. Who would you involve in identifying the specific problem?
4. What alternatives would you consider to resolve the conflict?
5. What would be some potential benefits of communicating with the entire team on the evening shift?

## REFERENCES

Arnold L, Mills J, Willoughby TL: Nursing assistants' attitudes toward dying patients in a long-term care facility, *Top Geriatr Rehabil* 4(1):40–49, 1988.

Baron J: Confusion of group interest and self-interest in parochial cooperation on behalf of a group, *Journal of Conflict Resolution* 45(3):283–296, 2001.

Barton A: Conflict resolution by nurse managers, *Nurs Manage* 22(5):83–86, 1991.

Beauchamp MR, Bray SR: Role ambiguity and role conflict within interdependent teams, *Small Group Research* 32(2):133–157, 2001.

Becker-Beck U: Methods for diagnosing interaction strategies: an application to group interaction in conflict situations, *Small Group Research* 32(2):259–282, 2001.

Brandt MA: How to make conflict work for you, *Nurs Manage* 23(11):32–35, 2001.

Butrin J: Cultural diversity in the nurse-client encounter, *Clin Nurs Res 1*(3): 238–251, 1992.

Caprioli M, Boyer MA: Gender, violence, and international crisis, *Journal of Conflict Resolution 45*(4):503–518, 2001.

Cloke K, Goldsmith J: *Resolving conflicts at work: a complete guide for everyone on the job*, San Francisco, CA, 2000, Jossey-Bass.

Collyer ME: Resolving conflicts: leadership style sets the strategy, *Nurs Manage 20*(9):77–80, 1989.

Crate M: Nursing functions in adaptation to chronic illness, *Am J Nurs 65*(10): 72–76, 1965.

Davidson MN: Know thine adversary: the impact of race on styles of dealing with conflict, *Sex Roles 45*(5/6):259–276, 2001.

Douglass LM: *The effective nurse: leader and manager*, ed 4, St Louis, MO, 1992, Mosby.

Easterly W: Can institutions resolve ethnic conflict? *Economic Development and Cultural Change 49*(4):687–706, 2001.

Gibson D: Theory and strategies for resolving conflict, *Occup Ther Mental Health 5*(5):47–62, 1985–1986.

Gordon C, Arian A: Threat and decision-making, *Journal of Conflict Resolution 45*(2):196–215, 2001.

Gruen L: *Conflicting values in a conflicted world: ecofeminism and multicultural environmental ethics*, Women & Environments, Fall 2001. Available at www.weimag.com.

Hasselkus BR: Rehabilitation: the family caregiver's view, *Top Geriatr Rehabil 4*(1):60–70, 1988.

Hendricks W: *How to manage conflict*, Shawnee Mission, KS, 1991, National Press Publications.

Jeong HW (editor): *Conflict resolution: dynamics, process, and structure*, Aldershot, UK, 1999, Ashgate Publishing.

Jones K: Confrontation: methods and skills, *Nurs Manage 24*(5):68–70, 1993.

Kubler-Ross E: *Death and dying*, New York, NY, 1969, Macmillan.

Mallory GA: Turn conflict into cooperation, *Nursing 10*(3):81–83, 1985.

McCaughan EJ: Violence, inequality, and the "civilized" world, *Social Justice 28*(3):39–40, 2001.

Morris, MW and Fu HY: How does culture influence conflict resolution? Dynamic constructivist analysis, *Social Cognition 19*(3): 324–349, 2001.

O'Connell JF: The NLRB at the grassroots, *Journal of Labor Research 22*(4):761–774, 2001.

Parker Roerden L: The resolving conflict creativity program, *Reclaiming Children and Youth 10*(1):24–28, 2001.

Sandler T: Economic analysis of conflict, *The Journal of Conflict Resolution 44*(6): 723–729, 2000.

Smith MH: Staffing: what's your legal obligation? *Nurs Manage 33*(8):19–20, 48, 2002.

Ting-Toomey S, Oetzel JG, Yee-Jung K: Self-construal types and conflict management styles, *Communication Reports 14*(2):87–104, 2001.

Tracy K, Ashcraft C: Crafting policies about controversial values: how wording disputes manage a group dilemma, *Journal of Applied Communication Research* *29*(4):297–316, 2001.

Wilson CN, Hamilton CA, Murphy E: Union dynamics in nursing, *J Nurs Admin* *20*(2):35–39, 1990.

# CHAPTER 8

# *Receiving and Giving Change-of-Shift Reports*

## GETTING ACQUAINTED WITH CHANGE-OF-SHIFT REPORTS

Continuity of care has a long history in nursing practice. Nurses assume responsibility for **continuity of care**; that is, they expect to work toward coordinating care through scheduled episodes of communication with each other for the benefit of clients. When sufficient continuity of care is provided, client satisfaction increases (Stubblefield and Murray, 1999, p. 356).

Whether in acute, long-term, or home care settings, no one nurse can provide all the care needed by the client over time (Anderson and Helms, 2000, p. 15). The primary care nursing model was designed to increase personal care continuity (i.e., care provided to the client by the same nurse). This has become known as *"front stage" continuity*, where the client sees the same nurse day after day. Continuity of care as the underlying function of change-of-shift reports is more than the personal care provided by a primary nurse; it relates to nursing efforts on a system level to coordinate consistently the personalized, specialized care needed by the client throughout the episode of care (Krogstad et al., 2002, p. 36) and has been described as *"backstage" continuity*. It is crucial that the information exchange involved in change-of-shift reports occurs where clients do not see or hear the process. Continuity of care depends on nurses to accomplish the required coordinated communication confidentially (Cochran, 1999, p. 45). Similarly, nurses coordinate communications needed to provide continuity of care when clients move from one provider to another (e.g., from one type of service to another, such as intensive care to intermediate care or from one health-care agency to another). The major component of continuity of care involves tracking the client's progress in achieving desired outcomes (Hansten and Washburn, 1999, p. 25; Parkman et al., 2000, p. 74).

Client care managers receive and give **change-of-shift reports** to provide for continuity of care. Staff focus on exchanging information about each client's status, current care plan, responses to current care, and what needs further nursing attention to provide consistent follow-through. The **form** and **style** of the change-of-shift report depend on agency policies and preferences of nursing unit work groups (Monahan et al., 1988, p. 80; Reiley and Stengrevics, 1989, pp. 54–56; Richard, 1989, pp. 63–64). The form of the report varies with the nursing service delivery pattern and the preferences of involved staff (i.e., change-of-shift report evolved in inpatient settings in acute and long-term care). Staff also need to provide continuity of care in ambulatory care settings as well. In addition to maintaining current client clinical records, staff employed in ambulatory care settings need to adapt the nature of intragroup and intergroup reports to suit the client population served and patterns of communication between staff. These reports aid the staff to organize work for a specified period and communicate concerns to enable the health-care providers to provide consistent follow-through or, at least, reduce fragmentation of care. Although the forms of change-of-shift reports vary, the face-to-face taped forms are most common in inpatient settings, and this chapter focuses on these types.

The registered nurses (RNs) assigned responsibility for care of individual clients typically give the reports, although some patterns of service delivery require associate nurses, who might be licensed practical nurses, to report on their assigned clients under the supervision of the RN. The RN finishing a shift typically gives the change-of-shift report to his or her counterpart beginning a shift. The reporting nurse bears a legal responsibility to communicate all facts relevant to the continuity of care of her or his assigned clients. With practice, client care managers learn to exchange efficiently information about their assigned clients' care that meets the needs of the oncoming shift. To give an effective report, the client care manager provides information to oncoming staff that is pertinent, current, and accurate.

## Function of Change-of-Shift Reports

Change-of-shift reports are used to provide for and promote continuity of care. A method of imposing order on seeming chaos, this type of report is a regularly scheduled, structured information exchange. It consists of **summaries of individual client progress** for each client assigned to an RN. Its primary goal is to exchange effectively and efficiently information between groups of nursing staff about client responses and changes in treatment programs. As described by Wolf (1988, p. 238), "Change-of-shift report was a scheduled, three-times-a-day opportunity for nurses to come together to discuss nursing care and patient progress." Although the report does not include all the details contained in clinical records, it provides accurate, current summaries of individual client progress. The change-of-shift report should strive not to duplicate information that is documented in detail in the client's clinical record.

## Focus of Change-of-Shift Reports

The change-of-shift report focuses on information about the anticipated needs of individual clients within the next 24 hours. The reporting nurse describes client care events that occurred during the previous shift and nursing activities anticipated during the next shift. The information exchange helps the nurse receiving the report monitor clients' signs and symptoms of disease, discomforts, and their management. The reporting nurse describes client progress in completing laboratory studies and diagnostic tests and related specimen collections. In this way, the change-of-shift report prepares nursing staff to carry out dependent functions efficiently. In addition, nursing responses to clients' needs are included, as are those of other multidisciplinary work group members. The change-of-shift report includes discussion of medical, nursing, and other multidisciplinary actions aimed at resolving actual or potential client problems.

The information provided in the change-of-shift report helps the nursing staff anticipate activities needed to coordinate the client's care during the next shift. Sometimes the reporting nurse describes "unfinished" nursing activities to enable staff on the next shift to complete needed client care.

## Organizing the Information Exchange

The information exchange has several key features. Typically, nurses use several **communication tools** to gather the needed information. In many inpatient settings, nurses use the **Kardex** as a communication tool, which, when kept current, contains summaries of the clients' statuses, treatments, and care goals. A typical Kardex is a written description of a client's personal care needs, individualized treatment goals and related desired outcomes, and nursing interventions; it often includes a list of prescribed drugs and medical treatments. Sometimes the nurse giving the report updates details on the Kardex during the change-of-shift report to maintain efficiently its currency as a primary resource for exchanging information between nursing work groups.

More recently nurses have begun to use actual **care maps** or pathways as a framework for planning care, goals, and specific procedures involved in the client's treatment program. The information may be stored electronically and accessed using specific database procedures. Nurses need to be involved in developing such information resources to avoid duplication and maintain confidence of other nurses (Howard-Ruben, 2002, p. 9). Nurses need to know where specific information is stored within the documentation system so that they have confidence in the currency and accuracy of the information resources they use. As they gain confidence, nurses will be less likely to duplicate information and will shorten the change-of-shift report (Howard-Ruben, 2002, p. 9; Rewick and Gaffey, 2001, p. 25).

The **sequence** of client summaries in the change-of-shift report often is organized to correspond to the work assignment of the reporter or the nurse receiving the report. If two RNs working nights each cared for a group of clients, one nurse would report on those assigned to his or her care, while the other supervised the entire unit. When the first RN had completed giving change-of-shift report, the other RN would give the report while her or his counterpart supervised the unit. Sometimes the reporter organizes the report to correspond to groups of clients assigned to individual staff members on the next shift. Typically the nurse giving the report starts at the beginning of a Kardex and continues sequentially to its end, which helps the staff who are listening to anticipate when individual client summaries will be presented.

If the Kardex is not used, the nurse giving the report often uses a **client assignment work sheet** or a form that lists the clients assigned to her or his care. In addition, the nurse might use **progress notes, flow sheets**, or the care maps used to monitor a client's condition as a source of reliable information and clinical records to provide additional details.

## VARYING THE CHANGE-OF-SHIFT REPORT

To communicate efficiently and effectively to nursing work groups between shifts, client care managers vary the **form and style of the change-of-shift report**, depending on the nature of the client's needs, the anticipated frequency of changes in client conditions, the type of practice setting, and the pattern of nursing delivery. Client conditions determine nursing responses. If client conditions change frequently, requiring considerable collaboration with multidisciplinary staff, the change-of-shift report includes a summary of these changes. These changes are documented first in various parts of the clinical record (Swenson-Feldman and Brugge-Wiger, 1985, pp. 44–46). Rather than use the Kardex as the primary reference for a change-of-shift report, the nurse might refer directly to the client's clinical chart.

This approach, especially with automated information systems, enables the nurse to provide detailed information without duplicating it on other work sheets often used to organize information before giving the report.

Similarly, the nurse might use medication or treatment flow sheets in the clinical record as the primary reference when reporting about a client's signs, symptoms, and discomforts. Using these records in this way permits the exchange of detailed information about the timing and effectiveness of treatments provided and about patterns of the client's discomforts and responses. This information helps the nursing staff evaluate whether treatment plans should be continued or reviewed by the attending medical staff.

Each form and style of the change-of-shift report offers advantages. The form and style of the reports vary with agency policies and nursing work group preferences. The pattern of nursing service delivery and the nature of the clients' health needs also affect how nurses exchange meaningful information.

## Modifying the Change-of-Shift Report According to the Pattern of Nursing Service Delivery

The organizational method used to divide the work of caring for a group of clients affects to whom the nurse reports and how the change-of-shift report is given.

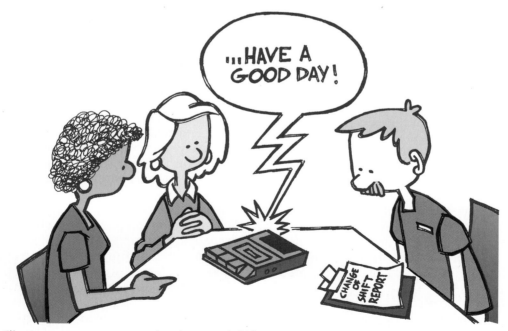

Client care managers vary the change-of-shift report's form and style to communicate efficiently and effectively between shifts.

### Functional Method

When the functional method is used, the RN from the previous shift usually reports to the RN responsible for the direct care of a group of clients within the nursing unit. If subordinate staff attend the report, the reporting nurse typically addresses a broader range of concerns so that the oncoming nurse uses less time to explain the special care needed by individual clients. Consequently the report may take longer at first, but less time is needed later in the shift to ensure that subordinate staff has current information about the details of the care they are expected to provide. Sometimes RNs report only to RNs to save time and to provide continued availability of subordinate nursing staff to clients as the report is being given. When this is done, the client care manager responsible for groups of clients is expected to "give report" to the subordinate staff to ensure appropriate follow-up for changing client needs.

### Team Nursing Method

The pattern of change-of-shift reporting might be similar to that just described when the team nursing method is used. If the clients' conditions are stable and corresponding nursing services are established, considerably less communication is needed. If client conditions are changing significantly from shift to shift, however, the work group leader or client care manager typically benefits from having all members of the oncoming shift attend the RN report from the previous shift. This approach reduces the amount of time and communication required to make timely changes in the nursing care provided. In these situations, the work group leader monitors individual client conditions more closely and seeks feedback from subordinate staff more frequently. This change in clinical nursing management routine enables the nurse to evaluate client progress, determine if changes are needed, and provide supervision in a timely manner.

### Primary Nursing Method

As discussed in Chapters Two and Three, trends in health-care financing have resulted in increased client acuity levels in acute and long-term care settings. Consequently, many health-care organizations have attempted to use primary nursing to respond to the changing needs of clients. When the primary nursing method is used, RNs assigned the direct care of individual clients on the previous shift typically give change-of-shift reports to RNs assigned the care of the same clients on the next shift. Often client assignments do not correspond to geographic locations or Kardexes. Primary nurses report directly to RNs assigned direct client care on the next shift. That is, a primary nurse might give a change-of-shift report to several different nurses, one at a time, according to their specific assigned clients. Primary nurses might give several change-of-shift reports concurrently. This method of exchanging information by change-of-shift reports typically takes less time than that required by one nurse to report to all primary nurses on the oncoming shift until all clients have been discussed.

### Case Management Method

As case management patterns of service delivery evolve, case managers are likely to conduct scheduled, structured discussions with the nursing and the multidisciplinary work groups. These discussions are likely to be held in addition to change-of-shift reports in inpatient settings. The change-of-shift report formats are likely to be similar to those used in team or primary nursing patterns of service delivery.

## Using Different Forms of Change-of-Shift Reports

### *Tape-Recorded Reports*

Sometimes the individual nurse tape records the change-of-shift report before the next shift is scheduled to receive the report. **Taped reports** are less time-consuming than face-to-face reports because there are no interruptions. Any break in concentration can result in omitting significant information. Interruptions also can distract the listener because the oncoming shift cannot anticipate as readily when specific individual client summaries will be presented. Because there are no distractions (e.g., answering questions) in a taped report, the nurse can be more systematic and thorough.

Taped reports may increase the reporting nurse's sense of control over the process of giving the change-of-shift report. This increased sense of control helps some nurses to organize the report more effectively. In addition, the nurse who has taped the change-of-shift report can complete other nursing activities while the next shift listens to the report. After the change-of-shift report has been heard, the reporting nurse often returns to clarify, answer questions, and update information that has changed since the report was recorded.

### *Face-to-Face Reports*

Other nurses prefer to give face-to-face reports. This method permits the reporting nurse to answer specific questions asked by oncoming staff. To increase its effectiveness and to reduce the amount of time needed to give and listen to the change-of-shift report while still providing sufficient detail, the content of the report can be varied according to the information needs of oncoming staff and whether they have had prior experience with individual clients. **Face-to-face reports** provide flexibility in reporting to many different nurses of the next shift. Nurses receiving the face-to-face report are asked only to listen to reports on their assigned clients, not on all the clients cared for by the reporting nurse. The face-to-face style of reporting allows greater flexibility in sequencing and pacing the exchange of information to match varied staff needs and client care assignments between shifts.

### *Electronic Reports*

As nurses increase use of electronic databases in the provision of care, they also will develop the electronic forms used to give a change-of-shift report. These forms will reflect the increased emphases on outcomes of care and specified lengths of stay. In addition, the **electronic reports** will incorporate nursing language, such as the terminology used in nursing diagnoses, interventions, and outcomes and the practice context (i.e., within the specific practice environment) (Howard-Ruben, 2002, p. 9). These developments are consistent with the evolution of nursing practice rooted in a common language and a cultural response to cost-effective care (Anderson and Helms, 2000, p. 25). Electronic reports may decrease the length of change-of-shift reports (compared with earlier formats) due to the decrease in duplication of information and the ready accessibility of detailed information when it is needed. Development and training costs will be incurred when transitioning to use of this type of change-of-shift report.

## Focusing the Change-of-Shift Report

The client care manager giving a change-of-shift report soon learns that listeners must remain interested. Listeners want to be informed about their assigned clients' conditions and what, if any, special care they need to provide. Consistent with their desire to complete their assignments in a timely manner, the listeners need to understand the nursing goals for each client and how their efforts will help clients meet these goals. All information exchanged during the change-of-shift report is provided to help the oncoming nursing staff. To consume valuable staff time addressing other concerns or discussing situations with which they are already familiar is neither a helpful nor a productive use of time.

Oncoming staff members appreciate a clear, concise change-of-shift report (Barbera, 1994, p. 41). They are not interested in listening to reports that repeat information they already have, such as descriptions of routines. Rumors or gossip about client circumstances can bias staff perceptions. Opinions and value judgments detract from quality client care. Descriptions of staff activities that do not contribute to increased understanding of client conditions (e.g., reporting normal findings that do not relate to the client's specific health condition, needs, or treatment) are irrelevant. Excluding these types of communications enhances the quality of the change-of-shift report and the effectiveness of the reporter.

## GIVING A CHANGE-OF-SHIFT REPORT

## Preparing to Give a Change-of-Shift Report

As **preparation** for giving a change-of-shift report for the first time, the client care manager reviews agency policies and whether the nursing unit has any guidelines for their form or style. The client care manager could confer with the first-line nursing manager (immediate supervisor) of the unit, who is often an excellent resource for insight about staff expectations about the style and substance of change-of-shift reports.

To maximize the efficiency of the information exchange, the nurse should plan to organize data gathered during the process of caring for assigned clients. Often, these data are collected for individual clients and in chronologic sequence. Some information received in the prior change-of-shift report is recorded on work sheets for use while providing care and for the exchange of information at the end of the shift. This information allows the nurse to compare data from a previous shift to evaluate client progress or lack of progress, which may indicate need for further medical evaluation. Data collected by the nurse in the process of completing an assignment often initially are recorded on a work sheet, then entered into the clinical record as care is provided throughout the day.

Typically the client care manager uses the Kardex or care maps and assignment work sheets as the primary references to give the change-of-shift report. Depending on the nature of the flow sheet and progress notes and the process of documentation within the nursing unit, the client care manager might refer to portions of the client's clinical record while giving the report. To the extent possible, copying data for the change-of-shift report is minimized to avoid errors and to reduce time required. The RN plans to give a report for each assigned client to the RN assuming responsibility for each client on the next shift. If working in collaboration with a licensed practical nurse as an associate nurse, the departing responsible RN participates in the shift report to ensure that all relevant facts needed to provide continuity of care are communicated.

## Presenting Individual Client Information

The client care manager should try to organize thoughts and information in a manner that helps the listeners anticipate the information that will be presented in the change-of-shift report. To the extent possible, the client care manager begins the change-of-shift report promptly as scheduled. The substance of the change-of-shift report generally consists of summaries of individual client progress. Each summary includes three **components**: client identification, medical plans, and nursing plans.

### Client Identification

**Client identification** is the first component of the individual summary. Often general information about the nursing unit census (e.g., number of clients admitted, transferred, or discharged) is given to help focus oncoming staff's attention. When beginning the report, each client should be identified by name and room and bed numbers. The next shift is informed if the client is not presently on the unit (e.g., if the client is in the recovery room or radiology department).

### Medical Plan

The **medical plan** is the second component of the individual client summary. To provide a broad perspective about the client's current health status, the admitting diagnoses and other major diagnostic or surgical procedures are noted, as are the dates the procedures were performed. Some agencies require that the client's attending physicians be mentioned, particularly if standing orders (routine medical directives) are in effect.

To identify collaborative concerns, pertinent information about the medical plan typically is discussed next. Physician's orders that have been discontinued or carried out in preparation for special procedures during the next shift are included. New orders to be implemented during the next shift also are included, especially if they are new, revised, or recently discontinued.

To help the next shift to plan for administering intravenous infusions, types of solutions and the medications added may be described. The rate of the infusion and the time that the current bag is scheduled to be completed also are indicated. If an infusion pump is being used, less information may be given, provided that the infusion does not contain specialty drugs (e.g., patient-controlled analgesia, insulin). To confirm the infusion schedule and to help the staff plan for timely addition of the next bag, the amount of solution currently remaining frequently is given within the context of the variations mentioned earlier.

The client's response to treatment is discussed, including any untoward effects that merit special nursing attention. The client's emotional response to her or his condition and medical plan are described. If the client's symptoms are being medically managed by PRN (as needed) medications, the drugs that were administered are named, and their effectiveness is described.

The client's progress in completing special procedures and diagnostic studies is described. The nurse explains which specimens have been obtained and which need to be collected during the next shift. In addition, if a client did not take medicines as prescribed, receive a treatment, or keep an appointment, the reasons are given.

### Nursing Plan

The third component of the individual client summary is the **nursing plan**. Several aspects of the nursing care plan pertinent to its continuity are included. As mentioned earlier, desired outcomes need to be emphasized (Hansten and Washburn, 1999, p. 25). Personalized nursing approaches used to enable the client to meet these goals are described, including use of special equipment, supplies, or special pacing of activities. If the client does not tolerate the prescribed diet or cannot ingest prescribed fluids orally, this information also is provided. If the client needs to change scheduled nonnursing therapies, these needs are communicated to the oncoming staff, who will inform the involved discipline or therapist.

The client's behavioral responses to his or her health status and treatment are summarized. If the client's behavior reflects denial, anger, frustration, or depression, it is described briefly without using negative labels. The focus should be on enabling the staff to help the client achieve his or her goals.

Nursing observations of vital signs, activity levels, and intake and output that pertain to the client's disease, postoperative course, and current status are described. New problems or concerns are identified. If new client outcomes or variances (changes or deviations from the established plan) have been added to the plan, they are described briefly, as are the approaches planned to meet them.

The client care manager also incorporates information about multidisciplinary plans and efforts. The client's response to special resources, referrals, and teaching programs attempted or in progress is described. Progress in implementing discharge plans is especially noteworthy (Anderson and Helms, 2000, p. 23; Lowenstein and Hoff, 1994, pp. 48–50) to allow sufficient time to complete interagency communication processes.

### Omissions

The previous discussion of the content of typical change-of-shift reports might seem to suggest that they exclude nothing. As alluded to earlier in this chapter, several common types of information about clients can be omitted. These **omissions** include descriptions of nursing routines, such as "A.M. or P.M. care." Personal opinions or value judgments about client conditions, behaviors, or lifestyles can distract staff from client goals and are omitted to avoid wasting valuable staff time.

Discussion of client idiosyncrasies not relevant to nursing care can be ignored in the client's best interest. Frequently, items already listed on the Kardex or care plan are omitted, especially if they remain unchanged.

## Questions and Communication Skills

When giving face-to-face reports, allow a brief period after completing a client summary for staff to ask questions. If the change-of-shift report is taped, whenever possible make yourself available to answer questions of staff on the next shift to promote continuity of care. If a regular pattern of presenting information is followed, staff can anticipate and focus attention. Similarly, if you use an outline while giving or taping the report, you are more likely to include all necessary information (Cox, 1994, p. 64). It is important to organize the information before giving the report.

Overall, the communication skills used to exchange information to provide for continuity of care improve with practice. By using the Kardex, care maps, notes on assignment work sheets, and integrated health information systems compiled in the clinical records, entry-level staff nurses learn to give clear, concise, accurate summaries of client progress. By presenting information in a logical, uniform manner, the client care manager helps the next shift to comprehend the change-of-shift report.

## RECEIVING A CHANGE-OF-SHIFT REPORT

## Preparing to Receive a Change-of-Shift Report

To promote efficiency, client care managers on the oncoming shift prepare to receive a change-of-shift report. At the beginning of a shift, the client care manager usually senses the "mood" of the nursing unit and gathers information about the number of clients and the number and type of staff available to provide care. The client care manager reviews data specific to the nursing unit, such as the number of clients on the critical list or classified as having high acuity; the number of clients to be admitted, transferred, or discharged during the shift; and which clients have unique needs (e.g., clients in the immediate postoperative period, clients receiving blood transfusions, and clients connected to special monitoring devices). These data are used to evaluate the adequacy of available staff and to assign responsibility for each client's care to individual staff members. Subsequently, when groups of clients are assigned to individual RNs, the client care manager receiving the change-of-shift report can begin to compile work sheets and the "things to do" lists mentioned in Chapter Four.

### Work Sheets

Before receiving a change-of-shift report, the client care manager begins to organize her or his thoughts and assignments. Depending on the type of service delivery pattern, the client care manager completes an assignment sheet that includes the names of various staff members under her or his supervision. Figure 8-1 illustrates a client care assignment work sheet that might be used in a functional or team nursing setting. If in a primary nursing or case management system, the client care manager begins to transcribe her or his assignment onto client care work sheets. Figure 8-2 illustrates a client care work sheet that might be used by staff using the primary nursing method.

### "Things to Do" List

The client care manager also begins a "things to do" list that identifies tasks to be completed during the shift, in addition to assigned nursing care. This list might

**CLIENT CARE ASSIGNMENT SHEET**

Date_____    Shift_____    Nurse leader_____

Unit A: RN_____/Assignment:                    Breaks:              Mealtime:

      LPN_____/Assignment:                    Breaks:              Mealtime:

NA:_____/Assignment:     NA:_____/Assignment:
Breaks:              Mealtime:            Breaks:              Mealtime:

NA:_____/Assignment:     NA:_____/Assignment:
Breaks:              Mealtime:            Breaks:              Mealtime:


Unit B: RN_____/Assignment:                    Breaks:              Mealtime:

      LPN_____/Assignment:                    Breaks:              Mealtime:

NA:_____/Assignment:     NA:_____/Assignment:
Breaks:              Mealtime:            Breaks:              Mealtime:

NA:_____/Assignment:     NA:_____/Assignment:
Breaks:              Mealtime:            Breaks:              Mealtime:


Unit C: RN_____/Assignment:                    Breaks:              Mealtime:

      LPN_____/Assignment:                    Breaks:              Mealtime:

NA:_____/Assignment:     NA:_____/Assignment:
Breaks:              Mealtime:            Breaks:              Mealtime:

NA:_____/Assignment:     NA:_____/Assignment:
Breaks:              Mealtime:            Breaks:              Mealtime:

FIGURE 8-1 Sample client care assignment form (functional or team method).

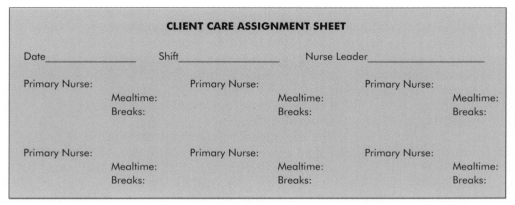

FIGURE 8-2 Sample client care assignment form (primary nursing method).

include requests for special equipment or supplies; special correspondence, such as transfer forms; or responses to requests for information from other departments, such as requests from the medical records department for additional information. The "things to do" list also could include similar tasks that might be delegated to subordinate staff.

### Record Identifying Client Information

To the extent possible, time before the beginning of the change-of-shift report can be used to write identifying client information on assignment work sheets. Some integrated health information systems provide an option of printing work assignment sheets for staff assisting clients with personal hygiene, treatments, or vital signs. These forms typically include the client's name, room number, clinical record number, attending physician's name, primary diagnosis, procedures done and planned, and drugs to be given for the next shift with special highlighting for special preparations. This information needs to be accurate and can be a big help to reduce the amount of writing that needs to be done. The nurse has more time to make written notes while listening to the report, without needlessly delaying the report's progress. This method also promotes efficiency by reducing the amount of time used to give and receive the report.

## Receiving the Report

Before beginning the report, the departing client care manager confirms that all oncoming staff expected to receive the report are present. If necessary, the sequencing of the presentation of the individual client information is noted to enable staff to anticipate information about their assigned clients. This approach helps reduce the need for interruptions and repetition.

Before beginning with individual client reports, the report typically starts with an overview of the entire unit. The overview usually includes the number of critically ill clients and clients with identified "fall risk," do-not-resuscitate (DNR), or other special classifications that are pertinent to all staff. As the report is given, the appropriateness of the client care assignments can be checked. That is, the oncoming client care manager can note whether all clients and specific activities are assigned appropriately to staff members. Principles for assigning client care appropriately are described in detail in Chapter Thirteen. The name and location of each client also can be noted to avoid errors related to client transfers within the unit or to other units within or outside the agency.

While listening to the report, the oncoming client care manager makes notes of key information about individual client conditions, progress, and responses to treatment that relate to the care needed during the next shift. To the extent possible, interruptions or distractions should be minimized. Questions need to be asked if the information received in the change-of-shift report is unclear. Questions designed to obtain information about an individual client should be addressed before proceeding to the next client summary when the reporter is present.

## SUMMARY

Client care managers receive and give change-of-shift reports as a method of exchanging information to provide for continuity of care. The form and style of these reports depend on agency policies, patterns of nursing service delivery, nursing unit guidelines, the preferences of members of the work groups, and the nature of the clients' needs. Frequently, common nursing communication tools, such as care maps, Kardexes, flow sheets, progress notes, and related portions of clinical records, are used to help organize the information exchanged during reports.

Tape-recorded and face-to-face change-of-shift reports can be given. Face-to-face discussions of information compiled in electronic databases also might be used as a form of change-of-shift report. Each style has its advantages. The specific style used depends on the needs of the individuals giving the report and those receiving it. Client care managers are expected to prepare for giving and receiving the report to promote an efficient and effective exchange of information. They complete assignment work sheets and "things to do" lists to help them organize their activities and ensure that the details of client care are attended to in efforts to promote continuity of care.

The substance of change-of-shift reports includes identification of clients and their locations, medical plans, and nursing plans. All pertinent information needed to provide for continuity of care between shifts is incorporated into these reports. Discussion of personal opinions about client lifestyles or value judgments can bias staff perceptions and detract from care. They are omitted to promote standards of care in the client's best interest and to avoid wasting valuable staff time.

With practice, entry-level staff nurses can learn to give clear, concise, accurate, and pertinent change-of-shift reports. By exchanging information between shifts in a logical, systematic manner, client care managers promote continuity of quality care.

## APPLICATION EXERCISES

1. Describe methods used to communicate client progress among nursing staff on your assigned clinical unit. Identify communication methods that supplement the change-of-shift report. Identify any communication methods that duplicate components of the change-of-shift report. How can the duplication be minimized?

2. Make a grid consisting of a list of the components of a change-of-shift report and a list of a group of clients. After listening to a change-of-shift report on each client, indicate which components were included. Note whether the information contained in omitted components was readily available elsewhere to the staff nurses.

3. Individual staff nurses use different sequences when giving change-of-shift reports. Identify individual differences that promote effectiveness or efficiency in providing continuity of care.

4. You are assigned to a busy unit using a modified primary nursing pattern of service delivery. A typical staff nurse assignment involves five to eight clients; the receiving staff nurse expects to spend no more than 20 minutes "in report." Describe what you would do to prepare and organize information before giving a change-of-shift report on your three assigned clients.

5. While receiving a change-of-shift report, before its completion the topic drifts to the personal lives of colleagues attending report. What would you do? Give reasons for your actions.

## CRITICAL THINKING SCENARIO

Imagine yourself as an entry-level staff nurse employed in a long-term care inpatient setting. Health-care reform is affecting the types of clients residing at your facility; in the past, the residents remained indefinitely; now most residents convalesce and return to less costly settings. The need for continuity of care and implementation of discharge plans has increased. Change-of-shift reports are consuming more staff time, but they often do not include information needed by the nursing and multidisciplinary work groups.

1. What would you do first?

2. Who are the stakeholders? What information do they need to provide continuity of care and carry out rehabilitation programs?

3. What change strategies would you use to reinforce desired changes?

4. Which clinical data resources would you use?

## REFERENCES

Anderson MA, Helms LB: Talking about patients: communication and continuity of care, *J Cardiovasc Nurs 14*(3):15–28, 2000.

Barbera ML: Giving report: how to sidestep common pitfalls, *Nursing 24*(9):41, 1994.

Cochran M: The real meaning of patient-nurse confidentiality, *Crit Care Nurs Q 22*(1):42–51, 1999.

Cox SS: Taping report: tips to record by, *Nursing 24*:64, 1994.

Hansten R, Washburn M: Seven steps to shift from tasks to outcomes, *Nurs Manage 30*(7):24–27, 1999.

Howard-Ruben J: Area nurses look for change in change-of-shift reporting, *Nurs Spectrum 15*(16IL):8–9, 2002.

Krogstad U, Hofoss D, Hjortdahl P: Continuity of hospital care: beyond the question of personal contact, *BMJ 321*(5):36–38, 2002.

Lowenstein AJ, Hoff PS: Discharge planning: a study of nursing staff involvement, *J Nurs Admin 24*(4):45–50, 1994.

Monahan ML, Bacha H, Phelps C, et al: Change of shift report: a time for communication with patients, *Nurs Manage 19*(2):80, 1988.

Parkman CA, Evans KJ, Cox R: Charting tips: mapping out care with TMAP, *Nursing 30*(8):74, 2000.

Reiley PJ, Stengrevics SS: Change-of-shift report: put it in writing! *Nurs Manage 20*(9):54–56, 1989.

Rewick D, Gaffey E: Nursing system makes a difference, *Health Manage Technol* August 2001, p. 24–26.

Richard JA: Walking rounds: a step in the right direction, *Nursing* 89:63–64, 1989.

Stubblefield C, Murray RL: Parents call for concerned and collaborative care, *West J Nurs Res 21*(3):356–371, 1999.

Swenson-Feldman E, Brugge-Wiger P: Promotion of interdisciplinary practice through an automated information system, *Adv Nurs Sci 7*(4):39–46, 1985.

Wolf RZ: *Nurses' work, the sacred and the profane*, Philadelphia, PA, 1988, University of Pennsylvania Press.

# *Transcribing Physician's "Orders"*

*When you complete this chapter, you should be able to:*

1. List the essential components of a physician's "order."
2. Describe each type of physician's "order."
3. Describe differences between verbal and written physician's "orders."
4. Describe the legal requirements for a verbal "order."
5. Compare a verbal "order" received in a face-to-face communication with one received by telephone.
6. Describe the legal ramifications of agency policy regarding nonphysician "orders."
7. Describe the principles of transcribing physician's "orders."
8. Describe the steps involved in transcribing physician's "orders" in the proper sequence.
9. Describe common errors made in transcribing physician's "orders."
10. Discuss advantages and disadvantages of computerized physician "order" entry.
11. Describe methods used to avoid errors in transcribing physician's "orders."
12. Describe the indicated communications with families when a client's condition changes.

transcription process
physician's "orders"/prescriptions
  essential components
  types
   standing
   PRN
   one-time-only or limited
   STAT
  style
   written
   verbal

face-to-face
  telephone
  electronic
physician's assistant and other
  nonphysician "orders"
principles of transcribing physician's
  "orders"
steps in the transcription process
common errors
communicate changes in a client's
  condition

## UNDERSTANDING THE CLIENT CARE MANAGER'S FUNCTION IN THE TRANSCRIPTION PROCESS

As client care manager, the entry-level staff nurse coordinates multidisciplinary work group efforts to address the diverse health-care needs of individual clients. As part of this function, client care managers transcribe physician's prescriptions for diagnoses and treatment, commonly known as *"orders."*

Depending on the agency's purpose and staffing, some of the activities required to translate written prescriptions into the agency's services might be delegated to a unit clerk. Generally, a nurse oversees and is accountable for the **transcription process**, however, as indicated by her or his signature when transcription of the "orders" is completed.

Although nursing practice acts vary from state to state, they often implicitly describe dependent nursing functions. Dependent nursing functions are nursing responsibilities and activities related to medical diagnosis and treatment of diseases, including related multidisciplinary functions. They are dependent nursing functions because the diagnosis and treatment of diseases remain within the province of medical practice and physicians, on whom the entry-level staff nurse depends for direction. For example, the nurse depends on a physician's "order" to guide body fluid replacement to specify the amount and type of fluids. Independent nursing functions are responsibilities and activities for which nursing is solely accountable. For example, the nurse is accountable for assessing the client's risk for pressure sores and prescribing preventive interventions. Nursing focuses on the human responses of individual clients to their health conditions (American Nurses Association, 1980, p. 9).

This competency relates primarily to dependent nursing functions, but the nurse might have to perform interdependent functions to maintain client safety. Interdependent functions require multidisciplinary interventions to satisfy client needs. The members of the multidisciplinary work group depend on each other's contributions in a collaborative manner.

It is essential that medical prescriptions for diagnosis and treatment be communicated consistently, accurately, and clearly so as to avoid errors in implementation. With the increasing public awareness of client risks related to medication errors, the importance of paying detailed collaborative attention to physician prescriptions and follow-through to promote safety cannot be overemphasized (Cohen and Winsley, 2002, p. 18; Curtin and Simpson, 1999, p. 5; Forster, 2002, p. 24; Jesitus, 2001, p. 31; Lott, 1997, p. iv; Napoli, 1999, p. 4). Task forces are making recommendations, external accreditation agencies are stipulating additional criteria, and new laws are being passed to address the public's concern about safe health care (Gebhart, 2000, pp. 58–59; Skuteris, 2000, pp. 16–17; Ukens, 2002, p. 34). No one discipline will be exempt from required changes in the health-care system, and information technology will not solve this persistent problem completely. The client care manager continues to accept the dependent and interdependent functions related to safe care.

Much of a client care manager's time and effort is devoted to meeting responsibilities associated with dependent and interdependent functions. Advanced practice nurses and other disciplines also legally prescribe treatment activities. Advanced practice nurses formulate nursing prescriptions, and dietitians formulate dietary prescriptions. Respiratory therapists frequently prescribe various breathing techniques to improve or maintain adequate ventilation. Physical therapists often prescribe exercise routines to be implemented by nursing staff to aid the client's mobility. Clinical psychologists prescribe behavioral therapies designed to enhance the client's coping skills.

**Physician's "orders,"** although broader in scope, are prescribed actions needed to diagnose and treat the client's symptoms or diseases. To be consistent with the client's legal rights, physician's "orders" more appropriately might be labeled medical **prescriptions,** directives, or remedies (Manthey, 1989, pp. 26–27). For the purposes of efficiency, prescriptions written by physicians and authorized nonphysician health-care providers are referred to as "*orders.*" The method to be used to determine who is authorized to give "orders" is discussed later in this chapter.

## ESSENTIAL COMPONENTS OF "ORDERS"

"Everyone is answerable for one's actions." Many types of "orders" are given to direct multidisciplinary staff efforts needed to implement medical remedies. Consequently a physician's "order" must indicate clearly what is to be done, to whom it is to be done, when, and how. Physician's "orders" vary, depending on how they are given (i.e., in writing, verbally, by telephone, or electronically), why they are necessary (i.e., to meet an agency requirement, to meet the client's dietary or activity needs, to complete diagnostic procedures, or to administer drugs), and when they are to be implemented (i.e., STAT [immediately], one time only or time limited, PRN [as needed], or continued until further notice). For example, if the physician's "order" is given to direct drug therapy, it must name the client and drug and specify the dosage, route of administration, and frequency it is to be given.

The **essential components** of a physician's "order" depend on the nature of the medical directive. To be complete, the physician's "order" must be dated (including time of day, if timing is crucial), indicate what the medical plan is, and direct when and how it is to be carried out. Who carries out the directive depends on the agency's purpose, services, and organization of functions or division of work. To communicate effectively and efficiently, the physician's "order" frequently is written, using abbreviations approved by the agency. Some agencies no longer accept prescriptions using "error-prone" (at high risk for misinterpretation) abbreviations (Dunn and Wolfe, 2002, p. 25; Lee, 2002, p. 42). The "order" must comply with agency policies and procedures. If specific agency policies or procedures are to be modified when the staff implements the "order," the deviation must be indicated explicitly. In this way, the "order" legally authorizes staff to address special client needs. For example, if the client is not to receive routine bowel preparations before a specific diagnostic procedure, this change is indicated by a physician's "order." Figure 9-1 illustrates a set of complete physician's "orders."

| HEALTH CARE FACILITY<br>Main Street<br>USA | | |
|---|---|---|
| | *Mrs. Alice Jones, age 87* | |
| | Addressograph Plate to Print Below This Line | |
| **PHYSICIAN'S**<br>PROGRESS AND PRESCRIPTION RECORD | | |

| Date | | Date | |
|---|---|---|---|
| 2/1/03 | Admit to general medical services | 2/1 | 87 year old ♀ c̄ HX of N+V |
| | STAT Med Profile 1 | | falls and dizziness for 3 days. |
| | V.S. q 4H | | Lives alone at home. |
| | Clear liquids as tolerated | | |
| | Bedrest with BRP | | |
| | EKG | | |
| | Chest x-ray | | |
| | IV fluids: 0.45 NaCl at 100 cc/hr; | | |
| | add 20 mEq KCl to every other liter | | |
| | Weigh in AM | | |
| | I + O. | | |
| | G. Brown M.D. | | |
| | | | |
| | **PHYSICIAN'S ORDER SHEET** | | **PROGRESS SHEET** |

FIGURE 9-1 Set of physician's "orders."

## TYPES OF PHYSICIAN'S "ORDERS"

To respond to physician's "orders" in a timely manner, client care managers distinguish four basic **types**.

### Standing "Order"

A **standing** "order" represents the physician's routine response to a client's symptoms delineating one course of action to be taken and remains in effect until it is discontinued or changed by another "order," generally one written by the same physician (Barnett, 1994, p. 74). Frequently, physicians express preferences in managing common health needs of clients. A surgeon may prefer that his or her clients be intermittently catheterized if they are unable to void 12 hours after surgery. This preference must be in writing, must comply with agency requirements, and must be entered on the client's record to be implemented when needed. Unless all of these conditions are met, the nurse is not authorized legally to implement the surgeon's preference.

Some health-care agencies have preprinted standing "orders," which are useful for nurses working during the night shift. These "orders" can be used without calling the physician for routine bowel elimination or nausea. When used, the "orders" need to be documented clearly.

### PRN "Order"

A **PRN** "order" is an "order" to be carried out when the client needs it. A PRN "order" often refers to drugs or treatments designed to promote client comfort. Similar to a standing "order," it remains in effect until it is discontinued or changed by another explicit "order."

### One-Time-Only or Limited "Order"

A **one-time-only or limited** time "order" is carried out only once or for a specified number of days, or doses, after which the "order" is discontinued automatically. Often controlled substances and antibiotics are discontinued because the agency has a policy limiting the number of doses or the time the "order" for the drug can be in effect without further medical evaluation. Depending on the client's progress, the nurse might confer with the physician to determine whether a particular limited medical directive should be continued. If so, another physician's "order" is written to indicate this change.

### STAT "Order"

A **STAT** "order" is to be carried out immediately. A STAT "order" often is written in an emergency and requires urgent nursing attention. STAT "orders" are transcribed first when they are listed within a set of physician's "orders." They are communicated to involved multidisciplinary work group members as soon as possible so that urgent client needs are addressed in a timely manner. Figure 9-2 illustrates a set of

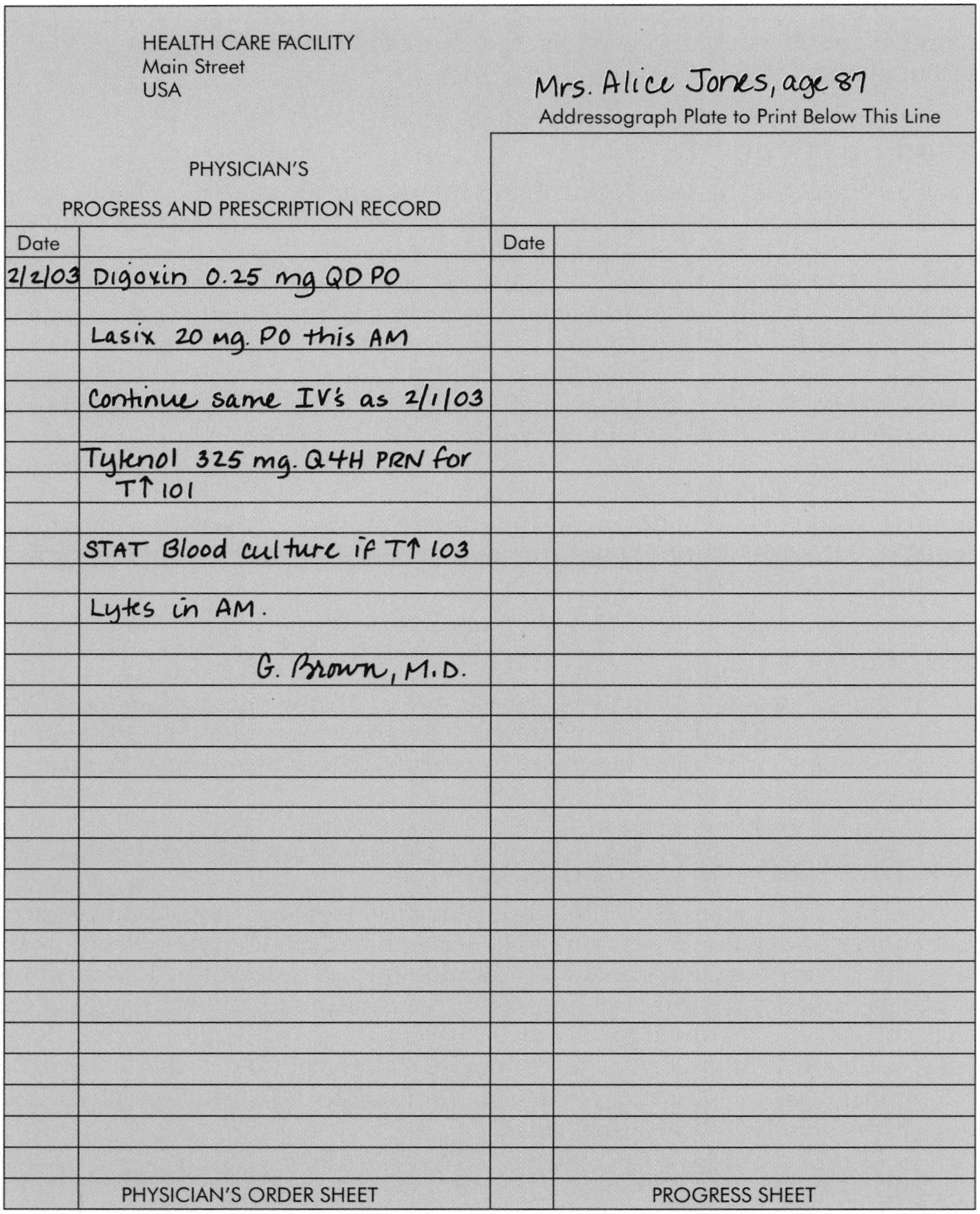

| HEALTH CARE FACILITY | | |
|---|---|---|
| Main Street | | |
| USA | | *Mrs. Alice Jones, age 87* |
| | | Addressograph Plate to Print Below This Line |
| PHYSICIAN'S | | |
| PROGRESS AND PRESCRIPTION RECORD | | |

| Date | | Date | |
|---|---|---|---|
| 2/2/03 | Digoxin 0.25 mg QD PO | | |
| | Lasix 20 mg. PO this AM | | |
| | Continue same IV's as 2/1/03 | | |
| | Tylenol 325 mg. Q4H PRN for T↑ 101 | | |
| | STAT Blood culture if T↑ 103 | | |
| | Lytes in AM. | | |
| | G. Brown, M.D. | | |
| | PHYSICIAN'S ORDER SHEET | | PROGRESS SHEET |

FIGURE 9-2 Various types of physician's "orders."

various types of physician's "orders" that might be written to respond to a client with diverse medical needs.

## Interpreting Medical Directives

The client care manager is expected to interpret the varied symbols used to communicate the medical directives efficiently and effectively, regardless of the type of "order." Accordingly the client care manager might use abbreviations approved by the agency to ensure a consistent interpretation. If at any time the physician's "order" is unclear or inconsistent with the safety of the client, the client care manager must seek clarification from the physician who wrote the directive (Langdon, 1984, pp. 23–25; Sullivan, 1991, pp. 65–66). If the physician confirms the "order," but implementing it would jeopardize the client's safety, the nurse must discuss the medical directive with her or his immediate supervisor (Langdon, 1984, pp. 23–24). Legally the nurse is responsible for the consequences of her or his actions, even though directed to perform them by a physician (Creighton, 1981, p. 111; Nurse's Reference Library, 1984, pp. 541–547). The nurse documents the client's condition and actions taken to resolve the question about the appropriateness of the "order." The nurse needs to communicate effectively and to apply steps of conflict resolution to ensure that the client's needs are met.

### STYLES OF PHYSICIAN'S "ORDERS"

The **style** or form of physician's "orders" varies. Sound nursing practice requires that all physician's "orders" be written in ink on the appropriate form of the client's clinical record; they usually are entered into the client's clinical record initially by physicians. Occasionally, client care managers enter physician's "orders," received only from those authorized to give them, into the clinical record to address client needs in a timely manner. The administrative staff of the agency determines who is authorized to give "orders" (Macdonald, 1994, p. 9); consequently, if the client care manager questions whether the medical student, physician's assistant, advanced practice nurse, clinical pharmacist, or dietitian is authorized to give "orders," he or she needs to seek verification from the nursing supervisor. Entry-level staff nurses also are expected to know the legal scope of their own practice within which they must work.

## Written and Verbal "Orders"

**Written** "orders" are needed to direct the medical plan. This type of "order" is dated, written on the appropriate agency form, and signed by the physician or other authorized clinician. In many agencies, the physician also may give a **verbal** "order" to a nurse authorized by the agency to receive it. Most often, these nurses are registered nurses who are responsible for evaluating the appropriateness of the "order" within the context of the client's condition and treatment plan. It is sound practice to repeat the verbal "order" to the physician to ensure its accuracy. To promote efficiency, the client care manager requests that the physician write the "orders" that are described in **face-to-face** conversations (Maher, 1989, p. 39). Receiving verbal "orders" for the convenience of physicians is generally not an effective use of the nurse's time (Doctor's verbal orders, 1986, p. 2). In situations in which the client's needs are urgent, however, sometimes the client is served better by the nurse writing the medical directive on the appropriate agency form.

The physician also might give a verbal "order" by **telephone** in accordance with agency policy. When medical directives are communicated verbally, the nurse should repeat the "order," with all its essential components, to confirm it. At the same time, the nurse must determine the appropriateness of the "order" (i.e., whether it is consistent with the client's condition and safety). The nurse seeks clarification if the medical directive is unclear or dubious. Then the nurse enters the verbal "order" on the physician's "order" sheet, beginning with the date, time of day, and medical directive, followed by the approved agency designation for telephone "orders," the physician's name, and the nurse's signature and title. Often, agency policies require that the physician countersign the "order" on her or his next visit or within 24 hours.

Many agency policies distinguish face-to-face verbal "orders" from "orders" received by telephone; others do not. Many agencies specify abbreviations to be used to differentiate face-to-face "orders" (e.g., *v.o.* for verbal "order") from those received by telephone (e.g., *t.o.* for telephone "order") when they are entered in the client's clinical record by the nurse.

Verbal "orders" received and written by authorized nurses must have all the essential components of "orders" written by physicians. They are transcribed and implemented in the same way as "orders" written by physicians. They need to be countersigned by the involved physician according to agency policy, as indicated earlier.

## Electronic "Orders"

With the increased development of automated integrated health information systems, physicians and other authorized clinicians enter their prescriptions or therapeutic directives directly into the system via computer. Many have reported that **electronic** "orders," or computerized physician "order" entries (CPOE), will help decrease the number of drug errors (Audet and Hartman, 2002, p. 3258; Bard, 2002, p. 46; Bates, 2000, p. 789; Doolan and Bates, 2002, p. 180; Freudenheim, 2000, p. c.1; Gryskevich, 2002, p. 38; McConnell, 2000, p. 50; Rochman, 2000, p. 24; Simpson, 2000, pp. 20–23), although not everyone agrees that the computerized physician "order" entry system is a panacea (Chordas, 2002, p. 99; Cohen, 2002, p. 28; Glaser, 2002, p. 44). Not all health-care agencies are investing sufficient resources into educating users of the systems to enable them to use this method properly and to work with situations that arise due to "bugs" in the system. Some believe that the process of "order" entry as a part of the total process of care needs reengineering to reduce errors, rather than continuing to do what always was done and resulted in too many errors.

As the electronic method of entering prescriptions increases, the need for multidisciplinary work group members to evaluate the appropriateness of "orders" and seek clarification as needed before implementation also will increase to prevent errors. Although the electronic system will transmit the "orders" quickly, the accountability for implementing "orders" safely, appropriately, and in a timely manner will remain with the health-care providers acting to carry them out. To use the electronic system effectively, everyone will need to use the readily accessible information to verify the appropriateness of the prescription to the client's identity and condition and determine the best (timeliness and cost-effectiveness) strategy for implementing the "orders." Implementing electronic "orders" often requires additional multidisciplinary communication and collaboration because the automated information system transmits information only and relies on the health-care providers for clinical judgment to ensure its appropriateness. Errors can be made entering the "order" on the wrong client's record, and nurses who are implementing the "order" need to verify that the prescription matches the client's clinical need.

## "ORDERS" WRITTEN BY NONPHYSICIANS

The client care manager's duty to implement medical directives given by physician's assistants or other health-care providers with expanded roles varies with state nursing practice acts and specified agency policies. **Physician's assistant and other nonphysician "orders"** are acceptable in some health-care settings. Physician's assistants have been authorized by some agencies to give "orders" as extensions of physicians. That is, they perform dependent medical functions. Their educational preparation might vary in length from 9 months to 5 years. Their actual practice depends on the needs of the supervising physician. Generally, physician's assistants are certified rather than licensed. Their scope of practice varies with the physician to whom they are responsible. To safeguard the quality of care provided to clients, many states and agencies may not permit physician's assistants to write medical directives because their educational preparation and certification vary widely. When implementing "orders" given by any authorized nonphysician health-care provider, the client care manager needs to know what constitutes a valid physician's "order" according to the agency's policy. The policy may direct the client care manager to implement the "order" after it is countersigned by the responsible physician.

With health-care reform and the increased emphasis on cost-effectiveness, a wide range of health-care providers with expanded scopes of practice have gained attention. Each state is responsible for defining the scope of practice of each type of professional health-care provider in its role to protect the public's health and safety. The agency is responsible for establishing policies and procedures for credentialing health-care providers consistent with state licensing laws and regulations. Reciprocally, each health-care provider is accountable for his or her practice and for knowing the scope and depth of practice within which he or she must function (Macdonald, 1994, p. 9). With the rapid expansion of various credentialing and privileging processes, the entry-level nurse is not expected to know what every health-care provider is authorized to do. In the interest of safe client care, however, if any question arises as to the authority of a health-care provider to give "orders" or prescribe, the nurse needs to obtain answers from her or his nursing supervisor.

The nurse is mindful that everyone is legally accountable for her or his own actions. If the physician's "order" complies with agency requirements but is unsafe or is inappropriate to meet the client's needs, it is not carried out (Fiesta, 1994, pp. 16–17).

## PRINCIPLES UNDERLYING THE TRANSCRIPTION PROCESS

The process of transcribing physician's "orders" incorporates several communication strategies. These strategies are designed to document medical directives efficiently to specific members of the multidisciplinary work group responsible for implementing them. Several **principles of transcribing physician's "orders"** are followed to maximize communication efficiency and minimize errors.

### Clearly Understood

First, the "order" must be clearly understood (Creighton, 1989, pp. 18–19; Cushing, 1986, pp. 1107–1108; Langdon, 1984, pp. 2325). The client care manager needs to know enough about the agency, services, departments, and staffing to be able to determine which department and member of the multidisciplinary work group are expected to carry it out. The client care manager also needs to know enough about the purpose of the "order" and its follow-through as it relates to the client to judge its safety and appropriateness (Cushing, 1990, pp. 29–30, 32). For example, is the client's current condition such that the "order" is a reasonable response to symptoms, concerns, and actual or potential health problems? That is, does the "order" fit? Does the "order," when implemented, place the client at unreasonable risk? For example, some types of bowel preparations might place an already dehydrated client at increased risk. If questions arise about the rationality, fit, or safety of the "order," they need to be answered before the "order" is implemented. The nurse should trust her or his instincts, which will develop with a few years of nursing practice experience, and follow through with interventions to ensure clarity.

### Legible

Second, every component of the "order" must be legible (i.e., written clearly enough that the reader can interpret every symbol accurately). The nurse should not make any assumptions. If any component of the "order" is unclear, each component that is not legible must be clarified. The client care manager does not have the privilege of guessing or making assumptions about what symbols were intended in the "order." To do either places the client at risk. The client care manager needs to pay particularly close attention to the exact symbols and letters used to communicate drug prescriptions to avoid errors related to the incorrect drug, dosage, route, or frequency. Numerous reports in the nursing literature describe the hazards of misinterpreting drug "orders" (Cohen and Winsley, 1991, pp. 48–49; Fiesta, 1994, pp. 15–17; Langdon, 1984, pp. 23–25).

A physician's "order" is often a combination of abbreviations and symbols. As mentioned earlier, most agencies have approved abbreviation lists to help ensure

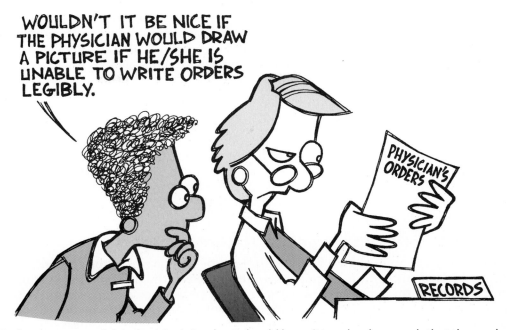

"WOULDN'T IT BE NICE IF THE PHYSICIAN WOULD DRAW A PICTURE IF HE/SHE IS UNABLE TO WRITE ORDERS LEGIBLY."

Each component of the physician's "orders" should be written clearly enough that the reader can interpret every symbol used.

that common abbreviations and symbols have the same meaning for all the people using them. This helps reduce misinterpretation of physician's "orders." In addition, the meaning of the abbreviations in the physician's "order" must be interpreted within the context of the client's medical needs. Some abbreviations can have different meanings, depending on the context in which they are used. For example, *HS* might mean "half-strength" or "at hour of sleep." The intended meaning of the abbreviation depends on the client's condition, health needs, and the other essential components of the physician's "order." If all the symbols are not interpreted as intended in the entry, the "order" will not be implemented safely. Some agencies restrict the use of abbreviations and symbols by established written policy in an effort to reduce errors; the client care manager needs to adhere to these policies when they exist. New prescription laws aimed at reducing drug errors require that numbers and commonly misinterpreted symbols be written out (e.g., 4×/day instead of QID and ml instead of cc).

## Communicated Exactly as Entered by the Physician

Third, the "order" needs to be communicated to others exactly as it was entered by the physician in the client's clinical record. This strategy promotes accurate interpretation of the physician's "order" by staff members responsible for carrying it out. When communicated in writing, the symbols are duplicated exactly, without interpretation. "Orders" are copied exactly on the care map, Kardex, or requisition forms. Each symbol and word is spelled exactly as it initially was entered. Some agencies use carbonless copy paper to avoid errors in duplication of "order" entries that need to be transmitted routinely to other departments, such as the pharmacy. Other agencies use electronic "order" entry, which eliminates errors of duplication.

## Varied According to Agency

Fourth, transcription procedures vary among agencies. The client care manager needs to use the symbols required by the agency policy to ensure consistency in interpretation. Some agency policies require the nurse to use check marks to indicate "orders" that have been transcribed; others might require that one line be drawn around the set of "orders" transcribed by the nurse.

## Varied According to Type and Nature of "Order"

Fifth, transcription procedures vary with the type and nature of the "order." If the "order" relates only to nursing, it is communicated to the involved staff members and written on the care map or Kardex or added to the medication administration form (entered here by pharmacy staff). If it involves drug or fluid therapy, it might be transmitted directly to the pharmacy, using the duplicate carbonless copy, and entered in the appropriate location on the Kardex or medicine administration flow sheet. If the "order" involves requisitioning diagnostic studies, it might require a signed consent form, scheduling, and special client teaching and preparations. Specific requisition forms may need to be completed with the client's name and identification numbers, and appropriate notations may need to be made on the care map or Kardex to inform all departments involved in the implementation of the "orders."

Similarly, computerized "orders" require different responses than noncomputerized "orders" (i.e., with computerized "orders," the emphasis is on checking accuracy versus writing the "order"). The transcription process varies, depending on the agency's interdepartmental communication methods. Generally the time the "order" was entered and when it was communicated to staff responsible for carrying it out specifically are noted, and the person involved in any special transcription procedures is identified.

## STEPS IN THE TRANSCRIPTION PROCESS

The nursing activities associated with transcribing physician prescriptions or directives for diagnosing and treating diseases are often complex, requiring effective communication with many different members of the multidisciplinary work groups and departments. Consequently, client care managers benefit from fostering effective working relationships within the groups by using communication protocols as described in Chapter Three. In addition, transcribing physician "orders" requires client care managers to comply with agency policies and the procedures involved in implementing these prescriptions. To avoid errors in communicating physician's "orders" to others, a specific sequence of **steps in the transcription process** is recommended. Box 9-1 summarizes these steps.

## Read the Complete Set of "Orders"

This review provides an overview of the medical plan and changes in the current plan. It provides information about the urgency of the "orders" and about what must be done to implement them. If clarification is needed before further implementation of the medical directive, the client care manager is required legally to obtain it (Fiesta, 1994, p. 17; Guarriello, 1984, pp. 19–21; Rhodes, 1990, p. 193; Tammelleo and Gill, 1984, pp. 13–14). This is the time for the client care manager to verify that the "orders" are entered on the appropriate client's record.

## Collect All Necessary Forms

This approach saves time, increases efficiency, and reduces the need to interrupt your concentration on the task at hand. It also helps you avoid distractions that increase the potential for omitting or duplicating more than one requisition for a specific "order."

## Complete All Requisition Forms for Diagnostic Tests, Treatments, and Supplies

This approach may help you to recall special requirements for specific studies, such as permits; preparations; equipment; supplies; client teaching; and compliance with restrictions on diet, activities, and elimination. It maximizes the time available to obtain specimen containers, equipment, and supplies needed to prepare the client for the study and avoids delays in completing the procedures. The client's name can be added to all requisition forms, saving time and avoiding errors related to client identification.

---

**BOX 9-1**

### Transcription Process

1. Read the complete set of "orders."
2. Collect all necessary forms.
3. Complete all requisition forms for diagnostic tests, treatments, and supplies.
4. Write the physician's "order" on the Kardex exactly as it was entered in the client's clinical record.
5. Complete the communication process needed to implement medication "orders."
6. Place telephone calls as needed to complete the physician's "orders."
7. Recheck your completion of each step to ensure accuracy and thoroughness.
8. "Sign off" your completion of transcribing the set of physician's "orders."

## Write "Order" on Care Map or Kardex, if Indicated

Write the "order" exactly as it is entered in the client's clinical record. This helps to keep the care map or Kardex current, which is crucial to its usefulness as a handy reference tool for staff. The entry helps staff members recall important components of the client's medical plan and progress in the diagnostic and treatment processes. More detailed information is available in the client's record.

## Complete Communication Process Needed to Implement Medication "Orders"

To complete this step, the client care manager needs to know the agency's drug administration procedures to complete the necessary forms. This ensures that every drug prescribed is transcribed and administered in a timely manner and documented properly. The drug administration procedure of some agencies requires the nurse to record all STAT drugs on "medication administration records" located in the client's clinical record or on the care map often located near the client's room. Other agencies require nurses to record STAT drugs on a "Medix" form located within the nursing Kardex to become a part of the client's clinical record after the client's discharge. Routine drug administration procedures might differ from those by administering "once-only" drug prescriptions. The client care manager needs to comply with the agency's drug administration procedures to transcribe these "orders" accurately and to ensure the necessary follow-through.

The fifth step might involve sending requisitions or the "order" sheet to the pharmacy or contacting the department by telephone if the client needs the drug urgently. In addition, it might require the client care manager to communicate the medication "order" verbally to other nursing staff members so that the change in the medical plan can be incorporated into their work plans for the shift.

## Place Telephone Calls as Needed to Complete "Orders"

As much as possible, to promote efficiency and accuracy and to reduce unnecessary interruptions of work flow of all departments receiving information (Rocereto and Maleski, 1984, p. 19), physician's "orders" are communicated through regular computer entry or by routine forms. If the client's need cannot be met satisfactorily with routine communication methods, use of the telephone is appropriate. Routine dietary changes can be communicated by completing forms and forwarding them in a timely manner. If the client has special needs not readily communicated in this way, conferring with the dietary staff by telephone is necessary.

## Recheck Completion of Each Step

Rechecking ensures accuracy and thoroughness. Client care managers encounter many interruptions and distractions in providing care. Rechecking lessens the possibility of omitting entries or details associated with specific "orders," and it reduces human errors that place the client at increased risk.

## Sign Off Completion of "Order" Transcription

This step legally confirms your completion of the transcription process. It informs others that these medical directives have been communicated to staff members who implement them. It is important to delay signing off on a physician's "order" until the transcription process is complete. Otherwise, you may omit "orders" that were transcribed incompletely. Figure 9-3 depicts a common method of confirming completion of the transcription process.

The policies of many agencies require the nurse to indicate the date and time the "orders" were transcribed and sign her or his full name and title in a specific color of ink. This helps readers differentiate the person transcribing it. If a computer is used to communicate "orders," the nurse often is required to enter identification, date, and time. If questions about the transcription of the "orders" arise, a specific person can be contacted for clarification.

## AVOIDING COMMON ERRORS

As in so many situations in health care, avoiding **common errors** in transcribing physician's "orders" is much easier than correcting them. In general, errors in the transcription process can be avoided by completing each of the recommended steps in proper sequence and by concentrating to "block out" distractions and interruptions, especially when identifying clients on computerized entries, requisition forms, care maps, and Kardexes before medical directives are transcribed. Basically, there are four types of errors: (1) incorrect identification of the client, (2) omission of words or symbols in the entry, (3) misinterpretation of words or symbols used in the entry, and (4) incorrect selection of the client's care map or Kardex (LaFleur and Starr, 1986, pp. 250–251).

The drug prescription and implementation process are documented on a legal document, the client's clinical record. Accordingly, proper documentation of error correction is required. Using error correction fluid (Wite-Out) is not permissible.

## Errors of Identification

The client care manager might err in transcribing physician's "orders" correctly by picking up the wrong client's imprinter or addressograph plate. An addressograph is used to print client identification information on clinical record forms. As a result, other departments would implement the medical directives for the wrong clients because they often do not review the actual physician's "orders." Similarly, computerized physician "order" entry errors can occur by entering the information in the incorrect client's clinical record. To avoid this type of error, individuals who transcribe "orders" must identify clients by matching exactly the information on the client's clinical record with that on the addressograph or imprinter, rather than by using the client's room number. Identification errors are likely to decrease when physicians enter their medical directives directly into computerized integrated health information systems. These systems reduce the need for client addressograph plates or separate client identification equipment.

HEALTH CARE FACILITY
Main Street
USA

Mrs. Alice Jones, age 87
Addressograph Plate to Print Below This Line

PHYSICIAN'S

PROGRESS AND PRESCRIPTION RECORD

| Date | | Date | |
|---|---|---|---|
| 2/2/03 9:00 A | ᵀ√ Digoxin 0.25 mg. QD | | |
| | ᵀ√ Lasix 20 mg PO this AM | | |
| | ᵀ√ continue same IV's as 2/1/03 | | |
| 2/2/03 9³⁰AM | ᵀ√ Tylenol 355 mg p.o. Q4 PRN for T↑101 | | |
| | ᵀ√ STAT BLOOD Culture if T↑103 | | |
| | ᵀ√ Lytes in AM | | |
| | Smith RN          G. Brown M.D. | | |

PHYSICIAN'S ORDER SHEET          PROGRESS SHEET

FIGURE 9-3 Confirming completion of the transcription process.

# Errors of Omission

Because of the urgency of many clients' needs and the illegibility of the writer's pen-manship, a nurse might misread a physician's "order." An "order" might be missed entirely in the transcription process, or part of an "order" might be left out. As a result, the client's medical plan might be implemented incorrectly or left unchanged when important changes were indicated. Errors of these types commonly include omission of a laboratory study, drug, or parenteral fluids. The incorrect procedure or route of administration could be used, or the medical intervention could be scheduled incorrectly. All of these errors could cause serious harm (Northrup, 1987, p. 43). Errors of omission can be avoided by making a special effort to read each word and symbol in the "order" and to use consistently symbols required by agency policy to indicate completion of various aspects of the transcription process. To avoid errors of omission, it is important for client care managers to use the same symbols used by unit clerks in the transcription process.

## Errors of Interpretation

Closely related to errors of omission are errors resulting from incorrect interpretation of a physician's "order." This type of transcription error occurs when words, common abbreviations, or symbols are incorrectly understood. For example, *QD* (every day) and *QID* (four times a day) often look similar, as do *QD* (every day) and *OD* (right eye). If the context and content of the "order" are not evaluated, misinterpretations can occur readily. This is particularly true if the "order" is written or entered hastily. To avoid incorrect interpretations of physician's "orders," the "order" must make sense in terms of diagnosing or treating the client's active health concerns. To make sense of a physician's "order," the nurse must understand the nature of the client's health problem and the anticipated consequences of the medical intervention. If it is a drug "order," the nurse needs to know the drug's action; dosage range, route, and frequency; and appropriateness for the client's condition. To proceed without this knowledge for any reason places the client at extreme risk. If the "order" is not clear, the client care manager is obligated to contact the physician for additional information.

## Errors in Care Map or Kardex Selection

Another common error in transcribing physician's "orders" occurs when the nurse selects the wrong client's care map or Kardex and writes another client's physician's "orders" on it without matching it with the identification on the chart. This error can be avoided by carefully matching the client's and the attending physician's names on the care map or Kardex with the names on the clinical record before duplicating the "order" and by ensuring that care maps and Kardex forms are returned to their proper location after use. Similarly the nurse might document incorrectly a drug administered by entering it on the wrong date. Table 9-1 lists precautionary measures that can be taken to avoid common errors.

## COMMUNICATING CHANGES IN CLIENT CONDITIONS

Client care managers are expected to **communicate changes in a client's condition** to the attending physician, the multidisciplinary work group, the client,

| TABLE 9-1 | |
| --- | --- |

## Tips for Avoiding Common Errors in "Order" Transcription

| | |
| --- | --- |
| Errors of client identification | Check that the "order" entry was written on the correct client's "order" form or matches the intended client's computerized clinical record.<br>Make a specific effort to check the name of the client on the forms where the "order" is being copied. Try to form a deliberate habit of starting *first* with matching the client's identification on each form used. |
| Errors of omission | Verify that the "order" answers what, where, when, by whom, and why. Note if any special procedures are inherent in implementation of the "order," such as client teaching, permits, or preparations. Does the process require special sequencing with other diagnostic studies or therapies?<br>If the "order" relates to drug therapy, check that it clearly states the name of the drug, the dosage, route, frequency, and any special restrictions on duration if indicated. Does this "order" make sense for this client?<br>Has each "order" been transcribed? |
| Errors of interpretation | Avoid abbreviations and symbols as much as possible to promote clarity.<br>Is implementation of the "order" consistent with the client's current health status and diagnostic and treatment needs?<br>Avoid abbreviations of drug names. Spelling the drug names promotes clarity and eliminates the need to interpret. |
| Errors in care map or Kardex selection | Match the client's and physician's identification on these forms. Return them to their proper location as a method of checking your work.<br>If the "order" is transmitted electronically, check to see that it is entered where you would expect to see it before its implementation. |

and the family or significant others. With the increasing acuity level of clients in acute and long-term care facilities, the likelihood is high that clients' conditions will change significantly. Often a change of condition indicates that the client is physiologically unstable and that related nursing attention is urgently needed.

## Complete a Nursing Assessment

Information about a change in the client's condition can come from various sources, including nurses' observations, reports from other staff, and the client or the client's family. In response, the client care manager completes a nursing assessment of the client's current status. This involves collecting information about vital signs, a detailed description of the client's symptoms and discomforts, and responses to the medical plan in effect. Some examples of changes in a client's condition that require additional nursing observation are responses to medically prescribed therapies, such as analgesics, dietary modifications, changes in fluid intake, weight gain or loss, and the inability to maintain functional abilities in activities of daily living. In addition to the client's concerns and perceptions, observations of multidisciplinary staff and family members are included in the nursing assessment. If the assessment leads to the conclusion that the client's physiologic status or functional abilities have changed significantly, medical evaluation is needed.

## Notify the Physician and Multidisciplinary Workgroup

The nurse has a responsibility to notify the physician of changes in the client's status in a timely manner. Depending on the urgency of the client's medical needs, if the physician does not respond within a reasonable time, the nurse should seek other sources of assistance as described by agency policy and division of organizational responsibilities. The client care manager informs the physician of the nursing assessment. Often the physician gives "orders" to remedy the client's problems. Transcribing these "orders" results in revisions of the client's medical and nursing plans of care.

Because the nurse is responsible for coordinating multidisciplinary efforts on the client's behalf, he or she is expected to inform the nursing and multidisciplinary work group members of the changes in the medical plan. Frequently, these changes involve several other departments (e.g., dietary, pharmaceutical, laboratory, rehabilitation services, or pastoral care).

## Contact and Inform Designated Family Member or Significant Other

The client care manager is expected to contact and inform the designated family member or significant other about the change in the client's condition and in the plans of care. Generally the family asks about the nature of the change, why the "orders" were changed, what actions have been taken to provide the needed care (e.g., medical evaluation), and what revisions in the medical plan have been made. The client and the family benefit from factual information offered in a tactful, sensitive manner (Mehn and Haas, 1999, p. 30). The client or representative is entitled to this information, and involvement in the interaction usually helps them to take an active part in addressing the problems confronting them. It is important to follow agency policies in relaying information to interested family and friends of the client so as not to violate the client's rights of privacy and confidentiality. It is important to know who of the client's support group is designated to receive confidential information before providing any information.

## Document Changes, Assessment, and Responses

The changes in the client's condition, nursing assessment, and responses need to be documented in a timely manner (Allen, 1989, pp. 62–64; Feutz-Harter, 1989, pp. 8–9). In addition to transcribing the physician's "orders," nursing progress notes must include the following information:

1. Date and time entry was made
2. Nursing assessment
3. That physician was informed and how (e.g., by telephone or pager)
4. Actions taken and revisions made in the plan of care
5. Information given and to whom (e.g., client and name of family member)
6. Responses of the client and family and any special requests they may have

Detailed documentation, as opposed to vague references, such as "physician informed of change of condition," helps nursing staff to provide the needed follow-up and to communicate with multidisciplinary staff when indicated. It also provides a complete legal record of care provided and client responses in the event of a legal dispute.

## SUMMARY

One type of dependent nursing function performed by client care managers is the transcription of physician's "orders" (medical prescriptions) or nonphysician therapeutic directives. Depending on the agency's purpose and staffing, unit clerks may share some of the responsibilities associated with transcribing "orders." The nursing activities associated with this function are often complex, requiring effective and efficient communication with many different members of the multidisciplinary work groups and departments.

To be complete, the physician's "order" must indicate clearly what the medical plan is and must direct when and how it is to be carried out. Who carries out the directive depends on the agency's purpose, services, and organization. To communicate effectively and efficiently, only approved abbreviations and symbols are used to promote consistent interpretation by all agency staff. To promote clarity, use of abbreviations and symbols is minimized.

Physician's "orders" vary in type and form. The client care manager complies with agency policies to ensure that the client's medical needs are addressed in a timely manner. Before transcribing any physician's "order," the nurse needs to verify that the correct client record is used; determine that it is consistent with the client's condition and safety; and seek clarification if the medical directive is unclear, ambiguous, or dubious. The client care manager also must comply with agency policy before transcribing "orders" entered by nonphysician health-care providers appropriately credentialed and authorized by the agency to prescribe therapy (i.e., advanced practice nurses, dietitians, pharmacists, physician assistants).

Principles for transcribing "orders" are strategies used to communicate efficiently and accurately. The transcription process is sequenced to ensure that the "orders" are communicated systematically to individuals who are responsible for implementing them without error or inefficiency. The steps are organized so that interruptions and distractions would not result in omitting any components during the transcription process. When computerized physician "order" entry is used, it is paramount that the correct client identification is verified as a first step.

Client care managers are expected to communicate changes in client conditions. Subsequently, they often transcribe physician's "orders" to make the needed revisions in the medical and nursing plans of care in a timely manner. In addition, the client care manager communicates these changes and revisions to the involved multidisciplinary work group, client, and family or significant others. Detailed documentation of the client care manager's coordination of activities helps the nursing and multidisciplinary work group provide the needed follow-up care.

## APPLICATION EXERCISES

1. You are admitting to a private room a client who has a wound with copious, foul-smelling drainage that may be infectious. Indicate whether you would (a) obtain a culture or (b) wait until you receive an "order" to do so. Give reasons for your actions.

2. Your assigned client with a history of chronic obstructive pulmonary disease quickly becomes dyspneic, disoriented, and ashen. You are unable to contact the attending physician immediately by telephone to discuss the client's change in condition. Identify your next intervention. Give reasons for your decision.

3. A physician writes an "order" for chemotherapy using abbreviations that are not approved at your agency. Describe what you are expected to do before transcribing it, according to your agency's policy.

4. A client questions you why she is unable to continue taking medicines she took before admission. She is worried she will get sicker. Describe your interventions to her nursing needs. Give reasons for your actions.

5. A client's condition has worsened, necessitating medical evaluation. The physician believes that the client needs multiple diagnostic studies and transfer to another unit. Describe the nursing responsibilities associated with transcribing such physician's "orders" at your assigned agency.

## CRITICAL THINKING SCENARIO

Picture yourself assigned to care for a 52-year-old married man reporting increasing (over the last 12 hours) spasms and difficulty breathing related to a chronic degenerative neurologic condition. His mother demands he be seen immediately (without an appointment) in your primary (ambulatory) care setting. His primary care provider is a nurse practitioner working with a collaborating physician. His wife is his primary caregiver but is unavailable due to employment commitments. He is oriented and thinks his mother is overly protective and exhausted from the multiple demands of his care during his wife's absence. Your agency's policy limits your discussion of your client's health needs to the client or significant other. The client has difficulty communicating by telephone.

*Continued*

## CRITICAL THINKING SCENARIO—cont'd

1. What would you do first? Give reasons.
2. With whom would you communicate first? Give reasons.
3. How would you proceed to obtain information needed to evaluate your client's health condition?
4. If neither the nurse practitioner nor the collaborating physician is accessible, would you obtain needed orders from the physician's assistant who also works with the collaborating physician but is not familiar with your client? Give reasons.

## REFERENCES

Allen AMB: Telephone documentation, *Orthop Nurs* 8(2):62–64, 1989.

American Nurses Association: *Nursing: a social policy statement*, Kansas City, MO, 1980, American Nurses Association.

Audet AMJ, Hartman EE: A 40-year-old woman who noticed a medication error, 1 year later, *JAMA 287*(24):3258, 2002.

Bard M: E-prescribing cuts costs and reduces medical errors, *Managed Healthcare Executive*, May 2002, p. 46.

Barnett C: Legal questions: when the choice is yours, *Nursing 24*(12):74, 1994.

Bates DW: Using information technology to reduce rates of medication errors in hospitals, *BMJ 320*:788–791, 2000.

Chordas L: Make no mistake, *Best's Review* August 2002, pp. 99–102.

Cohen MR, Winsley W: Avoiding errors caused by drug suffixes, *Nursing 21*(2): 48–49, 1991.

Cohen MR, Winsley W: Are all drug errors system errors? *Drug Topics* April 15, 2002, pp. 18–19.

Cohen MR: Not worth the time, *Nursing 32*(5):28, 2002.

Creighton H: *Law every nurse should know*, ed 4, Philadelphia, 1981, WB Saunders.

Creighton H: Nurse's failure to follow physician's orders, *Nurs Manage 20*(1):18–19, 1989.

Curtin L, Simpson R: Broken promises . . . or wasted efficiencies? *Health Manage Technol 20*(5):24–25, 1999.

Cushing M: Who transcribed that order? *Am J Nurs 86*(10):1107–1108, 1986.

Cushing M: Law and orders, *Am J Nurs 90*(5):29–30, 32, 1990.

Doctor's verbal orders and license revocation, *Regan Rep Nurs Law 25*(5):2, 1986.

Doolan DF, Bates DW: Computerized physician "order" entry systems in hospitals: mandates and incentives, *Health Affairs 21*(4):180–188, 2002.

Dunn E, Wolfe J: What's wrong with this prescription? *Drug Topics* May 6, 2002, p. 25.

Feutz-Harter S: Documentation principles and pitfalls, *J Nurs Admin 19*(12):7–9, 1989.

Fiesta J: Failing to act like a professional, *Nurs Manage 25*(7):15–17, 1994.

Forster J: Med errors: don't overlook the people part of the equation, *Drug Topics* July 1, 2002, pp. 24–25.

Freudenheim M: New technology helps health care avoid mistakes, *New York Times*, Corrective Medicine Column 02, c.1, Feb 3, 2000.

Gebhart F: New California law requires QA to cut drug errors, *Drug Topics* November 6, 2000, pp. 58, 60.

Glaser J: Knowledge management helps cut errors in half, *Computer World* July 8, 2002, p. 44.

Gryskevich R: Putting Safety First, *Health Management Technology* May 2002, pp. 38–39.

Guarriello DL: When doctor's orders aren't the best medicine, *RN 47*(5):19–21, 1984.

Jesitus J: Confronting medical errors: although new technologies will help, health plan personnel need to take leadership roles as well, *Managed Healthcare Executive* November 2001, pp. 28–32.

LaFleur MW, Starr W: *Health unit coordinating*, ed 2, Philadelphia, 1986, WB Saunders.

Langdon CLG: The legal burden of questionable orders, *Nurs Life 4*(5):22–25, 1984.

Lee S: Wis. Group launches attack on dangerous abbreviations, *Drug Topics* June 17, 2002, p. 42.

Lott LA: The conundrum of patient records, *International Journal of Health Care Quality Assurance incorporating Leadership in Health Services 10*(2): iv–vi, 1997.

Macdonald K: Regulatory considerations regarding accepting orders, *National Council of State Boards of Nursing 15*(2):9–10, 1994.

Maher VF: Your legal guide to safe nursing practice, *Nursing 19*(11):34–41, 1989.

Manthey M: What are doctors' orders, anyway? *Nurs Manage 20*(1):26–27, 1989.

McConnell EA: Clearing the way for a CPR, *Nurs Manage 31*(7):49–50, 2000.

Mehn J, Haas D: What to tell families about drug errors, *H&HN* February 1999, p. 30.

Melymuka K: Knowledge management helps cut errors by half, *Computer World* July 8, 2002, p. 44.

Napoli M: Public fearful of drug errors . . . with good reason, *Health Facts 24*(10):4, 1999.

Northrup CE: Don't overlook "routine" orders, *Nursing 17*(3):43, 1987.

Nurse's Reference Library: *Practices: legal risks, ethics, human relations, career management*, Springhouse, PA, 1984, Springhouse.

Rhodes AM: Carrying out physicians' orders, *Matern Child Nurs J 15*(3):193, 1990.

Rocereto LR, Maleski CM: Following orders . . . and other obligations: 8 legal questions, *Nurs Life 4*(6):18–19, 1984.

Rochman R: Real-time alerts! *Nurs Manage 31*(5):24–25, 2000.

Simpson R: Nurses—yes, nurses—improve physician "order" entry, *Nurs Manage 31*(9):20, 22–23, 2000.

Skuteris LR: Master five common medication administration questions, *Nurs Manage 31*(8):16–17, 2000.

Sullivan GH: Legally speaking: five "rights" equal 0 errors, *RN 54*(6):65–66, 68, 1991.

Tammelleo DA, Gill D: When following "orders" can cost you your license, *RN 47*(3):13–14, 1984.

Ukens C: Pediatric groups hail new med safety guidelines, *Drug Topics Health-System Edition* July 15, 2002, p. 34.

# MANAGING OTHERS

# Using Personal Strengths to Manage Others Creatively

*When you complete this chapter, you should be able to:*

1. Describe the application of human development theories in identifying employee motivations and needs.
2. Describe important characteristics of an organization's culture.
3. Describe phases of organizational development as stages of growth and change.
4. Describe types of power that staff nurses can use to influence others.
5. Describe characteristics of effective leadership.
6. Discuss common leadership styles.
7. Discuss major functions of nursing leadership.
8. Describe the nursing leadership function of providing role models.
9. Describe the nursing leadership function of providing staff direction.
10. Describe the nursing leadership function of providing feedback, including criticism and praise.
11. Describe nursing methods used to evaluate the success of the work group.

human relations management
human development theories
  continuities
  changes
characteristics of organizational
  cultures
  stages of development of an
   organization's culture
sources of influence
  power
   knowledge
   positional
   personal

leadership
  leadership style
   authoritarian or directive
   democratic or participatory
   laissez-faire or nondirective
nursing leadership functions
  motivate coworkers
  serve as role models
  providing feedback
   criticism
   praise
  evaluate the success
   of the work group

## Relationship of Management and Leadership

As described in Chapter One, the terms *management* and *leadership* are used interchangeably in some nursing circles. Actually the two terms have different meanings (Kotter, 1990, pp. 103–104). Nursing *management* refers to the judicious use of resources to achieve client goals. It includes responsibility for directing and controlling the process. Nursing *leadership* refers to skills used to guide others in such a way that followers accept direction voluntarily, without relying on an individual's organizational authority. Entry-level staff nurses use leadership skills to benefit themselves and their clients. That is, entry-level staff nurses use leadership skills to maximize their effectiveness as client care managers directly to benefit clients receiving care and indirectly to improve their nursing practice. As client care managers, staff nurses can learn to emphasize positive attitudes and personal strengths rather than negative perspectives or vulnerabilities to increase their effectiveness in helping others. Effective staff nurses manage others creatively by accentuating their own talents, strengths, and interests and those of their coworkers to provide quality care to clients. Client care managers need to balance concern for providing quality nursing care with concern for the people who do the work (Achenbach and Shepard, 1989, p. 76).

Client care managers achieve this balance in human interaction through use of communication skills that are rooted deeply in the culture. As the global economy continues to increase cultural diversity, greater attention will need to be paid to various cultures of clients and coworkers (Locsin, 2001, p. 3; Rashidi and Rajaram, 2001, p. 55). Not to attend to the effects of the growing cultural diversity is to invite conflict that would be difficult to resolve. Nursing staff members need to continue to value their cultural similarities and differences as people so that appropriate bridging of cultures needed to maintain workable human relationships can occur (Thomas, 2001, p. 44).

## Importance of Human Relations Skills

In today's evolving informational era, health-care environments confront staff with demands for complex changes deeply rooted in societal trends. The evolving cultures (patterns of interactions related to accepted values and behaviors) in these service-oriented work environments emphasize human relations skills. Consequently the client care manager's effectiveness depends largely on her or his **human relations management** skills. "Human management skill" was ranked as the most important criterion of effectiveness for chief nurse executives and middle-level nurse managers (Patz et al., 1991, p. 15). With the increasing emphasis on decentralizing organizations and the efficient use of scarce human resources, entry-level staff nurses also will be expected to use human management skills (Hendry, 1999, pp. 571–572; Manthey, 1990b, pp. 19–20). These skills relate to personal leadership characteristics. Consistent with the evolving emphasis on specified outcomes as integral to quality of care, client care managers will continue to be expected to develop scarce human resources (Blancett, 1990, pp. 4–5).

## Applying Human Development Theories

To gain insight into client behavior, nurses learn to apply human motivation theories. Many nurses are familiar with Maslow's theory and other theories used to describe human development throughout the life span. Similarly, nurses apply these theories to learn about the motivations of the people with whom they work and to identify factors underlying an employee's behaviors and perceptions of work experiences. Because most members of the nursing work group are adults, nurses can apply **human development theories** that address the concerns of adulthood to understand coworkers' motivations. If the entry-level staff nurse understands a coworker's motivations, he or she is likely to be able to identify that person's personal strengths, on which meaningful relationships can be established.

### *Developmental Continuities and Changes*

The knowledge of human development can be applied to gain insight into the motivations of coworkers and clients. A brief review of a developmental psychology textbook reveals many current human development theories. Basically, each theory describes predicted developmental continuities and changes typically occurring throughout adulthood. More recent theories place increased emphasis on cultural influences and historical background so that each generation of individual human development differs from all others (Dien, 2000, p. 1; Goodnow, 2001, p. 160; Phinney, 2000, p. 27; Prawat, 1999, p. 72; Sawyer, 2000, p. 59).

These theories help the nurse to anticipate biologic, psychological, and social continuities and changes that affect coworkers. Adults are influenced by the biologic continuities of their genetic inheritance and by biologic changes associated with increasing chronologic age. Table 10-1 lists common biologic, psychological, and social **continuities** and **changes** associated with adult human development.

The common continuities and changes of adulthood need to be considered to gain insight into the motivations of coworkers in an effort to maximize their individual productivity. For example, an individual whose basic values are consistent with self-esteem and respect for the rights of others is likely to continue to hold such values throughout adulthood. Similarly an individual who gained great personal satisfaction from fulfilling the role of a parent is likely to continue to value that role for as long as it is feasible to do so. Common social changes include loss of roles, such as worker, spouse, or friend, and decreased personal resources, such as body function, positive self-image, and income. The client care manager can use these insights to identify the coworker's strengths and vulnerabilities. This approach also might increase the client care manager's sensitivity to the concerns and needs of individual members of the work group.

## Becoming Acquainted with Important Characteristics of an Organization's Work Culture

The culture or ecology of the work environment strongly influences the behavior of members of a work group. The culture of a work group derives from its values; techniques; particular ways of doing things; and its basic beliefs and inherent assumptions, goals, practices, and concerns of its members (Jameton, 1990, p. 443–445).

TABLE 10-1

## Common Continuities and Changes During Adulthood

| Continuities | Changes |
|---|---|
| **Biologic** | |
| Genetic background | Decreasing function related to disease or disuse |
| Adaptation within limits of physiologic reserves | Decreased immune response to cellular deviation |
| Increasing individual differences due to "wear and tear of living" | Decreased endocrine response to maintain metabolic rate, reproduction |
| **Psychological** | |
| Continuation of personality structure | Increased introspection |
| Consistent or increased intelligence, especially verbal | Increased response time to stimuli |
| Continued patterns of perception or cognition | Increased caution in the interest of accuracy |
| **Social** | |
| Persisting basic values | Increased social losses (e.g., of friends and family) |
| Continuing basic roles within personal limits and resources | Decreased personal resources Body function Positive self-image Income, economic |

This influence has become increasingly clear as the safety issue has become publicized with the need to change the organizational culture from one centered on blame to one designed to promote client safety (Smith, 2002, p. 6). The culture of a work group can be defined as the "ways of thinking, behaving, and believing that members have in common" (Thomas et al., 1990, p. 18) and usually reflects the values for which workers are rewarded (O'Connell, 1999, p. 65). The nature of the work environment makes social demands on each member of the nursing work group. The culture of the work environment usually involves organizational values supported by administrative staff, norms, and interpersonal strategies (Coile, 2001, p. 226; del Bueno, 1986b, pp. 15–20). By gaining insight into the work group's values, norms, and expectations, client care managers can identify norms or social forces that motivate the behaviors of its members. This information provides useful insight in helping to make desired organizational changes and in helping individuals identify how they "fit" in the work group.

Individual employees have unique characteristics and motivations. In the same way, the **characteristics of organizational cultures** or patterns of interrelationships within work groups differ. Coeling (1990, pp. 26–30) described how entry-level nurses can use information about organizational cultures to adapt their behavior to various dimensions of the work environment. The culture of the nursing work group is rooted in its history and traditions. The group's values are reflected in deliberate or unintentional choices. A culture might value physiologic client needs over needs that are primarily psychological or emotional in nature. The leadership style used by key members of the work group provides clues about how decisions are made by the group.

Patterns of helping each other or working together to complete assigned client care indicate the group's commitment to teamwork rather than individual competition and achievement. Entry-level staff nurses need to be sensitive to how the members provided positive and negative feedback to the group. They need to notice how much emphasis key members place on following routines, policies, and procedures and how much on learning new methods and using flexibility and creativity. These patterns of behavior, or norms of the work group, are used to judge the acceptability of members' behaviors, including behaviors of new graduates joining the group. If entry-level nurses are unaware of or insensitive to work group culture, they are unlikely to change their behavior to meet prevailing expectations and less likely to remain with the work group. Adapting to the work culture is not easy for some people. Not fitting in with the work group culture also increases the potential for conflict. The questions listed in Box 10-1 can be used to become familiar with the organization's culture and to guide the nurse's adjustment to it. Effort expended to identify the characteristics of one's work group culture is likely to be very worthwhile.

## Relating Organizational Development to Work Group Culture

### Develop Desired Values and Norms

Work environments of health-care organizations vary widely. With the increasing interrelatedness of organizations and their corresponding competitiveness, much has been written about creating cultures that provide high-quality customer service (Curtin, 1990, pp. 7–8; Hicks and Silva, 1984; Kramer and Schmalenberg, 1991b, pp. 51–55; Manthey, 1990a, pp. 16–17; Peters and Waterman, 1982). These authors emphasized various methods of developing desired values and norms to increase employee productivity and effectiveness. More recently, increased emphasis is placed on responding to the need to change work environments to empower nurses or redesign units in a response to the integration of health care (Burke and Greenglass, 2001, p. 10; Comack et al., 1997, p. 32; Gifford et al., 2002, p. 13; Greenwood, 2000, p. 374; Havens, 2001, p. 258; Laschinger et al., 2001, p. 7; Newhouse and Mills, 2002, p. 65). Findings of these studies continue to support the need for organizational cultures that promote nursing autonomy in clinical practice and increase the quality of nursing work life.

### Identify Work Group Rules

Coeling and Wilcox (1988, pp. 16–22), in a study of two nursing units, identified work group "rules," by analyzing what the group members said and did (i.e., verbal

> **BOX 10-1**
>
> ## Questions to Describe a Nursing Work Group Culture
>
> ### Physical/Psychological/Cultural Focus
> Is it considered more important *first* to meet clients' physical needs, psychosocial needs, or cultural needs?
>
> Is it *more* important to be organized and efficient or flexible and creative to meet client needs?
>
> Is it very important to understand the client's point of view and to respect the client's values?
>
> ### Large/Small Power Distance
> Is the nurse manager more likely to reinforce rules and policies or reward staff input and participation in decision making?
>
> Who (coworkers or supervisors) tells another staff nurse what to do?
>
> Are some nurses more powerful than others? What sources of power do they use?
>
> ### Individualism/Collectivism
> Does the client care manager or the whole work group tend to decide what nursing care a client needs?
>
> Do nurses tend to work alone to complete their assignments?
>
> Do nursing staff members work together to finish the work of their shift?
>
> Is it acceptable to leave some tasks for the next shift if it benefits clients?
>
> Do fellow nurses openly compete with each other? Does the focus of the competition directly benefit clients?
>
> ### Criticism/Approval
> Do nurses tend to criticize each other publicly or privately?
>
> Do nurses typically give each other feedback directly or in a roundabout manner?
>
> Who gives positive approval publicly?
>
> ### Strong/Weak Uncertainty Avoidance
> Do the managers of client care tend to respect and continue past ways of doing things or get excited about learning and trying new approaches?
>
> Does the unit manager believe it is very important to follow policies and procedures?
>
> Do nurses tend to believe there is one right way to do things?

Adapted from Coeling HV: *Nurse Educ* 15(2):27, 1990.

and nonverbal behaviors). The researchers paid careful attention to the characteristics of the nurses who "fit in" and those who did not and what values were important to each work group. In addition, they identified various rules for working together, for telling others what to do, for following established standards, for organizing and using time, for taking the client's perspective, and for change (i.e., attitudes toward learning and improvement) (Coeling and Wilcox, 1988, p. 17).

Information about differences in rules among nursing units is invaluable for recruiting and orienting new work group members and for designing effective plans for change that promote professional nursing practice (Hill, 1989, p. 78; Hines, 1994, pp. 113–119; Thomas et al., 1990, p. 24; Thorsness and Sayers, 1995, pp. 197–209). These work group rules frequently are not written but are communicated to new members through face-to-face communication. It is important to attend to these rules and work toward understanding them.

### Analyze Stages of Development of Organization's Culture

Analysis of the **stages of development of an organization's culture** provides insight into the work group culture. When members within an organization agree on its norms, it becomes more resistant to change (Hannan and Freeman, 1989, p. 68; O'Connell, 1999, p. 65). The actions of individual members of the group can influence the organization significantly, however. The actions of individual workers matter more to the subunits of an organization than to the organization as a whole (Hannan and Freeman, 1989, p. 40). As members of a subunit of the health-care organization, entry-level staff nurses as members of work groups on specific nursing units influence its culture and can change it (Esler and Nipp, 2001, p. 56). They can support desired changes without eroding the organization's strengths. If they do not change to fit the work culture, they also can weaken the work group's cohesiveness or increase conflict. On the basis of information about the development of the organization's culture, they can identify which aspects contribute to its success and need to be continued and which are sources of conflict and require revision. It is crucial that all persons involved in the changes participate in developing the desired approaches and know what his or her part is. Communication is crucial and cannot be overdone. Whether the organization is growing, trying to maintain itself, or decreasing in size, when the contributions of all involved are respected, the changes can be made successfully.

### Understand Organizational Age, Gender, and Societal Influences

An organization's age influences its history and its patterns of response to management problems and principles. The evolving emphasis on decentralization in health-care organizations helps explain the ineffectiveness of many centralized systems that were less responsive to the increasing complexity of health care. Similarly, evolving shared governance organizations reflect organizational needs to sustain employee confidence in a period of rapid societal changes (Havens, 2001, p. 258; Laschinger et al., 2001, p. 7; Peterson and Allen, 1986, pp. 9–12). With staff downsizing that occurred concurrent with the increased emphasis on controlling costs, many nurse administrators experienced periods of mistrust by staff nurses. This atmosphere of mistrust made it difficult to develop cultures rooted in staff nurse confidence in clinical decision making. Gender differences in management styles also affect nursing work group cultures (Ronk, 1993, pp. 65–67).

### Analyze Rate of Growth and Change in the Health-Care Industry

Health-care organizations are influenced by the rate of growth of the health-care industry. Witness the popularity of downsizing as health-care costs have escalated.

Periods of relatively smooth expansion occur if there is increased demand for services. Periods of marked changes in methods of operating are difficult to delay when demand for services significantly declines, such as in the current paradigm shift from tertiary care to primary care and health maintenance. Client care managers need to understand the historical background of the organizational culture in which they work to predict better the likelihood that it will change markedly or continue without substantially altering the processes it uses to provide client care.

By analyzing the historical features of health-care organizations, the client care manager can gain insight into the processes of change occurring within them, and he or she can appreciate that solutions used during growth stages of organizational development sow seeds for the problems that give rise to restructuring or downsizing stages. Change is the only constant in organizational development of health-care agencies, and nurses need to be mindful that their professional practice and management of client care likely will remain a core component of such change.

## Developing a Personal Leadership Style

Using nursing leadership skills is an integral part of the client care management process. The leadership characteristics used and corresponding activities vary with the personal management style of the nurse, the setting, and the characteristics of client needs. Staff nurses as client care managers use various **sources of influence** or power to lead others. They use personal talents, strengths, and leadership skills to maximize scarce human resources to provide high-quality care. Each nurse communicates personal power differently to influence others and to motivate them to provide the needed client care. One nurse might use charisma to guide others. Another nurse might use self-confidence in nursing knowledge and skills to relate effectively to other members of the work group.

The nature of the work environment and work group culture influences the types of leadership skills that enhance the client care manager's effectiveness. The nursing leadership skills used to complete many concrete tasks in a busy surgical unit are likely to differ from the skills used to care for clients in a rehabilitation setting. In addition, because of differences in acute and long-term care staffing mixes, leadership characteristics vary with the composition of the work group, the pattern of service delivery, and the organization's priorities and work group cultures (Smith, 1987, pp. 513–514). The beginning staff nurse needs to seek feedback from others to develop awareness of her or his leadership skills and influence. As Tornabeni (2001, p. 1) aptly stated, "leadership is a matter of influence not position, influence that results from being both respected and liked. People follow because they want to, not because they have to. Everyone wins."

### Power

Hillman (1995, p. 30) described **power** as "the capacity to get work done." To mobilize the resources required to complete client care activities within the nursing work environment, staff nurses use power from several sources. Although power is difficult to define specifically without reference to situational variables, it generally refers to the staff nurse's "ability to do [what is necessary] to achieve nursing objectives" (Gorman and Clark, 1986, p. 129; Klein, 1998, p. 289). Basically, staff nurse power or ability to influence others in the work group stems from three major sources.

### Knowledge

As a result of his or her education in nursing, the client care manager has developed a source of power based on nursing **knowledge**. Application of knowledge is very influential (Curtin, 1989, p. 7). It enables the nurse to understand client situations and what must be done to meet clients' needs. Organizations that strive to provide quality health care and reward excellence in providing it typically are influenced strongly by applications of professional knowledge. Consequently, nurses who have more knowledge and apply it typically gravitate to more influential positions within health-care environments. For example, clinical nurse specialists often exercise considerable power in mobilizing resources for clients they serve. Similarly, some patterns of nursing service delivery using differentiated practice rely on applying greater nursing knowledge as the primary justification for differentiating levels of practice.

The image of nurses as knowledgeable professionals is evolving, albeit slowly. The perceived power of nurses as a function of their professional knowledge is creating an increasingly positive image of nurses among members of other disciplines and arenas, such as administrators, physicians, and the public, and among nurses themselves (Kramer and Schmalenberg, 1991a, pp. 52–54).

### Positional Power

The client care manager's position within the organization is another source of power. This source of power often is referred to as organizational authority or **positional** power. Within centralized organizational structures, persons occupying positions near the top have greater positional power than persons providing direct care. Within decentralized organizations, client care managers gain the positional power needed to provide effective care directly, including legitimate clinical decision-making authority. del Bueno (1986a, p. 125) referred to this type of influence as political power. To benefit from this gain in organizational power, the client care manager needs to use it consistently to provide needed nursing services in a timely manner according to agency and professional standards of practice. Typically the staff nurse strengthens positional power by corroborating with members of the nursing and multidisciplinary work groups to achieve common client care goals (Kerfoot, 2001, p. 29). This use of power requires careful communication and insight into the sources of power used by coworkers "to get what the client needs done."

### Personal Power

Another major source of influence is **personal** power related to an individual's characteristics. These characteristics include verbal and nonverbal communication skills and personality strengths. The client care manager's appearance is an example of the use of nonverbal communication skills to influence others. The importance of personal appearance often is communicated to nursing students by dress codes, although this frequently is not stressed as a component of personal power available for influencing others. The individual's choice of clothing, including fit, style, and cleanliness, influences the perceptions of coworkers and clients (Curran, 2000, p. 229). Clothing also conveys messages about the nurse's sense of self-esteem and worth. Other nonverbal communication skills include eye contact, body language, facial expressions, and use of touch and silence. These techniques can be used to communicate interest and concern for others and enthusiasm for providing needed client services.

Another aspect of personal power is the individual nurse's verbal communication skills. To communicate competence, the nurse should use proper terminology within the health-care setting and at all times avoid use of vulgar language, even though it may be common in his or her personal life, because of its great potential for offending clients, families, and coworkers. For the same reasons, written documentation should incorporate proper terminology. To support a positive image of her or his competence, the client care manager needs to pay special attention to accurate spelling, punctuation, and legibility. The nurse also must select carefully words that accurately describe her or his plans, observations, and actions taken to provide care.

The personality characteristics of client care managers are important sources of personal power. Each individual has personal strengths. Some individuals exude enthusiasm for nursing and exhibit considerable charisma in relating with others. Other nurses are soft-spoken and focus on meeting client needs by showing exemplary active listening skills. What is important is not that differences exist, but that every client care manager possesses strengths that can be used to influence others (Knippen and Green, 1990, p. 7) (i.e., to encourage others to do the right things or to do things right for clients). Focusing on these individual strengths helps identify and develop leadership skills. In this way, scarce human resources can be mobilized.

## Identifying Leadership Styles and Personal Strengths

### *Themes of Leadership*

Many scientists have attempted to define **leadership** and delineate the characteristics of people who are effective leaders. A universally acceptable definition has not been found, however (Yukl, 2002, p. 7). Themes of leadership needed now to enhance individual efforts within organizations were summarized by Yukl (2002, pp. 439–440). See Box 10-2 for a list of these themes as they have been adapted for the practice of client care managers. Yukl emphasized that (1) everyone in an organization can lead, and (2) the themes of leadership need to be felt profoundly by designated leaders (i.e., in nursing, client care managers). To lead, one has to bring out the best in people (i.e., work with strengths instead of emphasizing vulnerabilities). True leadership requires one to become more visible and known for interpersonal sensitivity.

### *Leadership in Client Care Management Context*

In the context of client care management skills, leadership refers to the nurse's ability to influence coworkers to behave voluntarily, without coercion, in desired ways

| BOX 10-2 |

## Themes of Leadership for Client Care Managers

1. Help interpret the meaning of complex events that are stimulating the needs for change. Help coworkers identify emerging trends and their associated threats and opportunities.
2. Work toward building agreement about what to do and how to do it, especially within nursing work groups. Try to reach agreement on client care goals, priorities, and strategies used to achieve them.
3. Promote enthusiasm for providing excellence in nursing service and commitment to meeting client needs. Show confidence that your work groups' efforts will succeed from day to day.
4. Strive to help coworkers understand each other, value their differences, and resolve conflicts in constructive ways. Foster mutual respect, trust, and cooperation between members of various work groups.
5. Make special efforts to help your work groups develop and maintain a positive identity. Plan to resolve issues with the membership in constructive ways that support the group's identity.
6. Expect to coordinate complex tasks to promote efficiencies of nursing and multidisciplinary work groups. Client care is a complex process, and you need to provide "the glue" (i.e., communications, including the setting of priorities and support needed to see that it all happens).
7. Plan to participate in continuous learning to meet client and work group goals. Expect to take the initiative in supporting the continued learning of others, sharing lessons learned and creating successful innovations.
8. Develop a keen awareness of what is needed to provide your assigned clients' care. Strive to obtain the administrative support, equipment, and supplies required to provide the needed care; encourage other work group members to develop such awareness and follow-up as well.
9. Expect that the people you work with need and desire leadership skills and that you can help them develop their strengths. As they develop these skills, your leadership skills will be enhanced.
10. Promote a work climate that is committed to fairness, compassion, and social responsibility. Protect individual rights and responsibilities and oppose unethical practices. Set an example.

Adapted from Yukl G: *Leadership in organizations,* ed 5, Upper Saddle River, NJ, 2002, Prentice-Hall, pp. 439–440.

(i.e., to do the right things in the right way). The client care manager leads (i.e., influences others to provide quality care). To say it differently, as described by Hillman (1995, p. 68), providing "good service . . . moves away from impersonal delivery toward a more personal and individualized touch . . . Good service by this standard simply wants `someone to talk with who can do well, and respectfully, what I ask for.' The five components [of good service]: a human person, with language and skills and sensitivity, adequate to the task, as judged by the recipient or customer." Providing these components in the current health-care arena is difficult but no less imperative than when resources are less scarce.

## Leadership Styles

**Leadership style** refers to the individual's pattern of relating to others or how the leader characteristically "gets along" with members of the work group. The leadership skills used to manage client care vary from nurse to nurse because they are rooted in personal strengths and exemplify the art of nursing practice. The individual leadership styles of client care managers reflect the skills used by each nurse to influence coworkers to do the right things correctly.

Three conventional leadership styles are authoritarian or directive, democratic or participatory, and laissez-faire or nondirective. Many other leadership strategies have been created to influence others. No one leadership style is best at all times. Rather the best leadership style is the one that most effectively influences others to do the right things correctly in a specific situation or context.

### Authoritarian or Directive Leadership Style

An **authoritarian or directive** leadership style is one in which the leader attempts to influence others through the use of positional power or organizational authority. An authoritarian leader directs others by telling them what to do and when and how to do it. This approach is usually effective in emergency situations in which the client depends on others to do the right things correctly within severe time limits. Little or no time is available for teaching, trial and error, or trying to reach a consensus among coworkers. In such circumstances, the staff nurse is obligated to be directive.

### Democratic or Participative Leadership Style

A client care manager using a **democratic or participatory** leadership style seeks and uses input in making decisions that affect others. A democratic leader using a participatory leadership style encourages others to take part in establishing the policies and procedures used by the group. To the extent possible, the leader strives to make decisions by reaching a consensus based on mutual agreement of the group members. This approach is often effective in developing work schedules and assignment plans in an effort to obtain the commitment of the workers involved.

### Laissez-faire or Nondirective Leadership Style

The **laissez-faire or nondirective** leadership style is characterized by a deliberate effort not to interfere or to intervene as little as possible with the activities of the work group. Although frequently criticized, this approach allows members of the work group to be flexible, self-directed, and creative in fulfilling their work responsibilities. It can be effective if members of the work group are highly skilled and self-motivated to do the right things correctly for clients. Such a work group may feel free to engage in and express creative thinking and address complex situations effectively. If some members of the work group are inexperienced or accustomed to directive leadership styles, they are likely to express dissatisfaction with this style. When a nondirective leadership style is used, minimally skilled members of the work group may not address client needs efficiently, or they may place clients at unreasonable risk because they rely on trial-and-error methods in the absence of adequate direction; workers may not even recognize urgent client needs.

Client care managers need to focus on meeting their client needs and protecting the rights of the clients they serve as well as their own. Although a democratic management style is frequently the most successful because it supports autonomous and accountable nursing practice, it may not be appropriate in all situations in which the human needs of clients and staff are priorities (Achenbach and Shepard, 1989, p. 76). As nursing work group leaders, their styles of leadership need to address providing a work environment that enables health-care team members to meet client needs in a caring, cost-effective manner (Boykin and Schoenhofer, 2001, p. 7; McNeese-Smith, 1993, p. 38). Client care managers need to promote sharing a common mission and goals and an involvement in teamwork and collaboration that builds relationships based on individual self-esteem, openness, and mutual respect (Lanser, 2001, pp. 7, 11; Schutz, 1994, p. 243). Such a working environment has unlimited potential for improving individual and organizational effectiveness.

### Being a Follower

This discussion of leadership characteristics and styles may seem daunting to a beginning nurse. The entry-level nurse might question correctly whether leadership skills can be applied by someone who has little practical experience as a client care manager. To the extent feasible, the entry-level nurse needs to avoid "mind talk" that minimizes her or his potential for leadership and to resolve to begin by developing effective follower skills. Being a courageous follower can be a sufficient challenge (Chaleff, 1995). Client care managers are expected to be effective followers in many traditional nursing organizations. Being an effective follower involves being able to think for oneself and take initiative in completing work (Kelly, 1988, pp. 142–148). Box 10-3 describes common characteristics of effective followers.

The staff nurse who strives to be an effective follower encounters opportunities to show personal strengths, knowledge, and organizational know-how and to practice leadership. Gaining experience as an effective follower is likely to prepare the staff nurse for future nursing leadership situations. The effective follower role is often a temporary, albeit necessary, position because every leader depends on followers. By being an effective follower of nursing leaders, the entry-level staff nurse frequently encounters opportunities to practice leadership skills. The formal organization depends on effective followership at the staff nurse level, which also includes use of leadership skills in managing care for a group of clients.

Some nurse leaders have articulated the need for nursing students to prepare to be effective followers when beginning their careers (Guidera and Gilmore, 1988, p. 1017; Murphy, 1990, pp. 68–69). This suggestion does not detract from the value of staff nurses. Rather, it acknowledges the need for staff nurses to function as followers to support effective leaders working toward the common goal of excellence in quality care. Effective followers can succeed without a strong leader, and they can

BOX 10-3

## Characteristics of Effective Followers

1. Demonstrate superb self-management skills
   a. Can think for themselves and know their strengths and vulnerabilities
   b. Can work independently without close supervision
   c. See themselves as equals of the leaders they follow; are apt to disagree openly with leadership unapologetically and are less likely to be intimidated by organizational structure
   d. Recognize that leaders are following the lead of others
   e. Try to appreciate the goals and needs of the team and organization
2. Demonstrate commitment to the agency's mission and goals
   a. Support leaders who are focused on the agency's goals instead of their own
   b. Are loyal to organizational needs
3. Develop competence useful to the organization
   a. Hold higher standards than are required by the work culture
   b. Value and participate in professional development activities
   c. Take on extra work after they complete their core responsibilities successfully
   d. Contribute to teamwork
   e. View coworkers as colleagues instead of competitors
   f. Often identify problems and take initiative in presenting solutions
4. Demonstrate courage, honesty, and credibility
   a. Establish a pattern of independent critical thinking
   b. Trust their own knowledge and judgment and consequently are trusted by others
   c. Stand up for what they believe in
   d. Are insightful and open in expressing their concerns to superiors
   e. Can keep leaders and colleagues honest and informed

Adapted from Kelley RE: *Harvard Bus Rev 66*:142–148, 1988.

help a leader to succeed. Leaders and followers need to promote client-focused organizational cultures. Being effective followers may be entry-level nurses' niche in the organization while they gain experience working with effective leaders. Effective followers readily exercise leadership qualities to help others get the right things done correctly for clients. Considerable savvy and expertise are needed to follow nursing leaders effectively and not dwell on negative features of the situation or sabotage the organization. Effective followers focus on common goals: They show commitment to providing quality care to clients and to sustaining nursing as a caring profession.

## PERFORMING NURSING LEADERSHIP FUNCTIONS WHILE MANAGING CLIENT CARE

Common **nursing leadership functions** performed by client care managers make use of the nursing process and corresponding clinical decision-making skills. The client care manager determines what clients need during the assigned period within the context of long-term goals, what resources are available to achieve these goals, and how individual client outcomes can be achieved best within the resource constraints of the situation. The nurse's leadership approach incorporates short-term and long-term client goals. The core leadership functions of the client care manager include the following:

1. Influencing staff to commit to individual client goals
2. Providing role modeling as a method of providing care
3. Providing feedback through constructive criticism and honest praise
4. Determining the extent of staff success in enabling clients to meet individual goals

## Motivating Coworkers to Commit to Individual Client Goals

By using power derived from applying nursing knowledge, organizational position, and personal attributes, client care managers contribute to the culture of the health-care environment and **motivate coworkers** to identify with the results of their work. The services provided need to be consistent with the agency's mission or purposes. The desired results are satisfied customers—clients who met personal goals, which often match the goals established by the agency's standards of care. Client care managers use leadership skills to organize and develop the people they work with while providing quality care for clients.

Entry-level staff nurses are expected to contribute to team building. In this role, they clarify priorities to help the work group focus their efforts to meet individual client care objectives. They encourage open communication, friendliness, and an atmosphere of having fun working together. They avoid punishing staff when conflicts arise, striving instead to resolve conflicts by retaining staff commitment to common goals of client care. They avoid blaming; rather, they collaborate with peers and colleagues, promote a spirit of cooperation, and attempt to increase or maintain self-esteem of individuals belonging to the work group. They use effective verbal and nonverbal communication skills when relating to members of the work group.

To help a work group resolve common problems, the client care manager focuses on individual client goals and identifies barriers to acceptable solutions. Specific communication strategies designed to promote constructiveness, openness, clarity, and trust are used. The nurse deliberately tries to emphasize positive gains. This approach does not mean that negative staff behaviors or client setbacks are ignored, but that communication focuses on helping staff improve care rather than on stopping undesired behaviors. Another communication strategy is to describe specific behaviors and suggest alternative approaches, rather than labeling the behavior or attacking the person. For example, if a staff member does not adhere to a client's plan of care, the client care manager might point this out. He or she then would follow with a discussion of reasons for carrying out the plan, rather than telling the staff member that he or she is uncooperative. In addition, comments about staff performance are offered frequently, privately, and as soon as appropriate to reinforce the desired behaviors. Only in urgent client situations in which danger is imminent does the nurse comment on inadequate staff performance in the presence of others; in these situations, the client's needs take priority over those of the staff.

The client care manager actively listens to expressed staff concerns and promotes open communication among group members. Nursing assessments of client needs and the interventions used to meet them within the limitations of available resources are central to communication activities. Client care managers focus on short-term client goals, while remaining mindful of the goals in effect for the long-term. They communicate by their actions that each staff member can contribute to meeting common goals and developing an enjoyable work environment.

## Serving as a Role Model

A common characteristic of nurses who positively influence coworkers is an ability to **serve as role models**. Role models consistently show positive attitudes and behaviors such as those described in the American Nurses Association's Code for Nurses. Their actions speak louder than words. Role models use their behaviors to teach others, realizing that what they do often communicates more clearly than what they say (del Bueno, 1989, p. 100; McNeese-Smith, 1993, p. 39). Consequently, what role models say must correspond to what they do and how they do it. Role models use nursing knowledge as the basis for their clinical decisions. They make a special effort to keep up to date with current practices and perform nursing procedures according to agency criteria and legal and ethical requirements. When they recognize limitations in their nursing knowledge or skills, they seek help from others. Role models present a positive image of themselves as individuals and as competent members of the profession.

As mentioned earlier, client care managers influence their work groups by their verbal messages and nonverbal behaviors. By deliberately serving as examples, they communicate their expectations to coworkers. Client care managers as leaders and their followers need feedback to determine their effectiveness. As leaders, client care managers soon "get the message" if their followers do not perform their work in desired ways. Without followers, client care managers are not leaders. Followers follow voluntarily, which explains why follower responses and feedback strongly influence leadership behavior. If a leader's influence does not lead to the desired responses, the leader should seek feedback from coworkers. Most nursing leaders actively seek feedback from their work groups to help them evaluate staff perceptions. Using the feedback enables them to continue to lead effectively.

## Seeking and Providing Feedback

Client care managers complete communication processes by regularly, informally **providing feedback** to the work group. The primary purpose of feedback is to help coworkers improve client care. Feedback is based on observations of client responses and staff behaviors. Formal feedback typically is given at infrequent intervals to meet agency requirements for employee performance evaluation. Informal feedback provided in various ways helps coworkers meet client care objectives. The nurse might communicate the feedback in face-to-face conversation or written messages or by encouraging coworkers to communicate directly with each other. Effective feedback relates specifically to client care and the specific behaviors of coworkers and does not judge the individual as a person. Feedback is generally more effective when it is given promptly after the behaviors are observed. It must be stated clearly in words the coworker can understand. Too much feedback at one time can overwhelm and threaten the coworker. The client care manager also avoids providing feedback in such a way that it is likely to humiliate, demean, or embarrass coworkers. If the feedback includes criticism of specific behavior, it needs to be provided in private.

Informal feedback is usually interpreted as either **criticism** or **praise** (Simpkin, 1991, pp. 4–5). The client care manager's pattern of providing feedback needs to include both. The type of feedback given depends on the coworker's behavior and its effects on client care. Generally, praise is given to reward desired behavior, whereas criticism is provided to suggest alternatives believed to result in more desired behavior.

## Using Nursing Process Skills to Help Coworkers Evaluate Their Effectiveness

As mentioned earlier, client care managers help coworkers clarify and comprehend individual client goals. Coworkers are expected to work toward helping clients meet these goals. This leadership function requires that the client care manager direct staff or clearly communicate expectations of coworkers, as well as nursing plans and the strategies to carry them out. Throughout the workday, client care managers seek feedback from coworkers and assess client responses. This information is used to determine which goals clients met and which require further staff effort. Client care managers treat coworkers as important members of the group and as participants who share responsibility for the care provided. An integral client care management leadership function is to **evaluate the success of the** nursing **work group.** In this way, they share successes and rewards with coworkers when client outcomes are met. More specific nursing strategies used to supervise and evaluate the work of coworkers are presented in Chapter Twelve.

### USING CRITICISM AND PRAISE TO STRENGTHEN COWORKERS' CAREGIVING BEHAVIORS

Client care managers are expected to contribute to a high level of morale among coworkers and to maintain coworkers' motivation to provide high-quality client care. How they accomplish these results depends on their effective use of leadership skills. Client care managers need to try to communicate creatively perceptions of coworker behaviors in a sensitive and tactful manner. The purpose of the communication is paramount, whether the feedback is in the form of criticism or praise.

## Providing Constructive Criticism

Client care managers are expected to provide constructive criticism to coworkers. Before giving feedback about a coworker's behavior, the manager must remember that the primary purpose of feedback is to help the individual provide better client care. If the feedback is given in such a way that it labels the behavior of the person, it is likely to be resented. If the criticism is given in a spirit of helpfulness, it is more likely to be heard and accepted.

It is important to learn the facts surrounding the coworker's behavior, which help identify situational factors contributing to the behavior. Factual information also helps to determine which factors were under the coworker's control and which were not. Insight into the situation surrounding an inadequate performance can help the client care manager suggest reasonable and realistic alternative approaches. Drawing hasty conclusions about what happened or criticizing the coworker's attitude is to be avoided.

The client care manager considers alternative possible causes for a coworker's inadequate work performance. As discussed earlier, the coworker may be motivated by common human developmental needs and by norms and values reinforced by the work group culture. The client care manager encourages the coworker to describe his or her perceptions of the situation and makes suggestions as to possible improvements. Frequently the individual brings up important points of which the client care manager was unaware. The approach also allows the individual to "save face" and maintain a sense of self-worth. Often the coworker can point out negative aspects of the behavior in question and suggest appropriate changes.

A key component of providing constructive criticism to most coworkers is to use a friendly approach and to listen actively (Luke, 1990, p. 7). One possibility might be simply to ask, "What happened?" The client care manager seeks clarification when the coworker's statements or suggestions are unclear, at the same time conveying confidence in the coworker's ability to make the needed changes. In addition, the client care manager needs to give reasons for the desired changes, using behavioral terms. For example, instead of saying, "You frustrate people," the client care manager might say, "Have you tried giving clients plenty of time to follow your directions? Some people feel very frustrated when their best efforts aren't fast enough." This approach ensures that the coworker's behavior is not a consequence of a lack of information about staff expectations.

Another advantage of using an open-ended question to seek clarification is that you might learn about a different perspective (i.e., "another side to the story") and discover environmental or organizational issues that led to the coworker's problem. These issues are more common and more difficult to resolve, whereas attributing the problem to a personal issue may seem to make it easier to solve.

To avoid giving criticism that causes embarrassment or is demeaning or threatening to the coworker, the client care manager carefully decides when and where to give it. He or she should observe the individual's demeanor for signs of frustration and examine herself or himself for signs of hurry or upset. Both parties need to be calm enough to hear and comprehend accurately what is communicated and ultimately to make behavioral changes. Anxiety or anger diminishes the likelihood of such comprehension. Unless a client's safety is at immediate risk, criticism of the coworker's behavior should be offered in private. This reduces the potential for embarrassment and the likelihood that the criticism will be interpreted as a form of punishment. Often the criticism is stated after opening with a genuine compliment or description of the coworker's typical performance, to preserve the individual's feelings of competence and self-confidence. This approach often prepares the coworker to listen carefully to the constructive criticism.

The purpose of constructive criticism is to prevent the recurrence of particular behaviors; to strengthen what the coworker is doing appropriately; and to promote the desired changes because the desired behavior is the right thing to do for clients, not merely because one wants to avoid punishment. Box 10-4 lists key considerations for giving effective constructive criticism.

## Using Praise to Build Coworker Strengths

Praise is a strong motivator because it addresses the common human need for recognition and approval (Luke, 1991, p. 3). The purpose of giving praise is to reward desired work performance. Client care managers are encouraged to use several strategies when praising coworkers to build on their strengths. Every member of the work group has strengths worthy of honest recognition.

It is a curious phenomenon that praise, which is a powerful reward and fun to give, is offered infrequently. Often client care managers hesitate to praise a coworker's performance because they believe it is common to the work group and want to avoid the appearance of favoritism. Generally, everyone who deserves praise should receive it. Perhaps the praise could be given in a group setting, where it is more likely to be fairly distributed. An individual coworker's work might be recognized in private or in the group, depending on the nature of the performance and its value within the organizational culture. Some staff members are uncomfortable receiving praise given openly. In any event, praise needs to be given frequently (i.e., often enough to ensure that good work is never taken for granted).

---

**BOX 10-4**

### Providing Constructive Criticism

1. Remember that the primary purpose of constructive criticism is to improve client care.
2. Select a time that corresponds to the needs of the giver and the receiver.
3. Learn about the circumstances surrounding the coworker's behavior.
4. Distinguish situational factors under the coworker's control from those that are not.
5. Suggest reasonable alternative behaviors.
6. Actively listen to the coworker's suggestions for change.
7. Use a friendly approach to communicate confidence in the coworker's abilities.
8. Explain reasons for the suggested changes in behavior.

Praise, similar to criticism, is necessarily based in fact. Frequently a manager's attention to details of complex client care situations and staff responses to them provides numerous opportunities for honest praise. Staff members are likely to be aware of their unique talents and strengths and use them routinely. Although these creative responses to client needs are seemingly commonplace, they should be recognized to ensure their repetition.

False praise or flattery should be avoided because it is insincere. It is often given to gain something rather than to reward desired behaviors. Flattery is likely to offend coworkers, rather than motivate them to continue to do good work.

Praise is an effective leadership tool when offered honestly and in such a manner that it increases workers' self-esteem. It is essential that the client care manager inform colleagues who are doing the good work if their wonderful work also is being described outside the group. It can be a powerful motivator, and it is far less costly than wage or salary increases. It rarely, if ever, has been overused in healthcare environments, where cost-effectiveness is often the preoccupation.

Rewarding special achievement is a method of helping positive work cultures evolve (Kerfoot, 2000, p. 264). Methods of communicating approval throughout the work organization are needed to reward the numerous effective responses made to meet client needs. Many new challenges depend on creativity and on effective clinical decision making on behalf of quality client care. Wouldn't it be fun to work

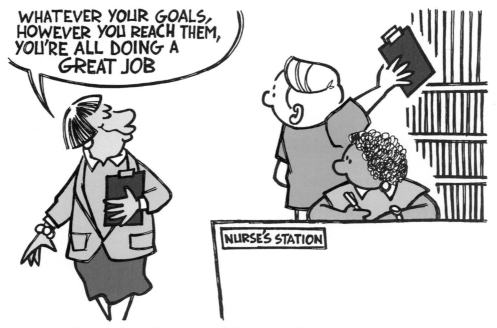

False praise or flattery should be avoided because it is insincere.

in a setting in which praise is given by and to coworkers as frequently as it is given to nursing staff by clients and families they serve?

## SUMMARY

Effective staff nurses manage others creatively by emphasizing their own talents, strengths, and interests and those of their coworkers. To help manage this process, they can apply human development theories to gain insight into the motivations and behaviors of coworkers. These theories help to identify common continuities and changes that occur during adulthood.

The organizational culture also influences staff behavior. Sensitivity to the norms, values, and expectations of the work group culture helps the entry-level staff nurse make the adjustments needed to succeed as a client care manager. Understanding the background development of the organization helps the staff nurse predict future growth and changes.

Entry-level staff nurses can use nursing knowledge, positional authority, and personal strengths as sources of power within the work environment to help the work group provide needed nursing care for the assigned group of clients. They also need to adapt their leadership styles to fit the nursing situation. Often staff nurses assume the role of effective followers to practice leadership skills and to support the organization and its leaders.

Common staff nurse leadership functions include motivating coworkers to make a commitment to individual client goals, serving as a role model, seeking and providing feedback, and contributing to team building. Staff members are encouraged to give praise and constructive criticism honestly, in a timely and tactful manner. Praise is an inexpensive tool that staff nurses can use to reward effective staff efforts and desired behaviors.

## APPLICATION EXERCISES

1. Interview a coworker. Identify the individual's stage of human development by reviewing his or her biologic, cultural, psychological, and social continuities and changes over the last 10 years.
2. Describe the nursing work group culture by answering the questions suggested in Box 10-1.
3. Identify the predominant leadership style you most frequently use to influence your nursing peers. Describe your sources of power.
4. A coworker's comments to a client about another colleague (in your presence) casts doubt on the colleague's competence. State what you would you do, where, and how.
5. The morale of your nursing work group is slipping. Members express feeling overworked, underpaid, and unappreciated. Describe what you would do to help without increasing financial costs.

## CRITICAL THINKING SCENARIO

Imagine yourself as the newest member to a work group providing care on a 1-day surgery unit in an acute-care, public, nonprofit facility. The health-care facility has been in existence for more than 125 years and consistently has emphasized values of excellence in quality care and staff as its most valuable resource. You have been appointed to an agency-wide nursing practice committee. Through the grapevine, you learn that the chair of this committee has evinced strong commitment to achieving its goals in a timely manner, frequently working "above and beyond" expectations to do so. You have become aware, however, that the chair has been excluded from any public recognition of the committee's achievements, which are extraordinary in a time of organizational turbulence. Nursing administration is displaying this committee's accomplishments to other departments as a prototype of the nursing department's progressiveness.

1. How would you feel about the norms of the culture?
2. Do you think the group will grow in its sense of worth and collegiality? Give reasons for your answer.
3. What would you do first? (*Clue:* Review Caroselli C: Assessment of organizational culture: a tool for professional success, *Orthop Nurs 11*[3]:57–63, 1992.)
4. What, if anything, would you do to change the situation to suit your style of nursing practice, leadership, and management? Give reasons.

## REFERENCES

Achenbach R, Shepard J: The study of management styles, *Nurs Manage 20*(6):76, 1989.

Blancett SS: Human development renaissance, *J Nurs Admin 20*(7/8):4–5, 1990.

Boykin A, Schoenhofer S: The role of nursing leadership in creating caring environments in health care delivery systems, *Nurs Admin Q 25*(3):1–7, 2001.

Burke RJ, Greenglass ER: Effects of changing hospital units during organizational restructuring, *Health Care Manager 20*(1):10–18, 2001.

Caroselli C: Assessment of organizational culture: a tool for professional success, *Orthop Nurs 11*(3):57–63, 1992.

Chaleff I: *The courageous follower: standing up to and for our leaders*, San Francisco, 1995, Berret-Koehler Publishers.

Coeling HV: Organizational culture: helping new graduates adjust, *Nurse Educ 15*(2):26–30, 1990.

Coeling HV, Wilcox JR: Understanding organizational culture: a key to management decision-making, *J Nurs Admin 18*(11):16–22, 1988.

Coile RC: Magnet hospitals use culture, not wages to solve nursing shortage, *J Healthcare Manage 46*(4):225–227, 2001.

Comack M, Brady J, Porter-O'Grady T: Professional practice: a framework for transition to a new culture, *JONA 27*(12):32-41, 1997.

Curran C: Creating a framework for patient centeredness, *Nurs Econ 18*(5):229, 262, 2000.

Curtin LL: Power: the traps of trappings, *Nurs Manage 20*(6):7–8, 1989.

Curtin LL: Creating a culture of competence, *Nurs Manage 21*(9):7–8, 1990.

del Bueno DJ: Power and politics in organizations, *Nurs Outlook 34*(3):124-128, 1986a.

del Bueno DJ: Organizational culture: how important is it? *J Nurs Admin 16*(10):15–20, 1986b.

del Bueno DJ: Our actions drown out our words, *RN 32*(8):100, 1989.

Dien DS: The evolving nature of self-identity across four levels of history, *Human Development 43*:1–18, 2000.

Esler RO, Nipp DA: Worker designed change achieves performance targets, *Nurs Econ 19*(2):56–61, 2001.

Gifford BD, Zammuto RF, Goodman EA, Hill KS: The relationship between hospital unit culture and nurses' quality of work life, *J Healthcare Manage 47*(1):13–22, 2002.

Goodnow JJ: Directions of change: sociocultural approaches to cognitive development, *Human Development 44*:160–165, 2001.

Gorman S, Clark N: Power and effective nursing practice, *Nurs Outlook 34*(3):129–134, 1986.

Greenwood J: Clinical development units: nursing's David? *Clin Nurs Res 9*(4):373–378, 2000.

Guidera MK, Gilmore C: In defense of followership, *Am J Nurs 88*(7):1017, 1988.

Hannan MT, Freeman J: *Organizational ecology*, Cambridge, MA, 1989, Harvard University Press.

Havens DS: Comparing nursing infrastructure and outcomes: ANCC magnet and nonmagnet CNEs report, *Nurs Econ 19*(6):258–266, 2001.

Hendry J: Cultural theory and contemporary management organization, *Human Relations 52*(5):557–577, 1999.

Hicks CR, Silva MA: *Creating excellence: managing corporate culture, strategy, and change in the new age*, New York, NY, 1984, New American Library.

Hill BM: The McAuley experience with changing compensation within the context of a professional nursing practice culture, *Nurs Admin Q 14*(1):78–82, 1989.

Hillman J: *Kinds of power: a guide to its intelligent uses*, New York, NY, 1995, Currency-Doubleday, pp. 66–82.

Hines PP: An interview with Moira Kelly, *Nurs Econ 12*(3):113–119, 1994.

Jameton A: Culture, morality, and ethics, *Crit Care Nurs Clin N Am 2*(3):443–451, 1990.

Kelly RE: In praise of followers, *Harvard Bus Rev 66*:142–148, 1988.

Kerfoot K: Leadership: creating a shared destiny, *Nurs Econ 18*(5):263–264, 2000.

Kerfoot K: The leader as synergist, *Nurs Econ 19*(1):29–30, 2001.

Klein G: *Sources of power: how people make decisions*, Cambridge, MA, 1998, The MIT Press.

Knippen JT, Green TB: Reinforcing the right behavior, *Supervis Manage 35*(4):7, 1990.

Kotter JP: What leaders really do, *Harvard Bus Rev 68*:103–111, 1990.

Kramer M, Schmalenberg C: Job satisfaction and retention: insights for the '90s, Part 1, *Nursing 91*(3):50–55, 1991a.

Kramer M, Schmalenberg C: Job satisfaction and retention: insights for the '90s, Part 2, *Nursing 91*(4):51–55, 1991b.

Lanser EG: A model workplace: creating an effective nursing environment, *Healthcare Executive* July/Aug 2001, pp. 6–11.

Laschinger HKS, Finegan G, Shamian J: The impact of workplace empowerment, organizational trust on staff nurses' work satisfaction and organizational commitment, *Health Care Manage Rev 26*(3):7–23, 2001.

Locsin RC: Culture-centrism and holistic care in nursing practice, *Holist Nurs Pract 15*(4):1–3, 2001.

Luke RA: How to give corrective feedback to employees, *Supervis Manage 35*(3):7, 1990.

Luke RA: Meaningful praise makes a difference, *Supervis Manage 36*(2):3, 1991.

Manthey M: Nursing: an ecological perspective, *Nurs Manage 21*(8):16–17, 1990a.

Manthey M: Three simple rules, *Nurs Manage 21*(12):19–20, 1990b.

McNeese-Smith D: Leadership behavior and employee effectiveness, *Nurs Manage 24*(5):38–39, 1993.

Miller KL: The human care perspective in nursing administration, *J Nurs Admin 17*(2):10–12, 1987.

Murphy D: Followers for a new era, *Nurs Manage 21*(7):68–69, 1990.

Newhouse RP, Mills MEC: Enhancing a professional environment in the organized delivery system: lessons in building trust for the nurse administrator, *Nurs Admin Q 26*(3):67–75, 2002.

O'Connell C: A culture of change or a change of culture? *Nurs Admin Q 23*(2):65–68, 1999.

Patz JM, Biordi DL, Holm K: Middle nurse manager effectiveness, *J Nurs Admin 21*(1):15–24, 1991.

Peters TJ, Waterman RH: *In search of excellence*, New York, NY, 1982, Warner.

Peterson ME, Allen DG: Shared governance: a strategy for transforming organizations, Part 1, *J Nurs Admin 16*(1):9–12, 1986.

Phinney JS: Identity formation across cultures: the interaction of personal, societal and historical change, *Human Development 43*:27–31, 2000.

Prawat RS: Cognitive theory at the crossroads: head fitting, head splitting, or somewhere in between? *Human Development 42*:59–77, 1999.

Rashidi A, Rajaram SS: Culture care conflicts among Asian-Islamic immigrant women in US hospitals, *Holist Nurs Pract 16*(1):55–64, 2001.

Ronk LL: Gender gaps within management, *Nurs Manage 24*(5):65–67, 1993.

Sawyer RK: Connecting culture, psychology and biology, *Human Development 43*:56–59, 2000.

Schutz W: *The human element: productivity, self-esteem, and the bottom line*, San Francisco, CA, 1994, Jossey-Bass.

Simpkin GD: Getting your staff to do what you want, *Supervis Manage 36*(1):4–5, 1991.

Smith AP: In search of safety: an interview with Gina Pugliese, *Nurs Econ 20*(1):6–12, 2002.

Smith MM: Getting ahead in the corporate culture, *Am J Nurs 87*(4):513–515, 1987.

Thomas C, Ward M, Chorba C, et al: Measuring and interpreting organizational culture, *J Nurs Admin 20*(6):17–24, 1990.

Thomas ND: The importance of culture throughout all of life and beyond, *Holist Nurs Pract 15*(2):40–46, 2001.

Thorsness R, Sayers B: Systems approach to resolving conduct issues among staff members, *AORN 61*(1):197–209, 1995.

Tornabeni J: The competency game: my take on what it really takes to lead, *Nurs Admin Q 25*(4):1–13, 2001.

Yukl G: *Leadership in organizations*, ed 5, Upper Saddle River, NJ, 2002, Prentice-Hall.

# Coordinating Care Provided by Nursing, Multidisciplinary, and Interdisciplinary Work Groups

## OBJECTIVES

*When you complete this chapter, you will be able to:*

1. Describe the types of work groups as clinical resources.
2. Distinguish between single-leader work group goals and interdisciplinary team goals.
3. Describe principles used to promote effective working relationships within work groups.
4. Describe barriers to work group effectiveness.
5. Describe contributions that a client care manager can make to enhance the efforts of multidisciplinary work groups.
6. Describe principles of coordinating priorities of work groups.

## KEY CONCEPTS

work groups
  multidisciplinary
  interdisciplinary
basic elements of effective work groups
work group types
single discipline, multidisciplinary,
  interdisciplinary work group styles
one-leader work group
teams
interdisciplinary team
interdependent work groups

culture of work groups
cooperation
collaboration
organizational provisions
  common language
  mission statement
  structured meeting time and place
interdisciplinary group goals
client priorities
role conflicts
value nursing contributions

culture of the multidisciplinary work
group

principles for promoting effective
working relationships
barriers

## INTRODUCTION TO WORK GROUP CONCEPTS

Health care is increasingly complex and requires work to be performed by groups of people who are interdependent (mutually dependent on each other), if quality care is provided in a comprehensive manner. Concurrently, nursing services remain at the core of health care. Consequently, nurses inevitably are required to accomplish complex client outcomes interdependently with multiple **work groups** (i.e., various medical and human service specialties for diagnoses and treatment). In addition, common patterns of nursing service delivery (i.e., team nursing, case management, and functional groups within complex vertically and horizontally integrated organizations) incorporate various types of nursing work groups. The realization that integration of health care requires several disciplines to combine their knowledge and skills has led some to perceive the need for increased interdisciplinary "teams." Careful analyses of the effectiveness of interdisciplinary teams result in questions about their effectiveness, however, in the face of vested interests in reducing costs related to "cross-disciplinary collaboration" (Gibson, 1999, p. 150; Hammond et al., 1999, p. 35; Higgins and Routhieaux, 1999, pp. 1–2; Hinojosa et al., 2001, p. 217; Reese and Sontag, 2001, p. 173; Schofield and Amodeo, 1999, p. 218; Slack and McEwen, 1999, p. 30; Sluzki, 2000, p. 350; Strasser et al., 2002, p. 122). The emphasis on cost-effectiveness in health care has promoted the study of the effectiveness of interdisciplinary work groups and their essential components. Important findings include the need to clarify terminology and what makes interdisciplinary groups effective (Katzenbach and Smith, 2001, pp. 3–4; Schofield and Amodeo, 1999, p. 217).

Schofield and Amodeo (1999, p. 217) recommended clarification of the terms *multidisciplinary* and *interdisciplinary* as follows: (1) **Multidisciplinary** refers to a work group in which a number of individuals from various disciplines are involved in a project (i.e., implementing a care pathway) but work independently, and (2) **interdisciplinary** refers to a work group in which representatives of more than one discipline work together in a coordinated group effort (i.e., share common goals to achieve desired client outcomes). An example of a multidisciplinary work group is members of various disciplines that provide care while following an established care pathway for a client who has undergone a total hip replacement. Each discipline involved has various representatives that implement the plan of care. An example of an interdisciplinary work group is the specific members from various disciplines that become involved in a complex care situation in which several members of a family are involved in serious trauma, requiring the complex skills of many disciplines to work together according to the priority needs of the clients as needs evolve. It is the nature of the complexity of needs that determines whether the skills of a multidisciplinary work group or interdisciplinary team are needed. Table 11-1 depicts work groups, styles and members' predominant mode of practice. These definitions help to identify important differences in the processes used by various work

TABLE 11-1

## Work Group Types, Styles, and Members' Predominant Mode of Practice

| Work Group Type | Style | Members' Predominant Mode of Service Delivery |
|---|---|---|
| Multidisciplinary | One-leader | Independently |
| Interdisciplinary | Team | Interdependently |
| Single discipline: nursing | One-leader or team | Independently or interdependently depending on specific work group and pattern of service delivery |

groups to provide needed care. To appreciate these differences, the client care manager needs to understand the basic elements of various work groups in which she or he will be a member.

Client care managers as nurses may be members of any or all types of work groups in a given day. If the client care manager does not pay attention to the specific work group and its style that he or she is participating in at a given time, it becomes apparent why confusion about role expectations is likely, especially in terms of one's decision-making authority and accountability for client outcomes. For example, a beginning staff nurse might be a member of a one-leader (case manager) nursing work group, a multidisciplinary work group, and an interdisciplinary team for one or more assigned clients with complex needs. Similarly a nurse might be a member of a primary nursing (pattern of service delivery) work group and a multidisciplinary work group. Different shifts in nursing may organize into different patterns of service delivery (e.g., primary nursing during the day or evening shifts and functional nursing during the night shift).

Katzenbach and Smith (2001, pp. 3–4) described five **basic elements of effective work groups**. See Box 11-1 for these basic requirements. Katzenbach and Smith (2001, pp. 4–12) further explain two basic **work group types** used to accomplish the work to be done: (1) one-leader style and (2) team style. *Each type of work group critically depends on the nature of work to be done for its success.* That is, can the work best be done by the work group's members working independently as individuals or as a group of people working interdependently toward a common goal for which the work group expects to share accountability?

The **one-leader style** of working together is common in health care (e.g., physician-directed diagnosis and treatment work groups or nurse case manager directed care). It is characterized by a leader who (1) makes the final decisions and communicates these decisions to the work group, (2) sets goals and individual responsibilities, (3) sets the pace and process of how the work group will get the work done, (4) evaluates the work group's progress and rewards individual contribu-

> **BOX 11-1**
>
> ## Basic Requirements of Effective Work Groups
>
> 1. Establish and understand reason and purpose for the work group.
> 2. Involve all work group members in constructive interactions in efforts to communicate and coordinate.
> 3. Establish clear roles and areas of responsibilities so that members can work independently (individually) or interdependently (together as a group).
> 4. Develop a set of expectations that promotes a time-efficient process (i.e., minimize wasted time and effort) for the work group.
> 5. Develop a sense of accountability (i.e., each member expects to answer for one's work or progress of the work group).

Adapted from Katzenbach JR, Smith DK: *The discipline of teams: a mindbook-workbook for delivering small group performance*, New York, NY, 2001, John Wiley & Sons, pp. 3–4.

tions toward its goals, (5) sets final standards and measurements of progress for the group, and (6) maintains control while working to clarify individual accountabilities and consequences (Katzenbach and Smith, 2001, pp. 5–6)

The **team style** work group differs significantly from the single-leader style. The team style is characterized by a small number of people (1) whose knowledge and skills complement those of other members; (2) who are committed to a common purpose, approach, and results; and (3) who hold themselves as a group answerable for their collective performance (Katzenbach and Smith, 2001, p. 7). The team style of group work is used best for the types of work that require members to work together to accomplish the results. By working together, shared skills produce the desired outcomes; team members expect to answer not only for the efforts of individuals, but also for performance as a group. One work group style is not more desirable in and of itself; rather, a particular style is more desirable when it will produce better results depending on whether individual or collective efforts are required to meet client needs.

## INTERDISCIPLINARY WORK GROUP (TEAM) AS AN ORGANIZATIONAL RESOURCE

Nurses frequently participate in multidisciplinary work groups and less frequently as members of interdisciplinary teams. Because interdisciplinary teams often are more cohesive than one-leader style work groups, client care managers might use their leadership skills to promote the development of **teams** from common multidisciplinary work groups. This may not be desirable for many work groups that require individual efforts to achieve the established client goals because it blurs role expectations and may mislead work group members as to their decision-making responsibilities. The focus of this chapter is to help entry-level staff nurses actively participate in work groups and use teamwork when it is needed to meet complex client outcomes requiring team style work group effort. This chapter describes the client care manager's role as a member of multidisciplinary work groups, while concurrently providing direct care as a member of nursing work groups. This chapter also is designed to help the client care manager contribute to team building consistent with **interdisciplinary team** functions, goals, available resources, and knowledge bases. The special efforts of interdisciplinary teams may be required to provide quality, cost-effective care to clients with complex needs not addressed by one-leader style work groups.

## Client Care Managers versus Traditional Case Managers

Entry-level staff nurses as client care managers need to distinguish elements of their role from those of traditional case managers. As described in Chapter Three and depicted in Figure 3-6, the client care manager role of entry-level staff nurses primarily involves direct service or providing care on a daily, shift-by-shift basis to clients. It is crucial that nurses who deliver direct care distinguish among the different roles they play in each organizational setting to increase the quality of bedside/clinical services (i.e., point of care) (Karpuik et al., 1994, pp. 41–42). In comparison, the case manager role typically emphasizes the coordination and monitoring of services provided by direct-service staff, including multidisciplinary groups, to "ensure that the agreed on services were provided" (Rheaume et al., 1994, p. 31). The case manager role involves far fewer, if any, direct services and much more coordination of direct services provided by other groups, agencies, or associations. The case manager links other service providers to provide continued care, reduce fragmentation, and promote cost-effective care to the client. The case manager typically communicates with various **interdependent work groups** (i.e., groups of individuals who depend on each other to provide specialized services in a timely and proficient manner). The case manager is often the leader of one-leader style nursing and multidisciplinary work groups.

## Interdisciplinary Groups

As more emphasis is placed on managing information in an evolving health-care arena with increasingly complex services, nurses became more interdependent with other health-care providers. Nurses know that "We can't know it all and we can't do it all" (Carrol, 1987, p. 43). This realization reflects the need for health-care organizations to support the efforts of multidisciplinary work groups. These groups are composed of members of several disciplines (e.g., clinical medicine, nursing, pastoral care, physical therapy, psychology, occupational therapy, respiratory therapy, social work, speech pathology) who rely on each other to meet priority individual client needs effectively and efficiently. Each multidisciplinary group's membership depends on the individual client's needs and the resources provided by the health-care agency based on its function. For example, the client care manager caring for developmentally delayed children in a long-term care setting is likely to work closely with special education teachers and occupational, speech, and physical therapists. A client care manager working with terminally ill adults in a hospice unit is likely to work closely with spiritual counselors, social workers, volunteer coordinators, and clinical pharmacists. This chapter describes components of the client care manager's role as a coordinator of multidisciplinary work group efforts on the client's behalf.

Although the concept of *teams* often is used synonymously with that of *groups*, there are significant differences between the two concepts. By understanding these differences, client care managers can contribute to work groups and teams as needed by clients. For the purposes of this chapter, a work group consists of two or more persons serving an individual client. They are members of the work group because of their participation in the individual client's care. The work group can be a team, but more often is a one-leader style work group. According to Katzenbach and Smith (1993, pp. 14–15), "Groups become **teams** through disciplined action," by using specific approaches and strategies that combine their efforts creatively so as to achieve results common to all members. "They share a common purpose, agree on performance goals, define a common working approach, develop high levels of complementary skills, and hold themselves mutually accountable for results" (Katzenbach and Smith, 1993, pp. 14–15). Katzenbach and Smith (1993, pp. 14–15) emphasize that a team is more than a group of workers with a common assignment. A team is connected permanently to its performance in meeting its common purpose. Team members accept responsibility for the team's performance collectively. No one member is more responsible than any other for the team's results (Katzenbach and Smith, 1993, pp. 44–45). This interdisciplinary commitment to a common purpose, although uncommon, is crucial and praiseworthy. Box 11-2 lists the essential criteria for an interdisciplinary team.

Typically a client care manager is more often a member of a multidisciplinary group rather than of an interdisciplinary team. A long-range goal of client care managers should be to strive to contribute to the development of interdisciplinary teams from multidisciplinary work groups (i.e., to participate in team building). Because many professional formal instructional programs do not include such preparation, in-service programs are likely to be needed. Because teamwork is preferable to group work when client needs are extraordinarily complex, development of teams from one-leader work groups can be a worthy management goal as a key strategy for maximizing use of available resources (Hammond et al., 1999, p. 28). If staffing shortages continue to increase or persist, the potential development and use of interdisciplinary teams will be severely challenged.

Client care managers coordinate nursing work group efforts to satisfy clients' nursing needs and may be the leader in one-leader style work groups. Because of their pivotal position within the health-care organization, client care managers also may contribute to the efforts of multidisciplinary work groups. They must identify the priority needs of individual clients, the agency resources available to meet them, and the process the organization uses to meet them effectively and efficiently. They need to know why clients' priority needs change throughout the treatment process and how these changes affect what attitudes, knowledge, and skills (competencies) are required to meet them. For example, early in a client's hospitalization, respiratory therapy might be needed to satisfy needs for adequate

BOX 11-2

## Essential Criteria for an Interdisciplinary Team

1. There is a common purpose (i.e., sense of direction) that members translate into specific actions and goals based on the team's common perception: a "compelling performance challenge" consisting of many collective work results.
2. It is small enough in number to be workable (i.e., able to communicate easily and frequently): *small size* (approximately 10 or less).
3. The team's performance is shared permanently among members to reflect and maximize performance potential. Outcome-based goals include individual and predominantly group results.
4. Skills crucial to team success are manifest (i.e., exist or can be developed) within group members: *comprehensive complementary skills.*
5. Every member contributes to and accepts responsibility for results: *mutual accountability.*
6. The team's commitment to its performance requires clear communication and conflict resolution: *common/clear language.*
7. There is agreement on approach to achieve desired results.

Adapted from Katzenbach JR, Smith DK: *The discipline of teams: a mindbook-workbook for delivering small group performance,* New York, NY, 2001, John Wiley & Sons, p. 12.

ventilation and to prevent complications. Later, physical therapy might be the highest priority to maximize mobility. Discharge planning activities might involve a variety of disciplines to enable the client to live at home with a chronic health problem. This background knowledge enables client care managers to anticipate evolving client care needs and to organize the multidisciplinary work group efforts to meet them.

## Coordinating Multidisciplinary Groups

Coordinating the diverse efforts of a multidisciplinary work group requires skills in human relations and group dynamics. Not only do individual client needs change daily, but also the composition of the multidisciplinary group is often in a state of flux. The culture of a health-care organization strongly influences what members expect of each other, who makes clinical decisions, how these decisions are made, and how treatment programs are carried out (Heinemann et al., 1999, p. 140). Each culture reflects what its multidisciplinary work groups and interdisciplinary team members perceive as their overall purpose and goals and how they are rewarded for success in their endeavors (Strasser et al., 2002, p. 115). In the past, employees typically were rewarded on their performance reviews for individual efforts. As a result of the increased complexity of client needs in current health-care settings, whether acute, long-term, institutional, or community based, the need for collaborative efforts is increasingly in demand (Marshall, 1995, pp. 6–9). The emphasis of employee performance has shifted to evaluating work group success in meeting desired client outcomes rather than the specific interventions taken to achieve them. Effective interdisciplinary teams are valuable resources. Without them, the health-care agency typically cannot efficiently or effectively provide complex quality care.

Entry-level staff nurses collaborate with members of multidisciplinary work groups as client advocates to meet established routine outcomes. Accordingly, client care managers play a key role in the success of multidisciplinary work groups. Coordinating multidisciplinary efforts provides staff nurses with numerous opportunities to influence the **culture of work groups** and the quality of care clients receive on a daily basis. Persistently organizing seeming chaos into goal-directed activities on behalf of clients is an arduous, demanding nursing function. Many client care managers learn to perform coordinating duties more effectively as they gain experience as a member of a specific nursing work group. They also might learn about the interpersonal dynamics involved in team building.

## Identifying the Multidisciplinary Group as an Organizational Resource

### Organizational Routines of Various Disciplines

Many health-care organizations, although not all, divide the work of client care along functional or departmental lines. Consequently, each discipline is organized formally as a unit or department with its own policies and procedures. These functional divisions of the work to be done should be consistent with the agency's overall philosophy, purposes, policies, and procedures. Each member of the multidisciplinary group has a primary identification with and commitment to a specific discipline and its knowledge, values, and skills. Each discipline's routines, which reflect its contributions to client care, guide its members in carrying out their functions and duties. The disciplinary routines of staff nurses entail providing nursing interventions in a timely manner that enables clients to adhere to other scheduled therapies, providing feedback to the other disciplines about client responses to treatment, and answering requests for specific follow-through on treatment programs that prepare clients for optimal self-management. For example, nurses frequently administer analgesics before various exercise therapies to maximize client participation; they may assist, teach, or supervise clients in the proper follow-through in the use of adaptive equipment to perform self-care activities; and they may discuss the clients' responses and difficulties experienced by the clients with members of multidisciplinary work groups.

### Cooperation and Collaboration

**Cooperation** and **collaboration** are key to multidisciplinary group work. As individual client needs change in response to treatment, multidisciplinary group members need to communicate and collaborate with each other to ensure that priority needs continue to be addressed. If communication and collaboration with the multidisciplinary group are inadequate, conflict occurs, and the quality of client care suffers. The larger and more complex the organization's work force, the more likely multidisciplinary conflict is to occur (Guy, 1986, pp. 111–112). Conflict can be avoided if there is open, timely communication between work group members about changes in client conditions and regular, scheduled conferences to communicate client progress, concerns, and evolving individual treatment programs.

### Common Language

Due to the interdependencies of various professions, many health-care organizations make several different types of **organizational provisions** (i.e., structured, scheduled multidisciplinary conferences) to enable their multidisciplinary work groups to address evolving client needs in an efficient and effective manner. Most disciplines use unique knowledge bases and language; to work together, however, the multidisciplinary work group needs a **common language**. At times, the same word or abbreviation has different meanings in different disciplines. For example, *mg* means milligrams to registered nurses, physicians, and pharmacists, whereas it might mean muscle groups to physical, occupational, and recreational therapists. If confusion of this sort is not clarified, errors or conflict can result. Building a work environment based on clear communication and a common language is difficult when melding a culturally diverse work force and client population. Striving to build an interdisciplinary team in such an environment is an important goal. Clear communication requires appreciation of core values, trust, and words as symbols of meaning. Multidisciplinary and interdisciplinary work group members must be encouraged to consult, collaborate, and evaluate group efforts without fear of retaliation.

### Common Purpose

Effective multidisciplinary work groups need a commonly understood purpose to guide them in setting priorities and identifying roles and responsibilities to clients within a specific setting. The **mission statement**, which defines the organization's overall purposes, reflects the multidisciplinary work group's overall goals. It guides a specific multidisciplinary group's effort toward specifying and accomplishing its most important purpose (i.e., to enable clients to maintain an acceptable quality of life or optimum self-sufficiency or to prepare clients to receive needed services in less costly settings). The interdisciplinary team translates this mission into its specific purpose (i.e., providing specialized services to clients with complex needs served by their unit [e.g., oncology, primary care, convalescent cardiovascular care]) as a basis for building a positive culture of working together. As the interdisciplinary team works together, norms or mutual expectations evolve that support an atmosphere of mutual respect supportive of team building. Members of an interdisciplinary team accept mutual responsibility for helping clients achieve common goals. The interdisciplinary team as a special work group maintains commitment to a common purpose mutually agreed on that helps members to identify with each other and as a meaningful group within the agency (Weiss, 1990, p. 5). As a work group, interdisciplinary team members share success and accept responsibility for lack of success. The team identifies areas in which it can improve its performance as a whole. Interdisciplinary team members readily acknowledge that their work

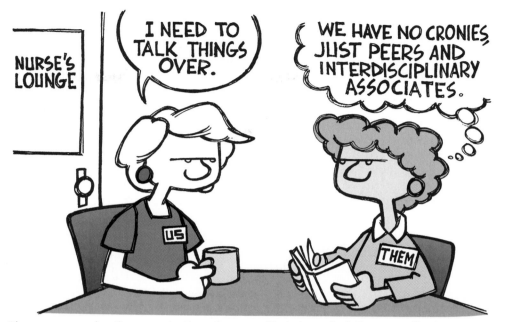

The more complex the organization, the more likely interdisciplinary conflict is to occur.

group is more likely to reach complex client care goals than they would be as individuals. This atmosphere promotes open, clear communication among members, including free expression of opinions and active listening.

### Structured Meeting Time and Place

An effective work group must have a **structured meeting time and place**. Health-care organizations need to provide meeting times and places for their work groups to communicate and collaborate (Moulder et al., 1988, p. 339) in addition to the day-to-day episodic interactions that occur while members of the work group provide care. Health-care organizations committed to effective work groups allocate resources so that group members can share information. When meetings are held, the nursing unit needs enough staff to cover a client care manager's clients while she or he attends the work group conference. Providing for meetings encourages the work group to discuss concerns and individual treatment responses to promote efficiency in addressing changes in client needs in a consistent and timely manner. Sharing knowledge of skills among group members often increases the value and credibility of the group and promotes creativity. Sometimes sharing expertise might entail continuing education programs and participation in in-service orientation programs (Reese and Sontag, 2001, p. 168).

Frequently, organizational support also includes developing staffing patterns that allow work group members to work together long enough to clarify roles and expectations and to become familiar with the common routines of the involved disciplines. Through a common understanding of the various disciplines represented

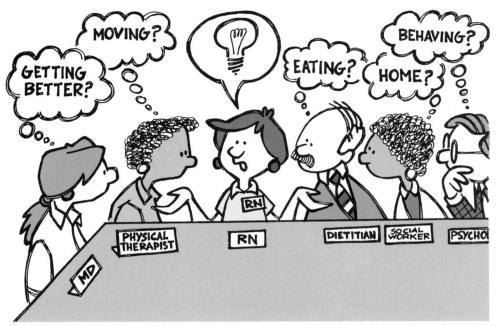

Effective communication is important to the interdisciplinary team.

in the group and the special talents of individual members, the work group is likely to identify a comprehensive range of treatment options available to meet common client needs in a cost-effective manner.

### Organizational Priorities

Health-care organizations use valuable staff time and human resources to support interdisciplinary work groups and to develop them into teams. It costs the agency money to provide time for group members to meet, confer, share, plan, and evaluate the extent of their success. Effective interdisciplinary groups and team-building efforts reflect the organization's priorities in providing complex client care and, when effective, are valuable organizational resources. To the extent that the organization supports structural changes needed by interdisciplinary groups, proactive work cultures, and collaboration between members, it increases work group productivity and competitive advantage over organizations that do not (Marshall, 1995, pp. 127–139).

## Comparing the Agency's Mission with Interdisciplinary Group Goals

A health-care agency's goals are likely to be stated in broad, general terms in a mission statement, as described earlier in this chapter. **Interdisciplinary group goals** reflect the special complex needs of the clients they serve and the knowledge and skills needed to meet those needs. The interdisciplinary group's purpose guides the formulation of mutual goals specific to individual client needs and activities.

The specific goals of individual clients mutually established by the interdisciplinary group and the client must be consistent with the agency's overall purposes and goals. If they are not, conflict is likely to result, and the group might not reach its goals due to lack of organizational support in the form of time, staffing, equipment, or supplies. To avoid unnecessary conflict, the health-care agency needs to communicate changes in its mission in a timely manner. Subsequently, the interdisciplinary team can incorporate these changes into their goals and activities to avoid conflict and frustration.

## Valuing the Contributions of Each Discipline

Due to the complexity of modern health care, every client is likely to use the resources of a multidisciplinary work group. That is, health problems that require care in an institutional setting are likely to require care from several disciplines. The composition of the multidisciplinary group corresponds to the type and complexity of services needed (e.g., diagnostic services, functional restoration, or supportive care). A client requiring primarily diagnostic services is likely to interact with a different group of professionals than a client who is receiving rehabilitation for a chronic health problem or a client receiving supportive care for a terminal illness.

**Client priorities** (i.e., the desired outcomes mutually agreed on by the individual client, family, and staff) also shape the contributions made by various disciplines. They determine how the client spends time in the health-care setting and how each discipline contributes to the client's well-being and achievement of desired outcomes. The interplay of these variables in the provision of individualized client care programs can cause confusion and **role conflicts** (incompatible or inconsistent expectations between multidisciplinary group members) if a common purpose, common goals, common language, norms for open communication, and accountability for results are inadequate.

Within the multidisciplinary group, different views of various disciplines as to who is to do what, when, and why for specific clients occur. To avoid multidisciplinary role conflicts, as evidenced by gaps or overlap in services provided, each member of the multidisciplinary group needs to understand what is expected of her or him and what reasonably can be expected of members of other disciplines. These expectations usually are determined by the following factors: the primary characteristics of the client's situation, type of setting, nature of client needs, group member's perceptions of the contributions of her or his discipline, and how these perceptions are communicated to other members. Specialized settings, such as settings focusing on psychiatric or rehabilitation services, require different disciplines (e.g., vocational rehabilitation specialists, counselors/substance abuse counselors, physiatrists) than are available in general hospitals or typical long-term care settings, where multidisciplinary work groups are more traditional in composition. Typical acute care settings usually provide more extensive diagnostic services than long-term care settings and might have more specialists available in this area of health care. In addition, communication among members of the multidisciplinary group is complicated by the fact that it occurs in various ways—face-to-face, by telephone, through automated information systems, or by written request forms.

Who does what depends on the nature of the client's needs and their complexity and the work group style (i.e., multidisciplinary or interdisciplinary). Often individual members of a specific discipline determine what is appropriate. For example, some physical therapists assist clients with exercises to strengthen upper extremities. Others might refer clients to other disciplines, such as occupational therapy. Some activity therapists might become centrally involved in developing spiritual programs, whereas others might assume a supportive role in such programs. To promote optimal effectiveness, these individual variations need to be communicated to the multidisciplinary group. A one-leader or team style work group should be selected depending on the nature of the client's needs and desired goals and the complexity of efforts and skills required to achieve them.

Because staff nurses frequently spend the most time with clients on a 24-hour basis, they often are expected to coordinate work group efforts. To do this, they rely on their knowledge of the client's needs and goals, the composition of the work group, and the special skills and talents of group members. In addition, they need to practice their assertiveness and collaborative work skills to advocate for individual clients in a timely manner. As norms evolve that support commitment to client goals and open communication, coordinating work group efforts may become less demanding and frustrating. Clients benefit from the work group's increased productivity (i.e., quality of service output per working hour) (Terry, 1992, p. 460). For example, a client with a recent amputation of a lower extremity must complete gastrointestinal x-rays needed to manage gastrointestinal distress. The client benefits from the nurse's effort to coordinate the scheduling of diagnostic studies requiring NPO (nothing per mouth) status and the therapies designed to increase mobility. Without this nursing coordination, the client's rehabilitation might be unnecessarily lengthened.

Staff nurses need to **value** their **nursing contributions** to work groups and to acknowledge verbally or respect behaviorally efforts made by members of other disciplines to satisfy client needs. These values are the foundation for building effective work groups and accountability for results. Many nursing students learn about the common contributions of various health disciplines early in their careers. Less frequently do they gain experience as a member of an interdisciplinary team that would help them to gain insight into the dynamics of such group work. Later, as entry-level staff nurses managing client care, they learn about special skills and contributions of individual members of interdisciplinary work groups. With a cooperative spirit, they need to communicate openly and collaborate with other work group members in an effort to meet specific, complex client needs. Effective teams are built by following through on identified special complex needs of clients and communicating concerns to other disciplines.

## PROMOTING EFFECTIVE WORKING RELATIONSHIPS IN WORK GROUPS

Client care managers are expected to promote effective working relationships among members of work groups to facilitate their success and promote team building (when teams exist). Persistent effort is needed to develop and sustain these relationships. As coordinator of multidisciplinary efforts, the client care manager has numerous opportunities to practice leadership skills and may contribute to team building.

## Clarifying Purpose

As mentioned earlier, each member of a work group needs a clear idea of the group's overall purpose to give meaning to the group's work. This principle emphasizes the importance of the group's goals and need for a language commonly understood by all members. Client care managers should not assume that everyone knows why the group exists and what is expected of its members. To do so is to invite conflict. By actively listening to the interactions of group members, the client care manager can identify differences in individual perceptions of the group's overall goals. These differences need to be clarified to avoid conflict within the group. As discussed in Chapter Ten, Coeling (1990, pp. 26–30) described five major categories of information that new graduates might use to analyze their work group cultures to help them adjust their practice to the norms and expectations of work groups common to nursing practice settings. Box 11-3 lists questions that nurses might use to analyze the **culture of the multidisciplinary work group**. Analyzing the answers to these questions also would help new graduates adjust their personal behaviors to the culture of the existing multidisciplinary work groups. Box 11-4 lists **principles for promoting effective working relationships** in interdisciplinary teams. Client care managers should apply these principles to develop interdisciplinary teams; these work groups are less common in nursing practice settings and will become increasingly more important in helping clients with complex needs. Accordingly, client care managers likely would benefit from participation on interdisciplinary teams.

## Meeting Group Goals

Each member of a work group needs to feel that he or she contributes to helping the group meet its goals. This need may seem obvious, but it can be difficult to fulfill, especially in rapidly changing work environments. Historically, nurses have struggled for professional autonomy, perhaps at the risk of decreased collaboration with others, especially physicians. Consistent with existing interdependencies, nurses appropriately emphasize cooperation and collaboration as strategies for interacting with various work groups. Rather than competing with each other, work group members need to determine priorities of care with clients and families, then plan how best to address them as a group with available resources. Although sometimes difficult to measure, every involved discipline's contribution to a client's care affects the plan's success in meeting desired outcomes. A discipline's authority to make decisions is not synonymous with the value of its contribution to client well-being. Collaborative efforts focus on making clinical decisions to achieve client outcomes rather than to further positional power or professional autonomy or control. Collaborative multidisciplinary work groups emphasize the contributions of participating disciplines to formulate and carry out a care plan efficiently and effectively.

BOX 11-3

## Questions to Ask to Understand the Culture of a Multidisciplinary Work Group

### Group Emphasis: Physiologic or Mental and Emotional Client Needs
Does the group consider it more important to address a client's physiologic or mental and emotional needs first?

How important is it to the group to be organized and efficient?

Does the group focus on the client's point of view and respect the client's values?

### Group Dynamics: Use of Power by Individual Members
Who can tell members what to do?

Who makes the decisions that determine what the work group does?

Does the group's leader use a more autocratic or democratic leadership style?

Are some members more influential than others? If so, what is the source of their influence?

### Group Spirit: Collaboration or Rivalry
Does a member or the whole group tend to decide what the multidisciplinary plan is for an individual client?

Do members tend to work alone to carry out their respective interventions?

How acceptable is it to compete with other members?

### Culture Building: Rewards and Discipline
Do members tend to criticize each other directly or indirectly?

Do members receive constructive criticism publicly or privately?

How are work group's efforts reinforced? By whom?

### Group Fashions: Tradition or Creative Change
Do members tend to value and stick to doing things in customary ways or get excited about learning and applying new approaches?

How important is it to follow policies and procedures? To what extent do members feel there is one right way to do things?

Adapted from Coeling HV: *Nurse Educ* 15(2):27, 1990.

It is hoped that as the emphases on increased productivity and cost-effectiveness persist, collaborative efforts are more likely to be recognized and rewarded. Subsequently, more interdisciplinary team building will occur.

Understanding the work group's culture is one strategy to help ensure that a client's goals are met. A work group culture includes norms, mores, and patterns of relating while the group focuses on common goals. Learning about the values of the work group culture helps the client care manager to gain insight into how the group sets priorities and implements collaborative plans of care. This information can be used to understand some of the bases for clinical decisions and patterns of commu-

> **BOX 11-4**
>
> ## Principles for Promoting Effective Working Relationships in Interdisciplinary Teams
>
> 1. Each member has a clear idea of the team's overall purpose in response to special complex client needs, which gives meaning to its work.
> 2. Each member feels that he or she can make or makes valued contributions that help the team meet its goals.
> 3. The team seeks and receives relevant, accurate, timely, and constructive feedback about its success in meeting its goals.
> 4. Group effort is rewarded (i.e., desired member behaviors are reinforced).
> 5. Members are encouraged to seek help regularly to develop skills needed to achieve the team's goals.
> 6. Members are encouraged to offer help willingly to develop other members' talents and skills.
> 7. Members share accountability for the team's success or lack of it as a group.

nicating and how the clinical services are scheduled and provided by various multidisciplinary work group members.

## Getting Feedback About Meeting Client Goals

The multidisciplinary work group needs relevant, accurate, consistent, and constructive feedback (i.e., factual information) about its progress in meeting client goals. To be most effective, feedback needs to be timely and given in such a way that it is understood by all group members. Through its form and style, feedback rewards positive behaviors while helping the group to avoid unproductive effort. Group members rarely tire of hearing about their successes when they are described accurately and sincerely. Typically the administrative staff and multidisciplinary work group members decide what data must be collected for program evaluation (i.e., continuous quality improvement), then how it will be made available to clinical staff. As mentioned in Chapter Ten, feedback helps the work group judge its effectiveness and identify areas needing further development. Information relating to the specific goals of individual clients also is collected. Often this information is gathered by analyzing data from relational databases, although additional data may need to be collected depending on the issues (e.g., equipment, supplies, staffing) being studied.

## Recognizing Positive Behaviors

The work group is strengthened when positive behaviors are recognized (i.e., when desired efforts toward the group's goals are rewarded). Rather than commenting, "You did a good job," one might say, "Your careful monitoring of M.T.'s discomfort helped her to avoid a serious reaction to the antibiotic." This is not to imply that group activities are not aimed at improving group performance, but that it is important to acknowledge regularly specific efforts that promote the group's success. More generally, open communication and expression of opinions free the group's creativity to identify healthy conflict within the group and identify new solutions. Using this creativity, the group may be able to solve old problems within the system that were interpreted earlier as individual performance problems.

## Sharing Knowledge and Skills

Developing mutual respect and effective collaboration among work group members is a complex process. Each discipline's unique knowledge base evolves in response to changing client needs, and the discipline's members are likely to be the most knowledgeable about these changes. Entry-level staff nurses need to acquaint themselves with multidisciplinary group members as individuals. They need to appreciate others' special interests in responding to various client needs. Members of the work group often need to be encouraged to seek help regularly from each other. Discussing client's responses reveals different perspectives that help the group to customize the planned treatment. For example, a child does not complain of pain caused by venipunctures. By comparing multidisciplinary observations of the child's behavior, the group is more likely to design strategies that better manage the pain and help the child cooperate to complete the procedures. Sharing special knowledge and skills promotes mutual respect, trust, and appreciation of the value of each other's contributions, which increases the value of the group's expertise. This approach also permits individual members to recognize limitations and seek help without risking a client's well-being. If multidisciplinary work group members are to keep pace with the information explosion and capitalize on the variety of interests pursued by individual members, sharing knowledge and skills needs to become an established norm in the work cultures of health-care organizations instead of being perceived as an ego trip. New knowledge and skills are likely to benefit clients and increase individual group member confidence and morale (Duffy et al., 2000, p. 780).

The opposite of seeking help is offering it. Most disciplines are willing to offer constructive help to each other. This sharing is likely to persist when group members trust each other and expect colleagues to receive help, without taking offense, when the goal is to improve the quality of client care. In such a work environment, offering help is likely to promote self-esteem and appreciation of the contributions of other disciplines. Sensitivity and tact are needed, as in all communications used to promote effective working relationships.

## Promoting Positive Relationships

Box 11-5 summarizes some "tried-and-true" approaches conducive to positive working relationships. Overall, strategies for working effectively with a nursing or multidisciplinary work group require staff nurses to show the value of nursing knowledge and skills by using them with confidence (Coker and Screiber, 1990, pp. 46–48). This encourages other members of the work group to respect nursing contributions. In addition, by seeking to clarify the roles and expectations of various other members of the work group, staff nurses can learn about the special knowledge and skills used by members of nursing work groups or by members of other disciplines in client care. By reinforcing positive behaviors, such as seeking and offering help, each member of the work group can maximize the effective use of available nursing or multidisciplinary knowledge and skills on behalf of clients.

Interdisciplinary team building proceeds at varying rates, depending on how much it is valued by the organization and how much support team members receive. With the increased emphasis on higher productivity as a means to help health-care providers remain competitive and cost-effective, more organizations may encourage team building.

## BARRIERS TO MULTIDISCIPLINARY GROUP EFFECTIVENESS

Given the complexities of client care and the variety of disciplines, work cultures, and individual personalities involved, it is not surprising that the multidisciplinary group sometimes is unsuccessful in increasing productivity. Considerable potential for conflict exists. Eliminating multidisciplinary groups is no longer an option due to the increasing complexities of health care. The interdependencies of the various disciplines involved in providing health care are likely to continue or increase in the future. Every discipline shares responsibility for enhancing multidisciplinary cooperation and collaboration for the benefit of clients. The skills needed to resolve interpersonal conflict described in Chapter Seven are useful for members of various groups.

Identifying common **barriers** to the effectiveness of multidisciplinary groups can help the client care manager improve productivity. Because a multidisciplinary

---

**BOX 11-5**

### Core Communications for Team Building: "There is no I in Team"

The six most important words:
  *"We appreciate your trying to help."*
The five most important words:
  *"You did a nice job."*
The four most important words:
  *"What is your recommendation?"*
The three most important words:
  *"If you prefer."*
The two most important words:
  *"Thank you."*
The most important word:
  *"We"*

work group is an expensive agency resource, its effectiveness merits thoughtful nurturing. Sometimes a health-care agency bears the expense of a multidisciplinary group without adequately evaluating the benefits clients derive from it. The health-care agency and the individual members of a work group share responsibility for success. While coordinating the group's efforts and acting as client advocates, client care managers often are aware of missed opportunities. By being aware of potential barriers to the groups' effectiveness, the staff nurse is in a good position to nurture its success.

In the hectic, stress-filled health-care work environment, clients often feel extremely vulnerable. Health-care workers try to do the best they can with the resources they have. In this environment, the care that clients receive can be fragmented and lacks focus even though the health-care work groups are highly motivated and skilled. Each discipline may be intent on providing the best care possible but lack an overall perspective from the client's point of view. Priorities of care often are not identified. Often, if the group has not worked together for long, there are no common goals. Unless the group has sufficient time and a place to meet and share concerns, it suffers from a lack of direction. Unless the agency's mission and overall multidisciplinary work group's purpose and goals are clear, its members often continue pursuing their respective disciplines' goals for clients. Clarifying the agency's mission or values can help to reduce conflict and identify and overcome potential barriers of this sort.

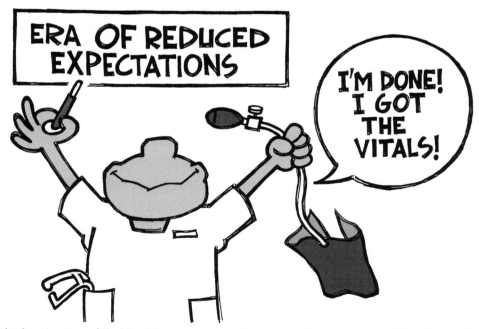

In the hectic, stress-filled health-care work environment, the care received by clients often is fragmented, even though the health-care team is highly motivated and skilled.

Each discipline is likely to observe the client in a slightly different situation. The approaches and treatment methods of the different disciplines lead to different perceptions of the client's suitability and responses to services provided (Hodes and Crombrugghe, 1990, pp. 73–75). To the client, these varying expectations may seem to be in conflict, when they merely may represent the different interpretations of individual work group members. Sometimes past experiences influence the values and attitudes of individual group members toward specific client situations. For example, a client experiencing difficulty controlling bowel elimination might be omitted prematurely from scheduled speech therapy sessions away from the nursing unit to avoid embarrassing "accidents." At the same time, other disciplines that regard speech therapy as a high priority might have made a special effort to adjust their interventions to enable the client to attend. The client is likely to experience frustration and difficulty in expressing his or her concerns to the group. The members of the work group need to communicate with each other and the client to avoid being distracted from the client's priorities. A special effort is needed to clarify goals, approaches, expectations, and values to enable the group to meet each client's health-care needs in a timely manner. When conflicts arise, it is crucial to analyze the situation rather than to attempt to fix blame on specific group members.

As technology evolves to permit the rapid transmission of information, health-care workers will continue to be confronted with the challenge of keeping up with current knowledge in their discipline. The need for a common language is likely to increase to meet these information needs. The specific, detailed information required to address a client's situation often is available only through automated systems (Swenson-Feldman and Brugge-Wiger, 1985, pp. 44–46). Staff nurses are expected to use automated systems to document care so that members of all disciplines have access to current information regarding client needs. Special effort is needed to communicate current information in a common language so that it is accessible to all disciplines. Client care managers, as coordinators, would benefit from the use of electronic integrated health-care information systems and computerized clinical records.

An effective multidisciplinary work group knows who is expected to carry out each part of the care plan for every client. Without a current written plan of care, avoiding overlaps and gaps in care is difficult, and evaluating the effectiveness of the group's contributions and the plan in general in nearly impossible. To prevent overlaps and gaps, each member of the multidisciplinary group must know what the plan is and what is expected of group members from each discipline. As technology evolves and knowledge bases expand, continued effort is needed to clarify the various roles of each discipline represented on the multidisciplinary group. Identification of individual client priority needs helps each discipline to anticipate what contribution it might make toward enabling the client to meet desired outcomes.

Marked differences in group members' personalities can interfere with the multidisciplinary group's effectiveness, but this type of barrier may be less common than often is thought. Before attributing the cause of the group's ineffectiveness to "personality conflicts," it is sound practice first to ensure that other barriers are not at fault. As the multidisciplinary group focuses on individual client goals and establishes effective communication processes to meet them, the norms of the work culture are likely to help members focus on major issues and concerns that interfere with the group's work instead of on individual idiosyncrasies.

If the individual idiosyncrasies of group members continue to result in interpersonal conflict, they need to be resolved using the suggestions discussed in Chapter Seven. No one is expected to change his or her personality. Rather, each member involved in the conflict is expected to try to change behaviors in an effort to provide quality client care in a responsible manner.

## PRIORITIES OF THE MULTIDISCIPLINARY GROUP

As the cost of health care escalates and the acuity of client health conditions increases, care during illness becomes more complex. The interdependencies of the work groups also increase. Clients depend on their caregivers to respond to their urgent needs in an effective and timely manner. In addition, because of the scarcity of human resources, a high value is placed on staff time and its efficient use to meet individual client needs. The client's well-being, if not survival, depends on early identification of urgent needs and their management as top staff priorities.

### Addressing Priority Client Needs

Client care managers are expected to help the multidisciplinary groups address priority client needs. To begin, each group needs to focus its efforts on individual client goals and assessed health problems. To ensure that the client receives services as planned, the client care manager must differentiate nursing priorities from the priorities identified by the multidisciplinary group to meet client goals. Often, owing to the complexity of the care needed, much nursing time and effort are consumed in addressing nursing care. The client care manager also needs to address multidisciplinary interdependencies, however, to ensure that the client receives the right care at the right time. For example, client care managers might place high priority on client comfort, whereas the multidisciplinary group might focus their efforts on increasing the client's physical mobility, endurance, and strength. It is not in the client's best interest, however, to support the lack of attendance at other high-priority therapies to avoid discomfort.

To avoid omitting important aspects of quality care, the client care manager needs to participate in multidisciplinary activities to help organize activities on the basis of client needs and priorities, rather than those of a specific discipline (Summers et al., 1988, pp. 665–670). By contributing to scheduled multidisciplinary group conferences, client care managers can obtain current information about client progress in various therapies. Desired client outcomes must be described in terms of long-term and short-term goals to avoid costly complications or inefficiency (i.e., establishing discharge dates and client needs that require continued treatment). Developing multidisciplinary care plans as critical paths or care maps likely will enhance the work group's effectiveness and efficiency by communicating expectations clearly (i.e., by specifying scheduled interventions) for group members. Defining long-term and short-term goals provides important time frames to help staff plan for changes in individual client treatment programs and to evaluate patterns of responses to treatment. These goals help the work group to plan continuing care and communicate as needed concerning available community resources in a timely way. Monitoring data about achieved client outcomes and variances within established care maps helps multidisciplinary groups evaluate their standards of care. Examples of established care maps are often part of integrated health information systems and might be described most simply in client education booklets and materials.

Given the hectic pace of health care, special effort is needed to identify specific plans and guidelines to measure the progress of individual clients. This planning helps nursing and multidisciplinary work groups to reduce inefficiencies and to ensure proper handling of life-threatening priorities of client care. To address this organizational need of multidisciplinary work groups, meeting times and places are structured to enable the group to communicate concerns about individual client goals at regular intervals and to revise plans in a timely manner.

## COORDINATING EFFORTS OF THE MULTIDISCIPLINARY GROUP

Individual client care goals and plans reflect multidisciplinary group priorities. Client care managers often are expected to coordinate the efforts of the multidisciplinary groups. This coordination entails knowing individual client care priorities and communicating them to the appropriate members of the multidisciplinary group in a timely manner. Coordinating does not include any decision-making authority, however, for other disciplines or on behalf of the client (Gadow, 1989, p. 541; Shaffer and Preziosi, 1988, p. 603). Rather, the nurse acts as a client advocate, helping to articulate concerns and communicate them to the multidisciplinary group (Prins, 1992, p. 78). By following several guidelines, the staff nurse can perform coordination duties efficiently and effectively.

## Maintaining Client-Centered Focus

To ensure that priority needs are met, the multidisciplinary work group needs to remain client-centered. The work group focus guides the focus of nursing. This focus of efforts is first and foremost on client needs; accordingly, staff scheduling, socialization, agency efficiency, and economizing rank no higher than second in importance. As changes in client needs occur, they are communicated to the members of the multidisciplinary work group whom they affect. Feedback helps the members to evaluate client responses to their plan and care.

## Sharing Responsibility for Desired Client Outcomes

As coordinator of the multidisciplinary group, the client care manager shares responsibility for enabling the client to meet desired outcomes of care. In this capacity, the client care manager frequently explains to clients, families, and staff why routine actions have been taken in the client's behalf. This accountability is shared with other individual members of the group. If a client has questions about the specific knowledge, skills, or methods used by members of another discipline to provide complex interventions, the nurse usually asks a member of that discipline to answer them. The nurse also might ask a group member to explain a complex treatment to ensure that the client has accurate information. These situations might arise when a client receives complex diagnostic preparations, drugs, dietary interventions, or specific exercises.

## Sharing Responsibility for Developing and Communicating Plan of Care

The case manager shares responsibility for developing the multidisciplinary plan of care and communicating it to involved group members. To succeed, the client care manager needs to understand what this plan is and be able to describe it clearly to others, using a common language. This responsibility includes promptly entering nursing information into the clinical record used by other disciplines to enable them to carry out the details of individual treatment plans. This information must be accurate, legible, and accessible when others need it to complete their activities in a timely manner. Changes in dietary plans associated with diagnostic studies are communicated to the nutrition department to ensure that the client receives adequate nourishment at appropriate times (e.g., when the client no longer needs to remain NPO on successful completion of a procedure).

## Supporting Group Effort to Carry Out Plan

The client care manager supports the multidisciplinary work group effort to carry out the plan. This support includes providing information and reinforcing explanations of the approaches used by other members of the group. Sometimes, to promote effective use of time, the nurse might assemble needed equipment and supplies. Each group member shares responsibility for performing all procedures and treatments safely. Consequently, each member of the group makes his or her needs for special equipment known to the agency staff expected to obtain them. In addition, the nurse frequently helps clients to prepare for scheduled procedures and treatment sessions so that members of other disciplines can provide them efficiently. This preparation often includes providing comfort measures in anticipation of the treatment, enabling the client to wear special attire, or scheduling activities to maximize the benefits the client derives from the procedures.

## Communicating Changes in Care Plan Goals or Interventions

The client care manager communicates changes in the goals or interventions of multidisciplinary care plans to affected multidisciplinary and nursing group members. Other disciplines often are brought up to date efficiently on changes when the group regularly schedules a time and place for this activity. Communication forms often are used to transmit routine information, but it can be transmitted electronically if the agency's information system is sufficiently automated. If scheduled sessions with the client need to be changed or discontinued on short notice, this should be communicated as soon as possible to enable members of other disciplines to revise their work plans and use available time effectively. The nursing staff shares responsibility for carrying out the multidisciplinary plan with other members of the group. A common example is the need to inform the physical therapy staff when a client is unable to attend a scheduled therapy session due to discomfort or activity intolerance.

## Evaluating Client Progress

The client care manager participates in evaluating the work group's success in enabling individual clients to achieve desired outcomes. To evaluate client progress, the client care manager needs to know what the multidisciplinary plan is, who is doing what to carry it out, and what time frame for outcomes is anticipated. Frequently the time frame corresponds to the client's insurance coverage program requirements. This information is invaluable to the client care manager in coordinating work group efforts and helps in planning for the client's continuing care. Client care managers often use information about the client's health insurance benefits to plan and evaluate outcomes of care and, if necessary, to refer the client to other less costly services available in the community.

## FUTURE AND TEAM BUILDING

As mentioned at the beginning of this chapter, simply because a group of people work together does not make them a team. The value of real teams in increasing productivity often has been underestimated, however. Real teams that permanently connect their performance with their purpose and share accountability for their results are powerful in transforming work environments. The evolving culture of teams is perhaps the least understood organizational resource for increasing work group productivity (Katzenbach and Smith, 2001, pp. 1–4; Marshall, 1995, p. 128).

Escalating health-care costs are likely to precipitate productivity crises, which may promote the development of collaborative work groups. These crises will encourage the development of real multidisciplinary work groups and interdisciplinary teams with a purpose consistent with the overall mission of the health-care facility. These groups need organizational support that provides them with structure, facilities, and equipment necessary for them to be able to confer, strategize, communicate, collect data, and evaluate their progress.

A team will develop only when a sense of trust exists and open communication occurs. Group members are likely to learn to work together as a group only by actually doing so ("on-the-job training") because few professionals obtain skills needed to be an effective interdisciplinary work group member in their formal preparation (Marotta et al., 2000, p. 26). Group members need to use leadership and group work knowledge and skills to develop commitment to the work group's goals and to prepare for the changes that will enable them to function collaboratively. All stakeholders in the change process need to be informed and involved to the extent feasible. Commitment to team goals will be tested when plans for change are carried out.

Given the availability of technology to gather and analyze data, the next phase of team development is likely to focus on the group's success in meeting its short-term and long-term goals. Typically, data are used to evaluate how well the team achieved its goals in meeting complex client needs in accordance with the agency's mission. Group members need to look realistically at progress, barriers, and the types and cost of resources needed to remain successful. True teams are likely to focus on their productivity instead of factors such as major restructuring or downsizing.

As teams increase their success, greater emphasis will be placed on sustaining their interdisciplinary productivity and facilitating their adjustments to required changes due to evolving trends affecting health care (Schofield and Amodeo, 1999, p. 218). These changes are likely to revolve around changing client population needs, agency mission, costs of health care, and availability of needed human resources. Considerable resources may be needed to sustain effective interdisciplinary health teams. The resources needed for this renewal include team-building skills for new members, continuing education, and personal and career development programs for team members.

Interdisciplinary team members are likely to participate on more than one team within an organization. This participation is likely to enhance the individual's skills and contributions if the person is not overly stressed or overwhelmed by demands placed on her or him.

The time for collaborative teams has come. By recognizing and accepting the need to maximize their productivity, members of various health-care disciplines can formulate plans for making positive changes in work cultures, processes, and outcomes. Technology will be used to collect and analyze data on effectiveness. As the costs of complex health care continue to escalate, collaborative teams will need time, facilities, and resources to address these demands and revise their strategies for maintaining or increasing their productivity.

## SUMMARY

The advent of the informational era has increased the interdependencies of work groups. To increase productivity, multidisciplinary groups will need to function more effectively as work groups. Client care managers are expected to coordinate the efforts of multidisciplinary groups to improve quality and reduce fragmentation of care on behalf of clients. They use skills in human relations and group work to succeed, emphasizing cooperation and collaboration.

Interdisciplinary work groups (i.e., teams) are a valuable organizational resource. They need a common purpose that is consistent with the health-care agency's mission, size, and common goals; complementary skills; mutual accountability; shared language; and a structured time and place to discuss common concerns, client priorities, and corresponding treatment plans. Each member of the group is committed to the values of a specific discipline, and his or her contribution reflects the unique knowledge and skills of that discipline. In addition to valuing their own disciplines, members learn to value the contributions of other disciplines to meet priority client needs and to develop new skills needed to accomplish the team's goals.

Client care managers should use their leadership skills to contribute to team building. They communicate their concerns and skills through what they say and do. Specific effort is needed to strengthen desired patterns of behavior and to provide feedback to the group about client responses to treatment programs. In the interest of providing quality care, work group members are encouraged to seek help from others and to offer it as well. By identifying barriers to multidisciplinary group effectiveness, client care managers can avoid destructive conflict. They can use communication skills to resolve conflict to enable the work group to focus on client needs and goals.

Client care managers use their nursing knowledge to help identify client priorities. They actively discuss plans of care and provide timely information when client conditions and plans change. By referring to individual client short-term and long-term goals, they help the group evaluate the effectiveness of a plan and make arrangements for the client's continued care as long as it is needed. Client care managers provide feedback to help the group identify successes and areas needing further development. The interdisciplinary work group is encouraged to collaborate and cooperate as colleagues rather than to compete.

Each discipline represented on the client's care work group believes it can help achieve outcomes desired by the client and family. Each group member approaches the client's situation from the perspective of his or her own discipline. Accordingly, each discipline has specific goals for each client, which need to be consistent with the group's overall goals for the client. Working toward common goals for individual clients requires cooperation and collaboration among members. Without open communication, neither cooperation nor collaboration is likely to occur. Nurses, similar to members of other disciplines represented on the multidisciplinary work group, need to make a specific effort to ensure that client needs and goals are understood and that accurate up-to-date references to them are readily accessible.

Client care managers need to make specific efforts to establish nursing goals with individual clients that are consistent with overall goals. These goals guide nursing staff activities and help the client care manager to coordinate the multidisciplinary group's efforts. Usually the long-term goals established depend on the client's length of stay at the health-care agency. The time involved varies, depending on the type of agency and the client's individual needs. Shorter term goals refer to gradations of client accomplishments required to succeed overall.

To increase effectiveness and efficiency, information about the client's responses and condition needs to be communicated to the multidisciplinary group at regular intervals. Unless a structured process for this communication is established (i.e., scheduled multidisciplinary work group conferences), the client's care is likely to be fragmented and deviate from the plan. In addition, opportunities to reinforce the client's progress can be missed, making it more difficult to sustain the client's motivation and group morale.

Feedback about the client's progress and the group's success is crucial in monitoring progress toward overall goals. Gaps and overlaps in group efforts often surface; frequently, they result from lack of information that exists but is not readily accessible or communicated to individuals affected by it. Group members need to concentrate their efforts on meeting client goals and avoid blaming one another. If conflicts arise, differences in goals and perceptions need to be identified and clarified. The group's plan is revised to meet priority client needs, in a spirit of collaboration and cooperation rather than competition among disciplines.

In the future, entry-level staff members are likely to be involved in collaborative teams. These teams will strive to increase productivity in response to the escalating costs of complex health care.

## APPLICATION EXERCISES

1. Give three examples of nursing or multidisciplinary group member behaviors reflecting cooperation and collaboration that promoted the recovery of clients for whom you have provided care. Describe your nursing contributions in these situations.
2. Make a list of five terms that you believe have the same meaning for all members of the multidisciplinary group. Verify the meaning of each of these terms with at least three different multidisciplinary group members.
3. Become acquainted with the work culture of the multidisciplinary group by systematically answering the questions suggested in this chapter. Identify any surprises.
4. Note communication patterns among multidisciplinary work group members while participating in a conference. Make a list of the ways that positive relationships among multidisciplinary group members were promoted. Describe two circumstances caused by communication barriers.
5. Compare your nursing priorities with the priorities of the multidisciplinary group for one of your assigned clients.
6. State the common purpose of a multidisciplinary group of which you were a member. Limit the statement to one sentence.

## CRITICAL THINKING SCENARIO

Imagine that you are a recently employed "new" member of a nursing and a multidisciplinary group in an extended care facility. Your clients typically are convalescing from multiple health-care problems that have reduced significantly their functional abilities to manage their personal care within their homes. The stated mission of the facility is to provide needed rehabilitation for the clients; the informal purpose is to provide rehabilitation for the length of stay "covered" in the individual's health insurance plan. Often the "covered" length of stay is over before the client reaches maximum benefit, causing the client to use personal funds or be discharged to another long-term care facility instead of home. The customer satisfaction survey results indicate declining quality of care. You notice that morale is low, direct service staff members are feeling stressed by the potential of being "laid off" due to decreasing census, and administrative staff members do not remain for longer than 2 years.

**CRITICAL THINKING SCENARIO—cont'd**

Effective, timely communication among disciplines and nursing work groups is the exception rather than the routine.

1. What would you do to clarify your employment status at this facility for the long-term?
2. What actions would you take to increase nursing and multidisciplinary group productivity?
3. What strategies would you use to improve communication between administration and the clinical staff? Among members of the nursing work groups? Among members of the multidisciplinary groups?
4. Would you plan to commit to team building for the "long haul"? Give reasons for your answer.

## REFERENCES

Carrol PF: Turf wars: time for a truce? *Nursing 87 17*(12):43, 1987.

Coeling HV: Organizational culture: helping new graduates adjust, *Nurse Educ 15*(2):26–30, 1990.

Coker EB, Screiber R: The nurse's role in a team conference, *Nurs Manage 21*(3):46–48, 1990.

Duffy MK, Shaw JD, Stark EM: Performance and satisfaction in conflicted interdependent groups: when and how does self-esteem make a difference? *Acad Manage J 43*(4):772–782, 2000.

Gadow S: Clinical subjectivity, *Nurs Clin North Am 24*(6):535–541, 1989.

Gibson CB: Do they do what they believe they can? Group efficacy and group effectiveness across tasks and cultures, *Acad Manage J 42*(2):138–152, 1999.

Guy ME: Interdisciplinary conflict and organizational complexity, *Hosp Health Serv Admin 31*(3):111–121, 1986.

Hammond K, Bandak A, Williams M: Nurse, physician, and consumer role responsibility perceived by health care providers, *Holist Nurs Pract 13*(2):28–37, 1999.

Heinemann GD, Schmitt, MH, Farrell MP, Brallier SA: Development of an attitude toward health care teams scale, *Eval Health Professions 22*(1):123–142, 1999.

Higgins SE, Routhieaux RL: A multiple-level analysis of hospital team effectiveness, *Health Care Superv 17*(4):1–13, 1999.

Hinojosa J, Bedell G, Buchholz ES, Charles J, Shigaki IS, Bicchieri SM: Team collaboration: a case study of an early intervention team, *Qual Health Res 11*(2): 206–220, 2001.

Hodes JR, Crombrugghe PV: Nurse-physician relationships: difference of perspective is one reason for continued nurse/physician conflict, *Nurs Manage 21*(7):73–75, 1990.

Karpuik K, Fjerestad T, Young S: Integrated care at the bedside: job description consensus, *Nurs Manage 25*(8):41–43, 1994.

Katzenbach JR, Smith DK: *The wisdom of teams: creating high-performance organization*, New York, NY, 1993, McKinsey & Co.

Katzenbach JR, Smith DK: *The discipline of teams: a mindbook-workbook for delivering small group performance*, New York, NY, 2001, John Wiley & Sons.

Marotta SA, Peters BJ, Paliokas KL: Teaching group dynamics: an interdisciplinary model, *Journal for Specialists in Group Work 25*(1):16–28, 2000.

Marshall EM: *Transforming the way we work: the power of the collaborative workplace*, New York, NY, 1995, AMACOM, a division of the American Management Association.

Moulder PA, Staal AM, Grant M: Making the interdisciplinary team approach work, *Rehabil Nurs 13*(6):338–339, 1988.

Prins MM: Patient advocacy: the role of nursing leadership, *Nurs Manage 23*(7): 78–80, 1992.

Reese DJ, Sontag MA: Successful interprofessional collaboration on the hospice team, *Health Social Work 26*(3):167–175, 2001.

Rheaume A, Frisch S, Smith A, et al: Case management and nursing practice, *J Nurs Admin 24*(3):30–35, 1994.

Schofield RF, Amodeo M: Interdisciplinary teams in health care and human services settings: are they effective? *Health Social Work 24*(3):210–219, 1999.

Shaffer FA, Preziosi P: Nursing: the hospital's competitive edge, *Nurs Clin North Am 23*(3):597–612, 1988.

Slack MK, McEwen MM: The impact of interdisciplinary case management on client outcomes, *Fam Community Health 22*(3):30–48, 1999.

Sluzki CE: Patients, clients, consumers: the politics of words, *Families Systems Health 18*(3):347–352, 2000.

Strasser DC, Smits SJ, Falconer JA, Herrin JS, Bowen SE: The influence of hospital culture on rehabilitation team functioning in VA hospitals, *J Rehabil Res Dev 39*(1):115–125, 2002.

Summers PM, Nadermann N, Turnis RM, et al: Quality management: program design—an interdisciplinary approach, *Nurs Clin North Am 23*(3):665–670, 1988.

Swenson-Feldman E, Brugge-Wiger P: Promotion of interdisciplinary practice through an automated information system, *Adv Nurs Sci 7*(4):47, 1985.

Terry JV: *International management handbook*, Fayetteville, AR, 1992, The University of Arkansas Press.

Weiss DH: Total teamwork: how to build an effective team, *Supervis Manage 35*(8):5, 1990.

# 12

# *Supervising and Evaluating the Work of Others*

## OBJECTIVES

*When you complete this chapter, you will be able to:*

1. Describe how client satisfaction influences an agency's definition of quality care.
2. Describe indications, characteristics, and goals of client advocacy.
3. Explain the functions of supervision.
4. Describe the characteristics of effective supervision.
5. Explain the principles of evaluating client care provided by others.
6. Describe the essential characteristics of the supervisory relationship between the client care manager and supervisees.

## KEY CONCEPTS

consumerism
quality care
 perspectives
  clients
  staff
  agency
 components
  structure
  process
  outcomes
client advocate
 paternalism

beneficence
maleficence
autonomy
supervision
 functions
  characteristics of effective
   supervision
evaluation of client care done by others
 standard of care
 criteria
responsibility for the action and
 nonaction of subordinates

## SATISFYING CUSTOMERS AS A FOCUS OF CLIENT CARE MANAGEMENT

Entry-level staff nurses supervise and evaluate the work of others with whom they share responsibility for providing quality care to clients. To fulfill the responsibilities of this component of the staff nurse's role, nursing services focus on satisfying client needs as the primary component of the health-care agency's purpose. To supervise effectively the work of others aimed at meeting client needs requires that the entry-level staff nurse, as client care manager, be a client advocate from time to time. While supervising the work of the nursing work group and coordinating the efforts of multidisciplinary groups, the staff nurse continuously evaluates the effectiveness of client services they provide. Satisfying customers—clients (external) and staff (internal)—is the focus of the staff nurse's efforts.

## RISING TIDE OF CONSUMERISM

**Consumerism,** a social movement that aims to protect clients or recipients from inferior or dangerous services, has intensified in the health-care industry with the increased publicity of unsafe care, medication errors, and emphasis on cost controls (Adams, 2000, p. 164; Smith, 2001, p. 293). Consumers, as key stakeholders, are demanding high-quality health-care services (Savage et al., 2000, p. 101). Consequently, client satisfaction is a prerequisite for a health-care agency's success. The staff nurse responsible for meeting client needs also is expected to promote client satisfaction with services received. Because it requires that client care managers address the health-care organization's needs and the client's needs, this responsibility complicates the supervisory process. The perspectives of clients and staff need to be respected.

With the evolution of the informational era, clients expect to choose how they will use their time, resources, and talents. This includes expecting to participate in making the decisions that affect how their individual health-care needs are managed (Larrabee, 1995, p. 10). As Toffler (1980, pp. 265–288) predicted, modern technology develops more options for individuals in many aspects of daily living, including health care. Increased availability of health-care information helps consumers obtain up-to-date information, think independently, and be assertive about their needs (Adams, 2000, p. 164). As a result, some health-care providers perceive that clients are justifiably more demanding than they were a decade or more earlier (Larrabee, 1995, p. 10; Sinclair, 1990, p. 63).

As health-care consumers, clients today have greater access to current information. Many clients learn about available health-care services, technology, and equipment from the mass media. Mass media has been used to create public awareness and pressure for increased expectations of treatment (Tomes, 2001, p. 544). Consumers expect providers to pay detailed attention to their individual needs. Concurrently, as a result of present health-care financing mechanisms related primarily to economic trends, clients personally pay a greater proportion of the costs of their health care. These trends influence health-care strategies. Many health-care providers compete to maintain or increase the number of clients they serve. Health-care organizations have responded by offering more programs and services than those traditionally provided. Most providers believe that satisfied clients are more likely to return to them for needed health care. Realizing that satisfied clients expect to participate actively in their care, providers involve them in decision making. Consumers are satisfied when their experiences match their expectations (Oermann and Templine, 2001, p. 240). Satisfaction with the quality of health care received is related closely to whether the client received the care that he or she perceived as necessary. Client satisfaction is an accepted and established measure of quality care (Goldstein and Schweikhart, 2002, p. 74; Larrabee, 1995, p. 12; Nelson et al., 1989, p. 185).

To help evaluate their services and measure client satisfaction, many health-care organizations request feedback from clients after discharge. Although the reliability of this approach should be questioned, this method has identified some important facets of client satisfaction that have been confirmed by more systematic study. Client perceptions of the amount of time spent waiting for services has been delineated as one key factor related to their satisfaction with health-care services received (Hildman and Ferguson, 1990, pp. 26–29). The findings of such studies are used to plan specific organizational efforts to increase promptness in providing services. Ultimately, focusing on client satisfaction with services received is a common method of improving the quality of care. In this way, the rising tide of consumerism in mainstream society is having profound effects on the quality of health care (Sower et al., 2001, p. 57).

In another study of client perceptions of quality care, Cramer and Tucker (1995, p. 66) reported that clients were better able to evaluate quality of care when they were guided by standards of care. Some strategies that are used to guide clients may be care paths or learning checklists with an emphasis on a partnership of clients and providers in establishing desired outcomes (Cramer and Tucker, 1995, pp. 56–62). In another report, Decker (1999, pp. 20–21) described customer service communication skills as a core competency required by all human service workers providing health care in hospitals. Nurses have established a long history of striving to provide client-centered care. By providing quality care, nurses will continue to be an integral part of health care in the future.

## DEFINING QUALITY CARE

**Quality care** (i.e., services that consistently produce desired results or outcomes) is a universal concern in health-care organizations. Because of their different vested interests as stakeholders, clients and providers perceive quality of care from different **perspectives. Clients** define quality care from their perspective: "They [providers] looked like they knew what they were doing"; "They explained things to me"; "I got better." The value of incorporating client perspectives into definitions of quality care has long been accepted by nurses and slowly is being recognized by other health-care providers (Geron et al., 2000, p. S259; Larrabee, 1995, p. 12; Lehmann, 1989, p. 227; Mayer and Cates, 1999, pp. 1281–1282; Nelson et al., 1989, pp. 185–186).

Health-care providers or **staff** define quality care from a perspective different from recipients of care, considering such factors as the acuity of the client's illness, availability of resources (staffing, equipment, and time required to address client needs), and standards of care provided compared with standards of practice they believe are essential for quality care. From the perspective of the **agency,** important issues include providing the resources needed by anticipated target populations; developing processes for delivering services; and creating explicit, established standards of care. The agency's perspective varies with the type of setting and predominant methods of financing (Docteur, 2001, p. 59; Griffiths et al., 2000, p. 529; Himmelstein et al., 1999, p. 159; Noble and Klein, 2000, p. 199; Torpy, 2002, pp. 177–178).

When considering crucial characteristics of quality care, it is necessary to remember that quality and evaluation always involve an element of subjectivity (del Bueno, 1990, p. 4). Evaluation involves ranking the importance of various benefits, or placing "value" on various aspects of quality care. Different components of quality care are measured, and corresponding data are collected and interpreted. Evaluation of care ultimately involves a subjective judgment by the evaluator and reflects the perspective of the specific stakeholder. When attempting to maintain or increase the quality of care, the measurements used need to quantify the aspects of care that staff can change (i.e., performance indicators versus health outcomes [e.g., preventive interventions in the home setting versus mortality in a facility providing tertiary care]) (Giuffrida et al., 1999, p. 94).

While supervising the work of others, staff nurses need to distinguish client perceptions, which often are based on personal experience, from perceptions of clinical staff, which usually are based on professional standards of practice and

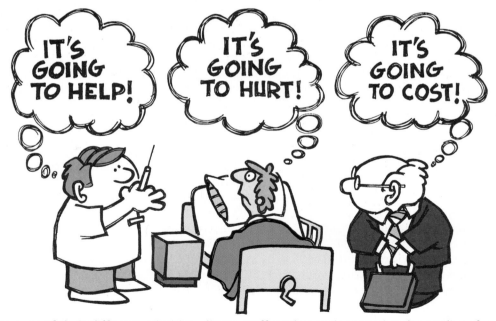

Because of their different priorities, clients, staff, and agencies perceive the quality of care differently.

institutionally established standards of care (Cramer and Tucker, 1995, p. 54; Patterson, 1988, pp. 628–629). Client care managers share responsibility for ensuring that every staff member understands the agency's definition of quality care. Sharing a common definition helps staff develop the system and language required to guide and direct service staff. Commitment to the agency's definition of quality care is so important that many health-care organizations consume considerable resources to make it explicit and explain its ramifications to staff. The staff uses this definition and related goals and standards as the basis for developing a system and process for providing quality care.

## Components of Quality Health Care

A universal definition of quality health care is elusive. Quality as a concept relates to the different expectations of various stakeholders (e.g., clients, staff, payers). Quality health care is believed to consist of three basic **components**: structure, process, and outcomes. The client population served needs to participate in each of the three components as partners with providers of their care.

### *Structure*

The **structure** of quality care is how the agency organizes its resources to match the specific needs of the client population it serves (Stewart and Lockamy, 2001, p. 50). Structure is reflected in staffing patterns and equipment and other agency resources made available to care for clients. The structure of quality care for acutely ill pediatric clients differs from that of chronically ill, middle-aged clients. The structure for pediatric clients would involve other key decision makers, whereas middle-aged clients are likely to make decisions about their own care. The basic parts of the service program are likely to differ in terms of staffing, equipment, and use of other agency services and resources. If the agency provides care only for pediatric clients, its purpose and mission and the methods used to address them differ from those of an agency whose client population includes persons of varying ages throughout the life span. The structure design needs to integrate flexibility into its responses to guide staff providing services for the wide variety of health problems presented by its client population.

An important component of the structure of quality care is the agency's explicit attempts to identify and distinguish its customers' expectations from their needs (Schneider and Bowen, 1995, pp. 19–84). They emphasize that the structure of quality service will satisfy customer needs for security (feelings of safety), justice (feeling fairly treated), and esteem (feeling competent to handle one's needs responsibly and able to solve problems with choices available). The perceptions of clients are important in designing the structure of quality health care.

Awareness of the need to develop a culture (i.e., work environment) of customer-oriented service is increasing. Such cultures value employees as people, as shown by the many and varied ways they are treated: "the culture employees experience will be the culture customers experience" (Schneider and Bowen, 1995, p. 240). Rather than developing unlimited policies and procedures to manage the providers of care, greater emphasis is placed on authorizing and enabling (i.e., empowering) employees who interact with clients to make the efforts necessary to satisfy client needs. More attention is likely to be paid to this relationship (Bergman, 1994, pp. 195–196; Decker, 1999, pp. 19–20; Sower et al., 2001, pp. 53–54; Torpy, 2002, pp. 177–178).

## *Process*

Closely related to the structure is the **process** used to provide quality care. The process depends on the nature of the client's needs and how the staff uses resources to address them. For example, an acutely ill client is likely to need more diagnostic services, whereas a chronically ill person is likely to require more monitoring, counseling, and support. The emphasis in the process of providing quality care is likely to change from admission to discharge. The changes in emphasis might be identified by reviewing care maps or critical pathways. The process of providing quality care is not synonymous with the nursing process, although the nursing process is used to promote quality care. The process of quality care encompasses broader agency activities. Nurses apply the nursing process to meet nursing practice standards, while meeting the agency's standards of care to provide quality care.

The process component of quality care varies with the client's health problems and responses to treatment. The client's perception of interactions with care providers affects his or her satisfaction with the services received. After the client has been discharged, many health-care organizations collect data about consumer satisfaction with various tasks of care and types of services received. These data are used to identify which patterns of staff activities promote client satisfaction and which merit further examination. This type of retrospective study does not help clients directly, and some dissatisfied clients are unlikely to describe their perceptions in writing. Relying on this method of evaluation alone is unlikely to promote accuracy or reliability.

Emphasis has been placed on decentralizing nursing service organizations. The need to focus organizational resources at the direct service level to plan the process of providing quality care is being realized more frequently (Albrecht, 1990, pp. 54–68). Where this is occurring, staff nurses are likely to gain organizational influence to develop systems of care that are responsive to individual client needs and to the needs of the staff providing the quality care.

## *Outcomes*

Health-care providers have given lip service, but without corresponding action, to client-centered care for many years. More recently **outcomes,** or results, indicative of quality care are receiving more attention. These outcomes include features of client (recipient) and staff (provider) perceptions and cost-effectiveness (payer) (Hoesing and Kirk, 1990, p. 11; Nelson et al., 1989, p. 185; Welch, 1989, p. 469). In the past, quality care often was believed to be ideal rather than realistic care. Consequently the actual results of services provided (i.e., client outcomes) and the costs of quality care were neglected. With increased concern about the costs of health services and increased proportions of expenses being paid directly by private individuals, client satisfaction and costs no longer can be ignored. Many health-care agencies use management information and decision support systems to delineate the costs and benefits of various strategies and desired outcomes within the context of available resources (Colton, 2000, p. 7; Nolan, 2000, p. 254; Zema and Rogers, 2001, p. 35). By focusing on desired outcomes that clients and staff agree on, health-care providers develop customer-driven services. The evolving methods of financing health care and the rising tide of consumerism and its associated competitiveness are stimulating continued focus on consumer interests and client-driven systems of quality care.

## Meaning of Quality Care

The benefits of developing a commonly understood language to discuss the components of quality care and what quality means to various members of the health-care work groups slowly are being recognized (Frankl, 1990, pp. 52–65). Developing a common understanding of quality care requires staff at every level of the organization to comprehend the agency's mission and priorities and the processes used to address them (Frederick et al., 1988, p. 1; Torpy, 2002, p. 177). Staff nurses need to comprehend the structure, process, and outcomes of quality care established by the health-care agency. When they comprehend the primary purpose of the agency, the clinical staff providing care directly to clients need to understand the crucial need to "do it right the first time." Attention needs to be paid to the details of care so that established protocols are followed and common errors are avoided to provide predictably safe care. Providing quality care requires that effective supervision be readily available to ensure that staff provide direct services reliably and accurately, identify client needs, and have the necessary resources to address them.

Quality care issues do not differentiate between the realistic and the ideal. Rather, quality care usually focuses on what clients perceive their needs to be and how the agency uses resources to meet them in a cost-effective manner (Hoesing and Kirk, 1990, pp. 10–15). Increasingly, emphasis is focused on involving the clients in identifying desired outcomes within the context of the agency's standards of care. Without satisfied clients, there is less need for specific health care agencies, including nursing services and, consequently, less need for nurses. The issues of quality care are complex and unlikely to disappear in the foreseeable future, particularly with the increasing involvement of the recipients of care.

## ACTING AS A CLIENT ADVOCATE

As a result of the persistent pursuit of quality care, the need for nurses to act as client advocates is likely to continue. Staff nurses use knowledge of the needs of the clients and the health-care agencies to provide care and oversee and coordinate services provided by others. Comprehension of the agency's definition of quality care usually strengthens the nurse's commitment to take independent nursing actions to respond to client needs in a timely manner. Staff nurses, as advocates, use their assertiveness skills to communicate client needs to other team members as often as necessary until they are addressed within the agency's predetermined parameters of quality care.

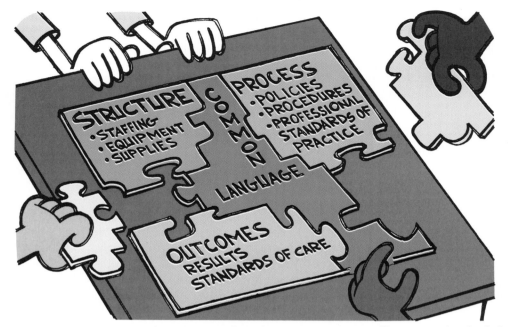

Developing a common understanding of quality care requires staff at every level of the organization to understand the agency's mission and priorities and the processes used to meet them.

Acting as a **client advocate** is not easy, smooth, or without risks, but it is crucial. Client advocates actively support client rights (as legally required) and make a special effort to defend client participation in decisions affecting them (Johnstone, 1989, pp. 31–34). Advocacy includes taking actions to secure the client's autonomy, or independence, in exercising one's rights. Client advocacy is needed in many types of situations. Clients are entitled to understand their rights as consumers of health care and to receive support in making decisions consistent with their individual goals, values, and lifestyles. Box 12-1 lists client rights in acute care settings. Box 12-2 describes client rights that nurses are obliged to protect in any setting. The primary purpose of client advocacy is to provide the client with information about his or her needs and available options. As Morrison (1991, p. 38) stated, "The advocate acts directly for vulnerable people and in many ways restores their basic rights of personhood and autonomy by acting in their interest as they perceive it and carrying out their wishes." When a client makes an informed decision, he or she reasonably can expect that the care providers will support these decisions in ways that enable clients to carry out the related plans of care.

## Advocate Responsibilities

An advocate helps clients obtain the information needed to exercise their rights. This information includes knowledge about the nature of individual health

## The Patient Care Partnership: Understanding Expectations, Rights and Responsibilities

When you need hospital care, your doctor and the nurses and other professionals at our hospital are committed to working with you and your family to meet your health care needs. Our dedicated doctors and staff serve the community in all its ethnic, religious and economic diversity. Our goal is for you and your family to have the same care and attention we would want for our families and ourselves.

The sections explain some of the basics about how you can expect to be treated during your hospital stay. They also cover what we will need from you to care for you better. If you have questions at any time, please ask them. Unasked or unanswered questions can add to the stress of being in the hospital. Your comfort and confidence in your care are very important to us.

### What to Expect During Your Hospital Stay

- **High quality hospital care.** Our first priority is to provide you the care you need, when you need it, with skill, compassion, and respect. Tell your caregivers if you have concerns about your care or if you have pain. You have the right to know the identity of doctors, nurses and others involved in your care, and you have the right to know when they are students, residents or other trainees.
- **A clean and safe environment.** Our hospital works hard to keep you safe. We use special policies and procedures to avoid mistakes in your care and keep you free from abuse or neglect. If anything unexpected and significant happens during your hospital stay, you will be told what happened, and any resulting changes in your care will be discussed with you.
- **Involvement in your care.** You and your doctor often make decisions about your care before you go to the hospital. Other times, especially in emergencies, those decisions are made during your hospital stay. When decision-making takes place, it should include:
  - *Discussing your medical condition and information about medically appropriate treatment choices.* To make informed decisions with your doctor, you need to understand:
    - The benefits and risks of each treatment.
    - Whether your treatment is experimental or part of a research study.
    - What you can reasonably expect from your treatment and any long-term effects it might have on your quality of life.
    - What you and your family will need to do after you leave the hospital.
    - The financial consequences of using uncovered services or out-of-network providers.
  Please tell your caregivers if you need more information about treatment choices.

*Continued*

BOX 12-1

## The Patient Care Partnership: Understanding Expectations, Rights and Responsibilities—cont'd

- *Discussing your treatment plan.* When you enter the hospital, you sign a general consent to treatment. In some cases, such as surgery or experimental treatment, you may be asked to confirm in writing that you understand what is planned and agree to it. This process protects your right to consent to or refuse a treatment. Your doctor will explain the medical consequences of refusing recommended treatment. It also protects your right to decide if you want to participate in a research study.
- *Getting information from you.* Your caregivers need complete and correct information about your health and coverage so that they can make good decisions about your care. That includes:
  – Past illnesses, surgeries or hospital stays.
  – Past allergic reactions.
  – Any medicines or dietary supplements (such as vitamins and herbs) that you are taking.
  – Any network or admission requirements under your health plan.
- *Understanding your health care goals and values.* You may have health care goals and values or spiritual beliefs that are important to your well-being. They will be taken into account as much as possible throughout your hospital stay. Make sure your doctor, your family and your care team know your wishes.
- *Understanding who should make decisions when you cannot.* If you have signed a health care power of attorney stating who should speak for you if you become unable to make health care decisions for yourself, or a "living will" or "advance directive" that states your wishes about end-of-life care, give copies to your doctor, your family and your care team. If you or your family need help making difficult decisions, counselors, chaplains and others are available to help.
- **Protection of your privacy.** We respect the confidentiality of your relationship with your doctor and other caregivers, and the sensitive information about your health and health care that are part of that relationship. State and federal laws and hospital operating policies protect the privacy of your medical information. You will receive a Notice of Privacy Practices that describes the ways that we use, disclose and safeguard patient information and that explains how you can obtain a copy of information from our records about your care.
- **Preparing you and your family for when you leave the hospital.** Your doctor works with hospital staff and professionals in your community. You and your family also play an important role in your care. The success of your treatment often depends on your efforts to follow medication, diet and therapy plans. Your family may need to help care for you at home.

## The Patient Care Partnership: Understanding Expectations, Rights and Responsibilities—cont'd

You can expect us to help you identify sources of follow-up care and to let you know if our hospital has a financial interest in any referrals. As long as you agree that we can share information about your care with them, we will coordinate our activities with your caregivers outside the hospital. You can also expect to receive information and, where possible, training about the self-care you will need when you go home.

- **Help with your bill and filing insurance claims.** Our staff will file claims for you with health care insurers or other programs such as Medicare and Medicaid. They also will help your doctor with needed documentation. Hospital bills and insurance coverage are often confusing. If you have questions about your bill, contact our business office. If you need help understanding your insurance coverage or health plan, start with your insurance company or health benefits manager. If you do not have health coverage, we will try to help you and your family find financial help or make other arrangements. We need your help with collecting needed information and other requirements to obtain coverage or assistance.

While you are here, you will receive more detailed notices about some of the rights you have as a hospital patient and how to exercise them. We are always interested in improving. If you have questions, comments, or concerns, please contact _____.

problems and the alternatives that might be used to manage or treat them. This information, which often is provided by various members of the multidisciplinary work groups, enables the client to decide on the treatment options that best match his or her goals, values, and lifestyle. Sometimes clients have difficulty understanding explanations due to language barriers. Sometimes time constraints, the process of care, and the nature of the services provided inhibit the transmission of information to the client (e.g., a client who is critically ill and anxious might not comprehend hurried or technical explanations). Certain procedures might be embarrassing or unacceptable due to a client's cultural or spiritual beliefs. These circumstances do not negate the client's right to understand available treatment options, however, and to make informed decisions about the plan of care.

Client care managers need to know and understand the rights of health-care consumers. In addition, they need to understand that **paternalism, beneficence,** and **maleficence** inhibit client **autonomy.** Paternalistic care providers act in a "fatherly" way, as if they know better than the client what is to be done.

BOX 12-2

## Nursing's Role in Patient's Rights

According to the NLN statement, nurses have a responsibility to uphold patients' rights:

To health care that is accessible and meets professional standards, regardless of the setting.

To courteous and individualized health care that is equitable, humane, and given without discrimination as to race, color, creed, sex, national origin, source of payment, or ethical or political beliefs.

To information about their diagnosis, prognosis, and treatment—including alternatives to care and risks involved—in terms they and their families can readily understand, so that they can give their informed consent.

To informed participation in all decisions concerning their health care.

To information about the qualifications, names, and titles of personnel responsible for providing their health care.

To refuse observation by those not directly involved in their care.

To privacy during interview, examination, and treatment.

To privacy in communicating and visiting with persons of their choice.

To refuse treatment, medications, or participation in research and experimentation, without punitive action being taken against them.

To coordination and continuity of health care.

To appropriate instruction or education from health-care personnel so that they can achieve an optimal level of wellness and an understanding of their basic health needs.

To confidentiality of all records (except as otherwise provided for by law or third-party payer contracts) and all communications, written or oral, between patients and health-care providers.

To access all health records pertaining to them, to challenge and correct their records for accuracy, and to transfer all such records in the case of continuing care.

To information on the charges for services, including the right to challenge these.

To be fully informed as to all their rights in all health-care settings.

From National League for Nursing: *Nursing's role in patients' rights,* New York, NY, 1977, Author.

Beneficent providers do what they think is in the client's best interest, not what the client thinks is best. The maleficent provider determines the care plan on the basis of avoiding harm or risk to the client, but again, the decision is not made by the client. The correct role for an advocate is to help clients obtain the information needed to make their own informed decisions about their care.

Another facet of advocacy in modern, fast-paced health-care environments requires that the client care manager communicate client responses to care in a timely manner. Services should match client needs, not agency routines or procedures or be restricted by predetermined care maps (Morrison, 1991, pp. 37–39). This ensures that legal requirements and the client's long-term interests are served and that shorter term, less cost-effective methods are not used in an attempt to meet client needs better. If the complexity of client needs conflicts with the staff's ability to respond to them or the agency's need to contain costs, the situation is prime for client advocacy. These situations require that the client care manager communicate the client's needs to the direct service staff and other involved multidisciplinary work group members. Often these efforts also require collaboration with staff from other agencies to analyze the client's situation and identify solutions that satisfactorily address the individual's needs. As mentioned in Chapter Seven, conflict resolution involves risk. To overlook or neglect client rights to avoid such risks or to take a path of convenience or expedience can jeopardize the longer term interests of the client and the agency.

One common situation that may require consistent and persistent advocacy is the increasing use of unlicensed assistive personnel (UAP). As the shortage of licensed nursing staff persists, some health-care organizations have opted to use UAP to fill the gap. In essence, this approach suggests that UAP can do what licensed nurses do without the requisite nursing knowledge and skills. In these situations, it is critical (legal requirement) that the client care manager perform all of the necessary nursing functions that clients require to meet their needs safely and delegate only the tasks that the UAP is prepared adequately to do. That is, the client care manager is legally required to assess, plan, implement, and evaluate the client's nursing plan of care and is accountable for the tasks delegated to the UAP in that framework. The principles of delegation (used to guide and supervise other licensed or credentialed nursing staff) apply. That is, the client care manager is accountable (i.e., expects to answer for one's practice of nursing related to specific individual clients and for the actions or nonactions of UAP that were delegated specific nursing tasks [e.g., recording intake and output or measurement and recording of vital signs]). If the UAP is not prepared to do the delegated tasks safely, the tasks cannot be delegated in the best interests of the client. The delegation expectations must be communicated clearly and follow-through monitored to ensure that safe, satisfactory care is provided. Principles of delegation are discussed further in Chapter Thirteen.

## EFFECTIVELY SUPERVISING THE WORK OF OTHERS

**Supervision** is actively monitoring or overseeing the activities of others. To supervise the work of others as a client care manager means to "oversee" client care activities. The function of supervision often is communicated (implied) to the work group by the organizational chart, position descriptions, or patterns of nursing service delivery. Having supervisory responsibilities often implies that the client care manager has a broader perspective on what needs to be done and different ("better" implied) methods of doing it based on nursing commitment, credentials, and authority consistent with the agency's purposes (Getz, 1999, p. 491). The primary **functions of** supervision include providing the desired perspective (i.e., attitude) and work environment that support agency goals and monitoring the extent to which these goals are met. Effective supervision helps the staff in several important ways.

## Characteristics of Effective Supervision

**Characteristics of effective supervision**, listed in Box 12-3, are reflected in the types of activities the client care manager performs to coach, monitor, and judge the effectiveness of work performed by nursing and health-care groups. To supervise others competently, the client care manager needs the proper attitude to guide others, the nursing knowledge and skills to provide the care needed by clients, and insight into the needs of the specific health-care organization (Arminio and Creamer, 2001, p. 35).

### *Maintain Suitable Working Conditions*

First, to supervise others, the client care manager takes an active part in maintaining suitable working conditions. He or she gives specific attention to the culture of the work group. Supervisees are encouraged to communicate concerns and questions to ensure that staff responsibilities can be met. The client care manager understands the language of the organizational culture and seeks to clarify misconceptions and agency goals. By reinforcing performance expectations, satisfactory effort can be recognized more readily and rewarded.

---

**BOX 12-3**

## Common Characteristics of Effective Supervision of Client Care

The client care manager actively provides suitable working conditions, including adequate staffing, equipment, and supplies.

The client care manager understands the needs of assigned clients and which agency resources are required to meet them.

The client care manager orients, teaches, and guides coworkers according to their individual learning styles and needs, consistent with their backgrounds, experience, and assignments.

The client care manager tries to stimulate desire for self-improvement in supervisees.

The client care manager encourages supervisees to use unique talents and develop special skills.

The client care manager demonstrates desired attitudes, skills, interests, and work habits.

## Understand Client Needs and Agency Resources

Second, the client care manager is expected to understand the needs of assigned clients and which agency resources are needed to meet them. To create a supportive environment to meet client needs involves supervisory responsibility to provide adequate equipment (Killian, 1990, pp. 34–35), supplies, and staffing. Supervisees are asked to report malfunctioning equipment, insufficient supplies, or help required to provide quality care safely. Often, to respond to the requests of coworkers, the client care manager needs to know how to operate equipment according to the manufacturer's specifications and how to troubleshoot when malfunctions are reported. To promote cost-effectiveness, the client care manager observes how coworkers use equipment and supplies and acts as a resource person to enable staff to learn to adapt client care to specific situations. The client care manager focuses on client needs within the context of agency guidelines and oversees the use of its resources in providing care.

A client care manager is likely to encounter certain common situations when supervising the work of others. A coworker might procrastinate instead of completing activities efficiently and have to complete key tasks late in the day or after the end of the workday. Conferring with this coworker earlier in the shift, the client care manager can inquire about the progress of various client care activities and suggest changes in the coworker's work organization or time management. For example, the manager might offer to help the coworker in ambulating clients earlier in the shift to ensure that client goals are met. Or the client care manager might anticipate that the coworker will need help from others and schedule early in the shift mutually acceptable times for performing these tasks.

Client care managers also are likely to encounter inadequate staffing to meet the variety of needs of the group of assigned clients. The client care manager must take the time and effort to listen actively to the expressed concerns and determine what type of help is needed by the group. Can client care activities be adapted to suit the work schedules better? Can the staff be taught different techniques for meeting client needs, such as sequencing activities to maximize exercise, comfort, and rest? Are additional staff members needed to provide safe and effective quality care in accordance with agency standards? Coworkers expect reasonable responses to their expressed concerns; if their concerns are minimized or ignored, they often learn not to communicate them or find different methods of responding to what they perceive as frustrating or unworkable circumstances.

## Teach Coworkers

Third, client care managers often are expected to orient, teach, and guide coworkers according to their individual learning styles and needs and consistent with their backgrounds, experience, and assigned client needs. Sometimes this supervisory responsibility involves selecting coworkers who are comfortable acting as desired role models. For example, the supervisee and another coworker can work together; the new employee can demonstrate skills while assisting the role model. The coworker acting as a role model is recognized for positive performance and encouraged to share her or his knowledge and skills with others. The client care manager

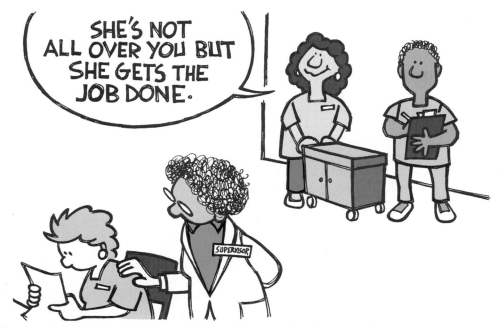

Characteristics of effective supervision are illustrated by the types of activities the client care manager performs to coach, monitor, and judge the effectiveness of work that the health-care work group performs.

should ensure that the planned learning activities enable the new employee to develop and demonstrate needed skills or competencies. He or she should make the expectations of all people involved in learning activities explicit so that they can be met. Orientation or competency checklists often are used to guide the supervisee and supervisor.

### Stimulate a Desire for Self-Improvement

Fourth, while supervising the work of others, client care managers try to stimulate a desire for self-improvement in supervisees. As mentioned in Chapter Ten, client care managers are more effective if they use leadership skills. While overseeing the work of others and interacting with them, client care managers are expected to praise and criticize coworkers to help them improve their work performance. Depending on the client care manager's leadership characteristics and communication skills, he or she often can use open, direct, tactful messages to stimulate a coworker's desire for self-improvement. As a role model, the client care manager can teach supervisees about the need for lifelong learning by conveying self-confidence, enthusiasm, and commitment to acquire new knowledge and skills on a daily basis.

*Encourage Use of Talent and Skills*

Fifth, client care managers guide supervisees in the use of talents and development of special skills. Within the limits of a coworker's position description and performance expectations, the client care manager teaches supervisees how to use unique talents and skills that enhance the quality of care. Some coworkers can convey empathy and concern to clients. Often they use active listening techniques that skillfully enable clients to reflect on their circumstances in a helpful manner. Recognizing and reinforcing the use of these skills enhances the quality of client care. Much can be gained by the supervisee when the supervisor recognizes and reinforces special capabilities.

*Act as a Role Model*

Sixth, while overseeing the work activities of supervisees, the client care manager has a superb opportunity to act as a role model and demonstrate desired attitudes, skills, interests, and work habits. The manager can provide an example of the desired attitudes and behaviors involved in providing quality care on a daily basis. This teaching method is powerful, but it is also demanding. As an imperfect human being and a lifelong learner, the client care manager functioning as a role model is in a vulnerable position. Sharing unique talents and skills with others in a sensitive manner reinforces the agency's goals, however, and enhances the quality of care.

## Meeting the Challenge

Providing effective supervision for coworkers is challenging. If coworkers do not perceive that supervision increases their effectiveness or efficiency, the resulting quality of care is not improved. That is, if the client care manager rewards or reinforces behaviors by emphasizing incorrect performance or inadequate effort while overseeing the work of others or if he or she attempts to change coworkers' behavior in health-care settings by coercion, work group performance suffers. In contrast, the client care manager needs to emphasize desired efforts to enable supervisees to improve their performance. Client care managers who provide effective supervision usually use a wide variety of teaching skills. These skills are based on knowledge of human motivation, communication, interpersonal relationships, and principles used to change behavior. Cameron-Buccheri (1986, pp. 16–25) reported findings of a study of the perceptions of 203 staff nurses and their perceived support of their supervisors. She noted that "a strong positive relationship was found" between job satisfaction and the amount of support the staff nurses perceived that they received from their supervisors. These staff nurses valued supervision and the associated influence, recognition, and communication that occurred with supervisory staff.

Supervisory skills are similar to the knowledge and skills used to teach clients. As a teacher of supervisees, the client care manager is sensitive to the motivations of individuals and the influence of the culture on the work environment. By remembering to combine the agency's mission, goals, and definition of quality care, the client care manager strives to help coworkers to develop and apply knowledge and skills used to care for assigned clients.

## EVALUATING CLIENT CARE PERFORMED BY OTHERS

Client care managers share responsibility for the effectiveness of care performed by others under their supervision and direction. As described earlier, to supervise the work of others effectively, the client care manager needs to know the clients' needs and what services and available resources are required to meet them. This nursing knowledge and skills cover proper use of equipment, supplies, and procedures. The client care manager needs to understand clearly the agency's definition of quality care, its established criteria for desired outcomes, its structure, and the standards of care used to guide staff.

Beginning staff nurses participate in judging the quality of work done by their peers and subordinates. They are expected to evaluate the effectiveness of peers and subordinates in helping clients satisfy health-care needs. This type of evaluation is different from formal employee evaluations in that it is done primarily to judge the success of an individual client's treatment program instead of the effectiveness of an employee's work performance. Entry-level staff nurses might be asked to provide feedback about the work performance of a nursing work group member. This section focuses, however, on evaluating success in helping a client to meet health-care goals.

## Evaluation Criteria

Evaluating the client care performed by others requires that the client care manager assess what clients need, determine the desired care outcomes within the context of the agency's standards of care, and determine the process for providing for them. Sometimes the evaluation process is facilitated by criteria specified in care maps or critical pathways. **Evaluation of client care done by others** requires knowledge of the agency's standards for quality care. The client care manager uses these standards to assess the adequacy of services provided and client outcomes. To evaluate the work of others, one must consider the client's entire situation in context, rather than examine various client characteristics (del Bueno, 1990, p. 6). The resulting judgment about the quality of care the client has received is likely to be more reliable, accurate, and enlightening. Nursing students often question the rationale for requiring them to develop varied skills. Without varied experience, they are likely to encounter difficulty when trying to determine the needs of a diverse group of assigned clients. It is difficult, if not impossible, to evaluate how effectively clients' needs have been met if the client care manager does not know what these needs are. Similarly, if the client care manager does not know the desired client outcomes and what is needed to achieve them, it is difficult to evaluate how effective other staff members are in meeting client needs. Concurrently, it is necessary to distinguish carefully between the results dependent on services provided from the results that are not.

### *Emphasize Strengths, Minimize Weaknesses*

The client care manager evaluates the work of others throughout the work day. He or she ensures that the supervisees have the knowledge and skills required to complete their work assignments and confers with them to obtain feedback and monitor progress. While meeting with supervisees, the client care manager makes a special effort to reinforce their strengths and minimize their weaknesses.

In most situations, emphasizing strengths has greater priority than minimizing weaknesses. Supervisees need the skills required to provide care safely. If a supervisee does not possess adequate skills, the client care manager needs to ensure that he or she acquires them. The client care manager then focuses on maximizing the supervisee's strengths and talents.

### Confer in a Private Area

When conferring with supervisees, it is always important to meet in a private area where open, direct communications can occur. Discussing client needs and care within earshot of clients, families, or visitors invites difficulty. Coworkers know that clients can misinterpret terminology or contexts, and they feel inhibited about engaging in open, forthright discussions in the client care areas. It is tempting to discuss concerns at the bedside while observing other aspects of the client's condition, but the client care manager must respect coworkers' privacy. This respect requires that detailed questioning and discussion occur in private so that the communication can be open, direct, and truthful. Depending on the nature of the discussion, subsequent revisions in the care plans may result to ensure that the client receives quality care suited to his or her needs. Effective (open and honest) communication cannot be ensured if it takes place in the presence of clients, family members, visitors, or other staff.

### Establish Criteria for Standards of Quality Care

The agency establishes standards of care, sometimes in the form of care maps or critical pathways, to guide staff. Each **standard of care** is a component of overall quality care as defined by the agency. Each standard is operationalized (defined in measurable terms) by **criteria**, clinical indicators that reflect the staff's current practices, a knowledge of relevant literature, and the opinions of clinical experts. The criteria depict elements of process and outcomes of quality care as they relate to specific client conditions and anticipated responses to treatment. Staff use these criteria to quantify or measure their effectiveness in achieving quality care and identifying areas that need further examination to improve services. A common set of criteria for a specific standard contains the following information about the client:
1. Knowledge of the health condition and its treatment
2. Skills (including various disciplines) needed to manage the situation
3. Knowledge of medications or nondrug or alternate treatment methods
4. Ability to adapt self-care behaviors, use of special equipment
5. Current health or physiologic state and rationale for parameters being used
6. Typical course of treatment or time frame for recovery
Information about the extent to which these criteria are met helps staff to judge the effectiveness of the structure, process, and outcomes of care.

### Evaluate Work Performance

Standards of practice and corresponding criteria are used to judge the work performance of staff. When overseeing the work of others, the client care manager must be flexible in determining acceptable variances in the work performance of supervisees. He or she must consider the context of clients' circumstances and compare agency standards for quality care. For example, the client care manager might consider whether client characteristics are atypical and might contribute to the client's short-term and long-term responses to treatment. Sometimes a client has a rare combination of diseases or symptoms that are difficult to treat, or the client experiences idiosyncratic responses to treatment. The client might not readily understand the nature of the health problems or might lack a support system. Client care managers accept responsibility for monitoring the efforts of supervisees to provide quality care as defined by the agency.

## Principles of Effective Evaluation

The goals of effective evaluation include maintaining or improving the quality of care provided and developing direct service staff capabilities. Client care managers apply several principles to provide effective evaluation. They often teach and coach coworkers (Davidhizar, 1990, pp. 42–44). In addition to role modeling positive and supportive attitudes, they actively help maintain the morale needed to sustain team efforts.

### Judge Work Performance

Client care managers are expected to judge the work performance of coworkers throughout the work day on a daily basis. The basic frames of reference for this evaluation are the pertinent standards of care and the specific employee's job description. The job description provides background information about the minimal requirements expected of a given category of employee. It typically includes descriptions of organizational responsibilities, quantity of work, knowledge, attitudes, and skills. This information is used to establish common expectations between the client care manager and the supervisee.

While monitoring client responses to care provided by others, the client care manager provides specific feedback about the coworker's work as it influences the quality of client care. Methods of controlling or reducing costs without compromising the effectiveness of care require constant attention. The manager provides concrete directions to the supervisee before, during, and after provision of care.

### Criticize Constructively

Constructive criticism is designed to maintain or improve the quality of care. Rather than offering general or vague comments, the client care manager, as an effective supervisor, describes behaviors or activities in concrete, observable terms. For example, the client care manager should not label the supervisee's behavior by saying, "Your clients are complaining about waiting. Can you organize your work better?" Instead, he or she might say to the supervisee, "Two of your clients didn't like waiting for your help with personal cares this morning. You usually use your time wisely. What might you do differently to care for them more promptly?" The client care manager needs to listen carefully to the supervisee's response and provide support. If the supervisee is unable to describe any possible remedy to improve performance, the client care manager might suggest alternative approaches. Specific suggestions are offered, based on the individual coworker's strengths, motivations, talents, and skills.

While providing constructive criticism, the client care manager should be prepared to receive it. Such a supervisory situation provides an opportunity to grow or improve, use humor, and be grateful. If this approach is taken, the supervisee learns that criticism should be received for the purposes it was given, rather than to sharpen defenses. Remember to role model the behaviors you wish to see in others.

### Understand the Organizational Culture and Reward System

As preparation for evaluating the work of others, the client care manager should understand the organizational culture, particularly how staff are rewarded for providing quality care (Casebeer, 1990, p. 42). When conferring with supervisees, the client care manager encourages them to evaluate their own work. Information gleaned from self-evaluation efforts helps the supervisor to gain insight into the individual's perceptions, attitudes, and goals. The experience might help the coworker to review old goals and set new ones.

### Reinforce Desired Behaviors

After minimal requirements are met, the focus of the evaluation needs to shift to accentuating the positive aspects of the coworker's accomplishments and reinforcing desired behaviors. Comparing the client care manager's evaluation with the supervisee's perspective sets up a learning situation. By negotiating differences, meaningful goals can be identified. Client care managers can learn a great deal from involving coworkers in solving client care problems (Schmieding, 1990, pp. 58–60), although this approach is not used as frequently as it could be.

By guiding the supervisee to take an active part in solving client care problems, the client care manager can help supervisees' self-esteem and self-confidence grow from seeing their ideas put into action. Combining active listening with an invitation to discuss ideas often helps the client care manager to focus on the needs of the coworker and client. When summarizing the discussion, alternative methods and goals can be described in measurable terms.

### Follow-Up on Response

To reinforce suggestions resulting from the evaluation of an individual's work, the client care manager needs to follow-up on the supervisee's response to the agreed-on plan. Withholding corrective actions until scheduled performance reviews should be avoided. Rather, constructive comments should be offered as soon as possible in a tactful, open, direct manner. Achievements need to be recognized, and positive feedback needs to be given. To maximize learning from the work experience, discuss what worked and what did not. Unsuccessful efforts also require recognition and revision, depending on clients' responses (Davidhizar, 1990, p. 44). Lack of such feedback diminishes the effects of the client care manager's efforts.

Seeking feedback from the client, family members, and support system is consistent with the advocacy component of the client care manager role. This feedback also is useful for determining the extent to which quality care was provided. A critical analysis of feedback is used to evaluate the client's total situation. Promoting meaningful communication patterns between direct service staff and their clients helps to evolve customer-driven health-care systems.

## ACCEPTING RESPONSIBILITY FOR THE ACTIONS OF SUBORDINATES

Effective client care managers accept **responsibility for the action and nonaction of subordinates**. When the client care manager provides effective supervision, certain conditions evolve and persist. Client care managers and their supervisees clarify expectations of each other. Each member of the work group learns to assume responsibility for assigned client care and expects to answer for what he or she does. These conditions are based on the assumption that the supervisor is

1. A resource person for clients and staff.
2. A teacher of clients and staff.
3. A loyal employee (Curtin, 1990, p. 7) (i.e., knows the organizational standards and expectations).
4. An accountable member of the nursing profession answerable for the actions he or she takes.

Before the client care manager as supervisor accepts this responsibility, he or she needs to ensure that the subordinates have four essential characteristics:

1. They need to know what care the client needs.
2. They possess the skills, equipment, and supplies needed to provide assigned client care services (Allen, 1990, pp. 14–15).
3. They need to know the goals of individual clients.
4. They need to provide feedback about client responses to the work group to provide for continuity of care.

If these characteristics are not present, liability for the actions of other health-care work group members and for one's own actions as a participant in the client's care may result. The client care manager needs to monitor supervisees to ensure that these criteria are met.

## SUMMARY

Client care managers accept responsibility for supervising and evaluating the work of others with whom they share responsibility for providing care to assigned clients. Within the context of the agency's definition of quality care, the focus of supervisory efforts includes satisfying customers and supporting and developing staff.

Client satisfaction has become an essential ingredient in quality care. Clients obtain considerable information needed to promote and maintain health from the mass media; they are becoming more sophisticated consumers. Due to the rising influence of client perceptions of the quality of health care they receive and changing mechanisms for financing and spiraling costs, more customer-driven systems are likely to evolve. To provide quality care, client and staff perceptions and cost-effectiveness criteria are incorporated into the agency's structure, process, and desired outcomes. To remain competitive, health-care agencies need to use valid and reliable methods to evaluate their success in providing quality care and to improve continuously the quality of care.

While fulfilling their supervisory responsibilities, client care managers are expected to protect client rights. The goals of advocacy activities include enabling clients to obtain information needed to exercise their rights and protect their autonomy in making decisions affecting individual plans of care. Advocacy activities often require the staff nurse to communicate client needs and concerns in a timely manner and to accept the risks involved in conflict resolution.

To oversee effectively the work of others who provide client care, staff nurses accept responsibility for maintaining a safe working environment in which staffing, equipment, and supplies are adequate. They support the agency's definition of quality care by comparing actual outcomes and services with established standards. They participate in the orientation, training, and incidental teaching of staff to ensure that needed care is provided safely, effectively, and efficiently. Another feature of effective supervision is the ability to stimulate coworkers to strive for continuous self-improvement by participating in self-evaluations of their performance. Closely related to these coworker efforts are the supervisor's recognition and reinforcement of special talents, knowledge, and skills. The client care manager also acts as a role model while providing care to teach desired attitudes and skills.

The client care manager evaluates client care performed by others. To promote accuracy and reliability in judging effectiveness, the client's entire situation needs to be considered in context. Feedback from clients, families, and support systems is used to evaluate the quality of care provided. This approach requires that the staff nurse know each client's needs and what resources are required to meet them. Standards of care are used as guidelines. Specific feedback is given in a place and a manner that reflects respect for clients and staff and promotes effective communication. To gain from the evaluation, the client care manager must follow-up with involved staff to ensure that indicated changes occur and desired behaviors are rewarded.

For a supervisory relationship between the client care manager and supervisees to be effective, supervisees must know what client services are needed, how to provide them using agency resources, how to communicate feedback about client responses, and the extent to which individual client health-care goals were met. When these conditions exist, the staff nurse can accept responsibility for the actions and nonactions of subordinates in providing quality care.

## APPLICATION EXERCISES

1. As consumers of health care, many clients pay for a portion of the costs of nursing services provided. Identify the specific phases of the nursing and management processes that provide opportunities for promoting client satisfaction. Describe how you would apply principles of customer service in these phases.
2. Describe specific components of quality care at your assigned agency in terms of the agency's structure, process, and outcomes. Are findings from client satisfaction surveys used to evaluate effectiveness? Are these survey results used to reward employees?
3. Give three examples of client advocacy that you witnessed while completing your clinical work assignments during the last week.
4. Observe the behaviors of a nurse supervising the practice of staff nurses. List the principles of effective supervision that you believe were reflected in the supervisor's behavior.
5. A "float" licensed practical nurse is assigned to your nursing work group. Describe what you would do as a staff nurse to demonstrate your acceptance of responsibility for her actions.

## CRITICAL THINKING SCENARIO

Picture yourself practicing in a relatively busy primary care/ambulatory care clinic setting within a large medical center. You spend most of your time with clients teaching, counseling, and collecting data used to compare client health maintenance. You also supervise five health-care technicians involved in respiratory care, conditioning programs, and health education activities, all of whom have worked in the inpatient setting. Although standards of care, related outcomes, and client outcomes are well established in the inpatient settings, they have not been adapted to your setting. You are aware of various groups who are developing care maps for common health maintenance needs (i.e., weight control, smoking cessation, diabetes management). At a staff meeting yesterday, you were asked to make sure that your supervisees were collecting data needed to monitor the achievement of client outcomes.

1. What would you do first?
2. Are the desired outcomes of clients served in the primary clinic different from those of clients in the inpatient setting? If so, describe.
3. Can the health technicians delineate the desired outcomes for the clients they serve? What resources would you suggest, if any? Give reasons for your answer.
4. Your supervisor requests that you list the desired outcomes for the clients served by the health technicians. What would you do?
5. How would you incorporate supervisory support, including the dimensions of influence, recognition, and communication, to promote the job satisfaction of your supervisees while completing this assignment?

## REFERENCES

Adams M: Road rage on the information superhighway, *Pharmaceutical Executive* September 2000, p. 164.

Albrecht K: *Service within*, Homewood, IL, 1990, Dow Jones-Irwin.

Allen AMB: Changing liability of the nurse over the past decade, *Orthop Nurs* 9(2):13–15, 1990.

Arminio J, Creamer DG: What supervisors say about quality supervision, *College Student Affairs Journal* 21(1):35–44, 2001.

Bergman R: The relationship between quality of care, quality of life, quality of work life and research, *J Clin Nurs* 3(4):195–196, 1994.

Cameron-Buccheri R: Nursing supervision: a new look at an old role, *Nurs Admin Q* 11(1):11–25, 1986.

Casebeer L: Personnel decisions "wheeling" toward better performance, *Nurs Manage* 21(8):42–44, 1990.

Colton D: Quality improvement in health care: conceptual and historical foundations, *Eval Health Professions* 23(1):7–24, 2000.

Cramer D, Tucker SM: The consumer's role in quality: partnering for quality outcomes, *J Nurs Care Qual* 9(2):54–66, 1995.

Curtin LL: Old loyalties in the new organization, *Nurs Manage* 21(3):7–8, 1990.

Davidhizar R: The manager as coach, *Adv Clin Care* 5(3):42–44, 1990.

Decker PJ: The hidden competencies of healthcare: why self-esteem, accountability, and professionalism may affect hospital customer satisfaction scores, *Hospital Topics* 77(1):14–26, 1999.

del Bueno DJ: Evaluation: myths, mystiques, and obsessions, *J Nurs Admin* 20(11):4–7, 1990.

Docteur E: Measuring the quality of care in different settings, *Health Care Financ Rev* 22(3):59–70, 2001.

Frankl KAJ: The language and meaning of quality, *Nurs Admin Q* 14(3):52–65, 1990.

Frederick BJ, Sharp JQ, Atkins N: Quality of patient care: whose decision? *J Nurs Qual Assur* 2(3):1–10, 1988.

Geron SM, Smith K, Tennstedt S, Jette A, Chassler D, Kasten L: The home care satisfaction measure: a client-centered approach to assessing the satisfaction of frail older adults with home care services, *J Gerontol Soc Sci* 55B(5):S259–S270, 2000.

Getz HG: Assessment of clinical supervisor competencies, *J Couns Dev* 77:491–497, 1999.

Giuffrida A, Gravelle H, Roland M: Measuring quality of care with routine data: avoiding confusion between performance indicators and health outcomes, *BMJ* 319:94–98, 1999.

Goldstein SM and Schweikhart SB: Empirical support for the Baldrige award framework in U.S. hospitals, *Health Care Manage Rev* 27(1):62–75, 2002.

Griffiths R, Jayasuriya R, Maitland H: Outcome measure for community nursing, *Aust N Z J Public Health* 24(5):529–535, 2000.

Hildman TB, Ferguson GH: Prompt service: a factor in patient satisfaction, *Nurs Manage* 21(12):26–29, 1990.

Himmelstein DU, Woolhandler S, Hellander I, Wolfe SM: Quality of care in investor-owned vs not-for-profit HMOs, *JAMA* 282(2):159–163, 1999.

Hoesing H, Kirk R: Common sense quality management, *J Nurs Admin 20*(10): 10–15, 1990.

Johnstone MJ: Professional ethics and patients' rights: past realities, future imperatives, *Nurs Forum 24*(3):29–34, 1989.

Killian WH: Equipment mishaps may result in lawsuits, *Am Nurse 22*(6):34–35, 1990.

Larrabee JH: The changing role of the consumer in health care quality, *J Nurs Care Qual 9*(2):8–15, 1995.

Lehmann R: Forum on clinical indicator development: a discussion of the use and development of indicators, *QRB 15*(7):223–227, 1989.

Mayer T, Cates RJ: Service excellence in health care, *JAMA 282*(13):1281–1283, 1999.

Morrison A: Clinical ethics: the nurse's role in relation to advocacy, *Nurs Stand 5*(41):37–40, 1991.

Nelson EC et al.: The patient judgment system: reliability and validity, *QRB 15*(6):185–191, 1989.

Noble E, Klein L: Quality assurance: the measure of quality culture in a managed care setting, *Total Quality Management 11*(2):199–205, 2000.

Nolan MT: Improving patient care through data competence, *Nurs Econ 18*(5):250–254, 2000.

Oermann MH, Templine T: Important attributes of quality health care: consumer perspectives, *Journal of Nursing Scholarship 32*(2):167–172, 1998.

Patterson CH: Standards of patient care: the joint commission focus on nursing quality assurance, *Nurs Clin North Am 23*(3):625–638, 1988.

Savage GT, Campbell KS, Patman T, Nunnelley LL: Beyond managed costs, *Health Care Manage Rev 25*(1):93–108, 2000.

Schmieding NJ: Do head nurses include staff nurses in problem-solving? *Nurs Manage 21*(3):58–60, 1990.

Schneider B, Bowen DE: *Winning the service game*, Boston, MA, 1995, Harvard Business School Press.

Sinclair VG: Potential effects of decision support systems on the role of the nurse, *Comput Nurs 8*(2):60–65, 1990.

Smith AP: Consumerism and efforts to regain the public trust, *Nurs Econ 19*(6):293, 2001.

Sower V, Duffy J, Kilbourne W, Kohers G, Jones P: The dimensions of service quality for hospitals: development and use of the KQCAH scale, *Health Care Manage Rev 26*(2):47–59, 2001.

Stewart LJ, Lockamy A: Improving competitiveness through performance-measurement systems, *Healthcare Financial Management* December 2001, p. 46–50.

Toffler A: *The third wave*, New York, NY, 1980, Bantam Books.

Tomes N: Merchants of health: medicine and consumer culture in the United States, 1900–1940, *Journal of American History* September 2001, pp. 519–547.

Torpy JM: Raising healthcare quality: process, measures, and system failure, *JAMA 287*(2):177–178, 2002.

Welch CC: Entering a new era of quality care, *ANNA 16*(7):469–471, 1989.

Zema CL, Rogers L: Evidence of innovative uses of performance measures among purchasers, *Health Care Financ Rev 22*(3):35–47, 2001.

# 13

# Assigning and Delegating Client Care Activities

*When you complete this chapter, you should be able to:*

1. Accurately distinguish licensed and unlicensed assistive personnel who are members of one's nursing work group.
2. Differentiate between assigning and delegating client care.
3. Describe principles of client care assignment.
4. Compare responsibility, authority, and accountability.
5. Define liability.
6. Contrast the two types of negligence.
7. Describe the relationship of accountability to client care assignment.
8. Discuss key concepts underlying effective delegation.
9. Describe principles of delegation.
10. Describe principles to be considered before delegating client care activities to less skilled staff.
11. Describe the relationship of delegation to accountability for client care.
12. Describe your rights and responsibilities when required to work mandatory overtime.
13. List three strategies that you as a client care manager can use to help reduce staff shortages.
14. Describe your obligations to agency nurses or nurses employed as temporary staff.

unlicensed assistive personnel (UAP)
assigning client care
nurse shortage
mandatory overtime
temporary staff
delegating client care
authority
principles for assigning client care
responsibility

agency staff
accountability
malpractice
liability
negligence
  commission
  omission
principles for delegating the work of
  client care managers

## DIRECTING THE WORK OF OTHERS

Entry-level nurses in the client care manager role direct the work of others who provide nursing care. This function usually entails assigning and delegating client care activities. This function requires the client care manager to know what one's obligations are to clients assigned to them and the types of nursing staff within the assigned work group. To fulfill these management responsibilities appropriately, the staff nurse needs to understand the nature of these functions and common strategies used to perform them. How client care is assigned often depends on the agency's organization and patterns of nursing service delivery and staffing. Careful consideration is given to individual employee credentials (licensure), qualifications, and capabilities. Proper delegation requires similar considerations.

Before making any decisions about assigning or delegating client care, it is essential to know what the nursing needs are of one's assigned group of clients and the number and types of nursing staff that are available to meet these needs during a specific period. In today's rapidly changing health care environment, the client care manager needs to anticipate changes in client conditions and who within the nursing work group is in the best position to respond appropriately (e.g., admitting, transferring, or discharging clients). As discussed in Chapter Four, the client care manager needs to maintain flexibility of the work group by careful consideration of the credentials and qualifications of each member of the nursing work group. Licensed nursing staff have established their legal status as nurses through educational requirements and licensure examination. It is important to understand the difference between the nursing knowledge base and skills of registered nurses (RNs) and licensed practical nurses (LPNs). Although the scope of nursing practice may vary from state to state, RNs are prepared to assess, plan, implement, and evaluate client care; LPNs are especially well prepared to function in the implementation phase of the nursing process under supervision. It is important to remember that certain tasks of data collection might be considered assessment, such as listening to heart and lung sounds. It is the RN's responsibility to analyze the available data as part of the client's overall assessment and evaluation of responses, determine what other data may be needed, formulate a plan of care, and identify interventions needed. If the client requires repeated, frequent assessments to provide safe care, often referred to as *less physiologically stable*, the client needs an RN to perform this type of function. If the client has complex tasks that need to be done frequently and documented according to agency policies and procedures, LPNs often are well prepared to perform them with supervision of an RN, who analyzes data gathered to monitor the client's responses and progress. This type of situation may require the RN and LPN to work together to meet a client's needs safely. Specific details of Nursing Practice Acts for each type of nursing staff typically are available within library reference holdings or can be obtained from the State's Board of Nursing or Department of Regulation and Licensing.

Nursing assistants (NAs) are another type of nursing work group member. NAs frequently are certified (versus licensed) by an educational agency from which they obtained their educational preparation. The amount and type of preparation vary, often in response to institutional requirements and types of facilities used to gain practical experiences to verify performance of needed skills. NAs might increase their knowledge and skills through additional in-service programs and specialized settings. NAs are one type of **unlicensed assistive personnel (UAP).** They may provide a large amount of personal assistance in activities of daily living to clients in various settings, especially long-term residential care facilities. Other types of UAP may be students, including nursing students, who are gaining experience working in health-care settings, with varying levels of educational backgrounds and experience.

## ASSIGNING VERSUS DELEGATING CLIENT CARE ACTIVITIES

Entry-level staff nurses frequently are expected to assign and delegate client care activities in an attempt to provide quality care with available resources. **Assigning client care** differs from delegating it in that licensed nurses have a licensed scope of practice and legal authority to perform the assignment. UAP, being unlicensed, do not have a scope of practice, and consequently do not have legal authority to perform the nursing activity or task until it is delegated. The nursing outcomes of assignment and delegation of nursing tasks are the same. Although these terms are often used synonymously, they are not the same.

Box 13-1 depicts components of assigning client care according to client needs. Care assignments are based on the complexity of nursing care that each client

---

**BOX 13-1**

### Assigning Client Care

**Work to Be Done Based on Client Needs**

Health condition:
  Unstable
  Unpredictable
  Infectious
  Complex
Environmental factors:
  Location of client to needed utilities
  Number and frequency of time-consuming tasks
  Interdisciplinary treatment schedules
Other needed agency resources:
  Equipment
  Supplies
  Physical plant
  Coordination of other therapies

**Staff Assignment Considerations**

Employee's scope of practice:
  Legal requirements
  Legal restrictions
  Employee's position description
Agency's division of work:
  Formal organization policies
Employee's characteristics:
  Need for in-service education to use safely and cost-effectively
  Skills and special talents
  Credentials, personality
  Related experiences
  Attitudes

needs and what the employee is licensed and employed (described in one's position description) to do with the agency's resources to meet them. Clients with unstable or unpredictable conditions require more complex assessment and monitoring than clients with stable conditions. Clients with complex needs for diagnostic or treatment procedures are likely to require more time and often more skilled care because they often require client teaching. Clients requiring special infection control measures typically also require more time.

## Assignment

Assignment refers to the client care manager's function of allocating the work required to care for a group of clients to available staffing. With the increasing demand for RNs and decreasing availability, fewer health-care agencies employ as many RNs as needed. The difference between the number needed and the number available commonly has become known as the **nurse shortage**. One common strategy used by health-care facilities is to provide a staffing mix (different combinations of various types of credentialed staff, i.e., LPNs, NAs, health-care technicians) to provide nursing care in combination with RNs. Frequently, staffing mixes are a response to the need to restructure organizationally to contain costs and better utilize and retain available RNs (de Ruiter, 2001, p. 40; Loquist, 2002, p. 33; Sheehan, 2001, p. 65). The agency assumes responsibility for providing administrative policies, educational preparation, and organizational systems including available orientation and in-service programs needed to use the staffing mixes appropriately. Consequently the agency, the RNs assigning care to available licensed and unlicensed staff, and the assigned staff all share responsibility for the quality of nursing care provided (Barter and Furmidge, 1994, p. 39). Crucial to assigning care, the manager must know each client's needs and what knowledge, skills, equipment, and supplies are required to meet them. The UAP depends on the licensed staff to delegate tasks appropriately. The accountability level of the client care manager is higher when UAP are used because they are unlicensed than when licensed staff comprise the nursing work group.

A growing concern with the shortage of nursing is the use of **mandatory overtime** as a method of providing adequate numbers of nursing staff. This strategy is appropriate when unexpected emergencies arise that increase the number of staff needed to address client needs. This approach has been found to decrease staff retention and patient safety, however. In response to the inappropriate use of mandatory overtime, many states have passed laws prohibiting its use as a fixed agency response to staffing shortages. Vernarec (2000, p. 72) advocated that every nurse know the key provisions of the Nurse Practice Act in the state in which he or she is practicing and ask, "Am I competent after an 8- or 12-hour shift to take care of patients and respond to an urgent situation?" If the answer is no, the Nurse Practice Act obliges the nurse to refuse mandatory overtime, even though doing so may result in getting fired. Vernarec (2000, p. 72) also listed several additional responses that may be indicated depending on the specific practice situation. To avoid such practice conflicts, many agencies have developed or are in the process of establishing systems that do not result in admitting more clients than there are available staff needed to provide safe care. Some agencies also hire "traveling" nurses or temporary nurses to meet anticipated staffing needs. **Temporary staff** need orientation and assistance in learning about the agency's policies, procedures, equipment, and supplies. In addition, the same principles of assigning and delegating care need to be applied when temporary nurses are members of the nursing work group (Fink, 2002, p. 32).

The agency is responsible for providing adequate numbers and quality of staff to care for its clientele; the RNs are responsible for quantifying the number and types of staff needed based on identified client needs and appropriately assigning (allocating the work to be done consistent with the agency's policies and procedures) and delegating care; and the members of the nursing work group are responsible for completing the nursing tasks as directed. Staff are paid to complete assignments in accordance with their credentials and position descriptions and, when feasible, their individual talents and preferences. When completed, assignments include a matching list of staff, clients, and other activities describing the work to be done on the nursing unit during a specified time. The list designates specific staff duties in meeting individual client needs and related nursing tasks. How the nursing work group is organized to complete their assignments depends on the available staff, quantity and complexity of client needs, and the pattern of nursing service used. Assigning client care is different from delegating it, although each is not mutually exclusive of the other. Some of the principles involved in assigning care apply to appropriate delegation of care.

When the client care manager assigns care according to established agency policies, procedures, and position descriptions, it is a form of delegation; the decisions about the appropriateness of the delegated acts have been made by authorized nursing staff (e.g., nursing managers, supervisors, or directors of nursing) or nursing practice committees at other levels of the health-care organization. These decisions result in shared responsibility or answerability for the consequences of the delegation. It is incumbent on every client care manager as an RN to know what the scope of practice is for each work group member to whom tasks are assigned and delegated. Nurses need to read carefully and understand the Nurse Practice Act of the state in which they are practicing as client care managers. The client care manager appropriately can delegate the performance of nursing tasks to UAP, but not nursing functions necessary for the provision of safe care.

Given that the function of assigning client care is a form of delegation, it is crucial that the client care manager know the commonly accepted "rights" that need to be granted. These rights include (1) right task, (2) right circumstances, (3) right person, (4) right direction/communication, and (5) right feedback/supervision/ evaluation (Habgood, 2000, p. 1058; National Council of State Boards of Nursing [NCSBN], 1997b). Further information about these delegation rights can be obtained from the website: http://www.ncsbn.org/public/regulation/delegation_ documents.htm.

## Delegation

Delegation involves transferring (often in the form of a verbal request) the authority to someone else to perform a task that is one of your responsibilities (NCSBN,

1997b, p. 2) or work that you are being paid to do. **Delegating client care** refers to the client care manager's authority in addition to leadership, resource management, and staff development functions. Proper delegation of client care activities requires that the client care manager consider the employee's position description, the employee's legal scope of practice, and the complexity of individual client needs. The delegated activity is not part of the employee's work assignment, rather an addition to it. The nature of the client care needed and the individual staff member's credentials, scope of practice, and individual characteristics need to be considered. In addition, the coworker must accept the delegated work voluntarily and be motivated to learn about it and perform it safely. Delegation emphasizes individual staff strengths and preferences.

A client care manager may delegate various activities to promote efficiency and cost-effectiveness. Clinical and nonclinical tasks can be delegated. For example, tasks needed to provide "bedside" care and tasks integral to marketing, public relations, or organizational health might be delegated to various members of the work group. Delegation can promote staff development and effective time management for the RN.

## Using Authority

**Authority** refers to one's source of power to act (NCSBN, 1997a, p. 1). The client care manager's authority for making assignments and delegating tasks of nursing care stem from his or her legal status as an RN and the agency's established policies, procedures, and pattern of nursing service delivery system being used.

The client care manager uses authority differently to direct staff when assigning care and delegating it. For example, a client care manager might assign an LPN to provide personal hygiene and dressing changes and complete the corresponding documentation for a group of clients under her or his supervision. This assignment is likely to be consistent with the LPN's position description and legal scope of practice. It would not be an appropriate assignment for an NA because of the need to understand principles of asepsis (to change dressings safely), which usually are not included in NA's legal scope of practice (if it exists). The client care manager also could delegate to an RN the responsibility of monitoring the vital signs of a client during the client care manager's lunch break. This delegation is contingent on acceptance by the RN, who must agree to complete the client care activity, in addition to completing her or his current assignment. If the RN has the knowledge, skills, and experience to provide the interim care safely, the delegation process can proceed. If not, the client care manager must ensure that the RN has the needed knowledge, information, directions, and instruction before delegating the client's care. The client care manager accepts ultimate primary responsibility for the consequences of delegated tasks.

Entry-level staff nurses usually have opportunities to observe more experienced (and licensed) staff nurses assign and delegate client care activities (in accordance with the agency's organization, context, and work group characteristics). These learning experiences often are provided as a component of an in-service orientation program before the nurses are expected to perform these functions independently.

## OTHER FACTORS TO CONSIDER IN ASSIGNMENT AND DELEGATION

### Environmental Factors

Many environmental factors can affect the nature of a work assignment. Generally, caring for clients located in the same area of the nursing unit requires less energy and time than caring for clients in rooms some distance apart. Clients with time-consuming needs, such as frequent monitoring of vital signs or collection of specimens, also require more effort. Special attention must be paid to clients with established treatment schedules involving other disciplines, such as physical, occupational, speech, or group therapies, so that nursing care can be completed within limited time periods.

### Agency Resources

Another factor that affects the amount of work to be done to meet a client's needs is the type of agency resources available. If equipment is shared by all, staff members must coordinate the use of it, which takes time and effort. The availability of supplies and the process for obtaining them also can affect how long it takes staff to complete assignments. The client care manager shares responsibility for making readily available commonly used supplies and supplies that are used less frequently, such as wound débridement trays used in assisting other disciplines in providing client care. The nature of the physical plant, such as the availability of toilets and sinks in private rooms or the lack of them in multibed wards, can place additional demands on staff. The use of other therapies in the client's overall treatment plan may increase demands on nursing staff, who ensure that the client is prepared and available to participate as scheduled.

### Agency Functions

Agency functions affect how the work involved in providing client care is divided. Critical care units expect to provide more highly skilled staff in lower ratios to clients than do long-term care agencies that provide convalescent or maintenance care. When assigning client care, the staff nurse designates which staff members are to care for specific individuals. This designation usually is based on responsibilities delineated in their position descriptions, legal scopes of practice, and educational backgrounds. An assignment implies an employee's responsibility to perform activities consistent with her or his position description, in accordance with legally accepted practices (NCSBN, 1997a, p. 1). The employee is expected to accept work assignments that meet criteria outlined as conditions of employment in her or his job description. Each employee assumes primary responsibility for completing the client care activities included in daily work assignments.

### Characteristics of Nursing Staff Members

The personal characteristics of nursing staff members need to be considered when making assignments. Clients with certain personality characteristics, such as anxiety or low self-esteem, often are managed more effectively when matched with staff members who are talented in responding appropriately to such characteristics. Sometimes staff members have special interests in common with clients, and matching them can add a special touch in care. Conversely, staff vulnerabilities need to be considered when clients require special approaches or procedures contrary to a nursing work group member's disposition. A demanding client who expects follow-through on every detail is unlikely to fare well with a staff member who readily acknowledges that he or she "can't stand sweating the small stuff."

## ASSIGNING CLIENT CARE

Experience in overseeing the work of others helps produce insights into the complexities of client care and the diversity of persons (and corresponding qualifications, skills, and talents) providing it. Generally the entry-level staff nurse gains experience supervising the work of others before being asked to assign client care activities. These experiences are designed to help the beginning nurse to gain knowledge about and insight into the competencies of various nursing work group members and how those knowledge and skills are used to meet client needs. Conger (1994, pp. 21–27) reported effective use of a nursing assessment decision grid in teaching staff nurses to identify tasks involved in providing nursing care and corresponding skills needed to assign appropriately LPNs the tasks delineated. (Remember that the assessment of client needs is done before assignment and is legally a function of RNs.) Conger (1994, pp. 21–27) noted that the staff nurse should allocate nursing staff resources only after she or he has identified the nursing tasks on the basis of nursing problems. She reported that the nurses' primary language affected their ability to identify nursing problems requisite to delineating tasks involved in the client's care. Further study of strategies for learning to assign care is needed.

## Principles for Assigning Client Care

Some **principles for assigning client care** can be followed to ensure that the group's work is allocated properly so that all needs are met satisfactorily. Box 13-2 lists guidelines for assigning client care.

### *Assess Clients' Needs*

First, the client care manager assesses the needs of all clients whose care will be assigned. This preliminary assessment might be done in several ways (e.g., from information obtained directly from the client and family or from the clinical record, the classification system, or the change-of-shift report). These assessments enable the nurse to determine generally what types of needs the group of clients have and how to meet them, how complex the care is, and approximately how much time is needed to complete it. On the basis of this information, the client care manager sets priorities for her or his assigned group of clients. For example, clients who are responding unpredictably, who are threatened by serious complications, who have infectious conditions, who require complex nursing procedures or time-

BOX 13-2

## Guidelines for Assigning Client Care

1. Determine the amount of nursing care time required and the complexity of the activities allocated.
2. Identify who, of the available staff, is best qualified to provide the client's care, considering attitudes, skills, demeanor, and efficiency.
3. Consider each staff member as an individual with a unique combination of needs, skills, and talents.
4. Strive to maximize continuity of care and reduce fragmentation.
5. Combine assignments to increase efficiency; consider treatment schedules and geographic location of clients.
6. Describe the assignment in measurable terms; be specific about expected results.
7. Designate one person or an absolute minimum number of staff to be responsible for each client's care.
8. Plan to provide additional help, direction, or instruction as necessary to match the needs of individual staff members.
9. Communicate assignments clearly, preferably in writing. Follow-up frequently during the shift to check progress and any changes in clients and subsequent changes in assignments.
10. Assign responsibility for holistic care: avoid assigning only nursing procedures.

consuming care, or who are experiencing high levels of anxiety receive special consideration. When assigning care, the client care manager attempts to maximize the available staff knowledge, skills, and time to address each client's care safely and satisfactorily. Special needs influence which staff are assigned to care for which clients. Physiologically unstable clients require more expertise and time to ensure that their needs are met safely. Nurses caring for clients who need extensive infection control measures require additional knowledge, skill, and time to ensure the safety of the clients and others in the immediate environment. To promote effective infection control strategies, a staff member is generally not assigned more than two clients requiring such care during any shift so that she or he can plan effective use of time and supplies.

### Consider Staff Number and Type

Second, the client care manager usually knows the number and categories of staff available to provide the needed care, either before or immediately after receiving the change-of-shift report. Agency policies, rooted in state laws that define and delimit scopes of practice, require that work assignments be consistent with the responsibilities, tasks, and activities included in corresponding staff position descriptions. The position descriptions for client care managers, as entry-level RNs, generally require that they accept responsibility for using the nursing process to determine client needs and establish, implement, and evaluate care plans to meet them. In addition, they often delineate dependent and interdependent nursing functions on the client's behalf. For example, RNs are expected to communicate effectively with multidisciplinary work group members and coordinate efforts made to enable clients and families to gain and maintain independence in self-care. In addition, after adequate preparation, client care managers perform a wide variety of nursing procedures using established guidelines provided by the agency or manufacturers of the equipment and supplies. As nursing establishes itself as a profession, RNs will assume greater responsibility for the scope of their practice, including accountability for individuals working directly under their supervision and direction. This role is likely to be demanding, yet essential to the success of the nursing work group (Ameduri, 1994, pp. 21–24; Evans, 1991, pp. 17A–20A), now and in the foreseeable future.

In comparison, LPNs and NAs depend on other professionals to assess client conditions, analyze the information gathered, and establish safe and effective plans to respond to the identified needs. Various categories of subordinate nursing staff rely on RNs to provide guidance and direction in responding to individual client needs. Consistent with their legal scopes of practice, each staff member is answerable for actions or nonactions taken to meet client needs. Accordingly, they share liability for any harm or injury they cause clients in the performance of their duties.

Generally, LPNs are prepared to implement established plans of care and to provide feedback about clients who are expected to respond predictably. They usually can be expected to perform procedures according to protocol, but they are not prepared to assess, analyze, or evaluate client responses to various treatments, particularly those that indicate unstable physiologic conditions requiring immediate attention. LPNs are prepared to perform various infection control procedures, apply principles of asepsis (sterile techniques required in various procedures designed to prevent or control infectious processes), and conduct established routines.

NAs, when assigned client care, have the most narrow scope of nursing practice (more often certified instead of licensed), which corresponds to their educational background. Typically, they are prepared to provide routine personal hygiene measures, especially those related to the clients' activities of daily living. These activities include bathing, dressing, transferring, ambulating, repositioning, toileting, and feeding clients. They also can record routine intake and output and other basic nursing routines that require them to perform specific hand-washing procedures and comply with universal precautions. NAs are not prepared, however, to apply principles of asepsis. They can be expected to perform basic nursing procedures for which they have been prepared, and they are answerable for such actions.

UAP need to be assigned using the same principles as NAs. UAP are assigned only those tasks for which they are adequately prepared and consistent with the agency's policies and procedures. Because they are unlicensed, they do not have a scope of practice and cannot be assigned nursing functions of assessment, planning, or evaluation.

When assigning client care, the client care manager determines who of the available staff is best able to provide each client's care. The agency is likely to use a classification system, policies, and position descriptions to match estimated client needs with available staff. These factors strongly influence the staff's expectations of their work assignments. It is important to establish high performance expectations and work together to meet them (Schaffer, 1991, p. 146). The client care manager uses her or his knowledge base, imagination, and creativity to assess individual staff capabilities to maximize client care. Some staff are more efficient because of skills gained from working with others in complex situations. Other staff members might be inexperienced, but be good listeners for clients with less complex physical, but greater emotional needs associated with undergoing extensive diagnostic procedures.

The client care manager needs to assign care primarily on the basis of client needs and demonstrated staff competence to address them. Without such a foundation, it is not safe to assume that the client will receive safe and satisfactory care. If there is any question about the adequacy of the staff member's qualifications and competencies to provide care, the situation must be clarified before assigning care. To enable staff to proceed safely, the client care manager asks questions, discusses mutual expectations, provides instruction when a staff member is unfamiliar with a specific approach or procedure, gives specific directions for adaptations, and plans with each member to ensure proper follow-through. The assignment is acceptable only when each staff member understands it and is prepared adequately to carry it out.

### Demonstrate Trust in Coworkers' Abilities

Third, the client care manager must respect or treat each coworker as an individual with specific needs, who contributes to the group's effort and is recognized for contributing. Unless there is a specific reason not to do so, the client care manager expects each staff member to perform all functions and tasks delineated in her or his position description. Although trust is difficult to manage, it is crucial (Manthey, 1990, p. 28). Each staff member should be trusted to follow through on a client care assignment. Not to trust a coworker, without justification, diminishes the person's sense of self-worth and decreases the individual's value to the organization. All client care activities are important. By assigning staff in a way that challenges them to use their strengths and maximizes their contributions to quality care, the client care manager promotes the agency's efficiency and effectiveness.

### Promote Continuity of Care

Fourth, to the extent possible, client care is assigned consistently to the same staff to promote continuity of care. Most clients benefit from receiving care from staff who have in-depth knowledge and experience. Although clients generally do not mind answering occasional questions when they need to be asked, they appreciate not being asked to answer the same questions repeatedly. Consistency in working relationships between staff and clients improves efficiency and effectiveness and increases client satisfaction.

### Avoid Disrupting the Logical Work Flow

Fifth, the client care manager helps staff organize work by assigning activities in similar locations and in combinations that are compatible with multidisciplinary treatment program schedules. Each staff member can be in only one place at a time. If they are expected to be in two places simultaneously to complete care according to the multidisciplinary work group's schedule, work flow is likely to be disrupted. In addition to frustrating clients, these disruptions often negatively affect nursing staff, other work group members, and departments.

### Describe Assignments in Detail

Sixth, after ensuring that nursing staff are prepared adequately to complete client care assignments, the staff nurse describes the desired care in concrete or measurable terms. Detailed information is usually available on individual plans of care or defined in nursing procedure manuals. If it is not, it is important that clarification be made. For example, it is not adequate to say, "Mr. J needs regular intermittent catheterizations." Rather the staff member needs to know the frequency of the intermittent catheterizations and the amount of residual urine that is to be reported immediately for further evaluation. This clarification helps the employee and the staff nurse evaluate the outcomes of care. To confirm that the assignee accurately comprehends the assignment, the staff nurse seeks feedback throughout the workday. Sharing mutual expectations about client outcomes provides a sound foundation for evaluation later. Specific information about the care provided and feedback about the client's responses to it provide clues to areas of continuing concern as well. The RN is responsible for evaluating the client's responses and progress in meeting desired outcomes.

### Assign All Aspects of Care

Seventh, although it almost goes without saying, **responsibility** for the total care of each client is explicitly assigned (Schaffer, 1991, pp. 147–148), including concrete tasks and overall functions involved in assessing, planning, and evaluating care. To ensure that customer-driven services are consistent with common nursing goals, the client care manager to avoid assigning only procedural aspects of client care. Frequently, only the nursing tasks (e.g., monitoring vital signs, dressing changes, personal hygiene measures) involved in a client's care are assigned. Knowledge and skills to analyze the data collected about client responses and to evaluate what, if any, revisions in the care plan also are needed. Assigning everything promotes caring attitudes and development of corresponding systems to divide the nursing functions and activities involved in providing the desired client care. In addition to completing nursing tasks, nursing routines evolve that provide for accurate and timely assessment of client needs, communication and collaboration required for continuity, and coordination of details of discharge planning and implementation.

To promote accountability for all of a client's care and manage resources of UAP effectively, the client care manager (RN) needs to ensure that all nursing functions are assigned and performed to provide the care, not only the tasks of nursing care. Nurses can delegate tasks that they do, but they cannot delegate what they know (Murphy, 1999, p. 277). These situations require that RNs be assigned concurrently with UAP. Not to do so jeopardizes the client's well-being and places the RN at increased risk of liability. Expectations are communicated in terms that enable staff to determine if the desired results were achieved successfully. Through an orientation that is unique to nursing, this method emphasizes the totality of the client's care.

An assignment method might involve two types of responsibilities: (1) those that must be completed during each shift and (2) those that occur over extended or indefinite periods of time. In primary care manager patterns of service delivery, a primary care manager is designated in combination with staff nurses who are assigned care each shift (Tremblay and Roach, 1994, pp. 5, 47). The staff nurses implement the plan and need to perform all nursing functions to ensure that urgent needs and timely revisions in the plan of care are made. The primary care manager assumes responsibility for managing the client's response and evaluates the need to make changes in the plan based on emerging needs that require attention. In a modified team or functional nursing pattern of nursing service delivery, several persons might be assigned to manage a client's overall plan of care. In addition, each client care manager also might be assigned another group of clients for an extended period. These assignments would involve monitoring client responses and striving to ensure continuity of care for a group of clients over the long-term.

By reviewing completed client care assignment sheets, a staff nurse should be able to identify who is assigned to complete each aspect of the client's care. The responsibility for completing client care assignments rests primarily with the staff members employed to carry them out. A manager can never delegate this responsibility totally to other staff, however; ultimately the client care manager accepts responsibility for nursing functions within only the RN's scope of practice to ensure the quality of care provided. The client care manager shares responsibility for the nursing tasks assigned to other nursing work group members as well.

### Consider Changes in Clients' Conditions

Eighth, to ensure that clients receive needed care, the staff nurse considers the time and complexity of the assigned or delegated activities, initially and throughout the workday. Clients' conditions change, requiring reassessment of needs and perhaps different knowledge and skills to meet them. Sometimes changes in client conditions are anticipated and incorporated in the initial assignment. Typically, staff with greater knowledge and skills are assigned to care for less physiologically stable clients. At other times, a client's condition changes unexpectedly. These clients require more monitoring and skilled responses by the client care manager, including changes in work assignments, to ensure that client needs are being monitored, assessed, evaluated, and addressed adequately.

### Consider Changes in Clients' Plans of Care

Ninth, changes in client conditions or plans to treat them can mean that staff need more help or instruction to ensure safe care. Equipment, supplies, or treatment modalities may be prescribed that staff are unfamiliar with or that are beyond their scope of practice. If the nature of the client care remains within the assigned staff member's scope of practice or competencies, the client care manager needs to provide the additional help or instruction. Sometimes the staff nurse initially learns about changes in a client's plan of care when transcribing physician's "orders." It is crucial that the client care manager communicate these changes accurately and in a timely manner to assigned staff on the client's behalf. If the changes in the client's plan of care exceed the assigned staff member's scope of practice, the client care manager must reassign the client's care and make the provisions needed to provide it.

### Assign Responsibility for Total Care

Tenth, the client care manager needs to assign all of the nursing effort required to provide the client's care, including time, knowledge, and skills needed to communicate with others to coordinate, collaborate, and resolve issues and concerns in a timely manner. To do this, the client care manager needs adequate current information about the client's diagnostic or treatment programs and insight into problem-solving strategies needed to implement them cost-effectively. The immediate tasks of care are readily apparent to the work group; the nursing functions are less apparent. If the nursing functions are neglected, efficiency, quality, and continuity suffer, and risks of liability increase.

## Legal Aspects of Assigning Client Care

Thus far, this discussion has emphasized the need to focus on assessed or identified client needs as an essential foundation for meeting the responsibility of assigning client care (Feutz, 1988, p. 10). The agency's resources, policies, procedures, or position descriptions cannot be used as the sole basis for designating which staff member reasonably can provide care; the clients' needs also must be considered. The agency depends on staff nurses to collect information on clients' needs and to determine what needs to be done to meet them during the work shift. If the staff nurse does not know what care clients need, she or he cannot match the available knowledge, skills, attitudes, and talents corresponding to those needs.

As mentioned in Chapter Three, staff nurses are expected to provide accurate information about client needs demanded by the agency's classification system to help it provide adequate staffing. In addition, they are expected to assign available staff correctly to match client needs. The health-care agency assumes responsibility for providing adequate staffing, in terms of numbers and qualifications (Calfee, 1987, p. 26). If available staffing is inadequate, staff nurses are expected to communicate their concerns (preferably in writing) to their supervisors immediately to ensure safe and adequate care (Creighton, 1986b, p. 14). If the response is unsatisfactory, copies of the expressed concerns and personal records detailing the situation should be kept. Identifying the problem of inadequate staffing does not permit the staff nurse to decrease the standard of care below that required by law (Rabinow, 1985, p. 29). Clients are legally entitled to minimal standards of care, whether or not the agency is staffed adequately. Client care managers share responsibility for ensuring that these standards of care are provided. Client safety is required (White, 2002, p. 195). Standards for safe practice are based on scopes of nursing practice as defined by state licensing agencies. In a court of law, these standards might be compared with actions that would be taken by a peer, or reasonable and prudent nurse, in similar circumstances.

The staff nurse, as client care manager, assumes responsibility for nursing judgments, decisions, and actions (Creighton, 1986a, p. 24). That is, the nurse expects to answer for situations that are under her or his control. In circumstances in which control is shared, responsibility also is shared. In previous years, when the nurse acted as an agent of the health-care organization, the agency was held accountable under the respondeat superior doctrine. The agency, as "master," was assumed to exercise control over the nurse's actions and was accountable for the consequences of the nurse's judgments, decisions, and actions. As nursing gains recognition as a profession, individual nurses are likely to be perceived as being personally answerable for their judgments, decisions, and actions.

The staff nurse has the authority to judge the nature of client needs and the adequacy of staffing and to take action as necessary to obtain staffing. In other words, based on nursing knowledge and skills, the nurse has the personal and positional power to determine client needs and the organizational power to request adequate staffing. The nurse also decides whether the qualifications of the available staff match the complexity of client needs. Qualified staff can recognize promptly and manage changes in clients' conditions (Feutz, 1988, p. 9). The more complex the client's needs, the more knowledge and skill are needed to assess and manage them. Inexperienced (recently graduated) staff, temporary staff, or **agency staff** (subcontracted by temporary staffing agencies) usually need supervision and often additional direction if clients with complex needs are to receive safe care. If minimal standards of care are not provided and client safety is at risk, the nurse needs to take immediate action to alleviate the situation.

## Accountability

**Accountability** refers to being answerable for actions or inactions, including results, of self or others in the context of delegation (NCSBN, 1997a, p. 1). The staff nurse is answerable for the consequences of decisions made and actions taken in meeting the responsibilities of client care. Similarly, the staff nurse also needs to answer for what was needed and not done and the inaction (not doing what needed doing) of self or others to whom nursing tasks were delegated. If the nursing task was delegated appropriately, accountability may be shared. The staff nurse's primary accountability is to clients, as stipulated in the standards of practice established by the profession. These standards are used as a foundation for judging the correctness and adequacy of care. Not to adhere to accepted standards of practice and place the client at risk or cause harm is **malpractice,** or professional misconduct. Nurses carry malpractice insurance to manage the risk of being accused by clients of causing them serious harm or injuries. Malpractice insurance reduces the risk or financial burden of resolving accusations (Bernzweig, 1990, pp. 379–380). The individual nurse's need for malpractice insurance is discussed in more detail in the Epilogue.

Secondarily the nurse is answerable to the agency and is expected to comply with its policies, procedures, and guidelines. Accordingly, to be accountable when assigning care, the staff nurse must know the agency's guidelines for determining the employee qualifications needed to respond adequately to various types of client needs. The agency depends on input from staff nurses about assessed needs and the adequacy of staffing. When staff nurses identify the problem of inadequate staffing, they are expected to communicate immediately specific information about the nature of the clients' needs and available staffing to their immediate supervisors. As mentioned in Chapter Four, attempting to complete an impossible assignment and consequently endangering clients is irresponsible.

**Liability** is legal accountability or responsibility for client risks, danger, and injury caused by the nurse's malpractice or negligent acts. **Negligence** involves either acts of **commission** (i.e., doing something that harms the client) or acts of **omission** (i.e., not doing something that should have been done to prevent client harm or injury).

When the staff nurse assigns client care, the agency expects that nursing knowledge, skills, and standards will be the basis for designating what work each staff member is requested to do. The client care manager is authorized to allocate resources consistent with client needs and agency goals. Improperly assigning client care increases the nurse's risk of liability resulting from one's actions or the actions of others (Rhodes, 1986, p. 315). If the nurse acts responsibly, in accordance with agency policies and professional standards, the agency, as employer, can be held liable for the consequences of inadequate staffing. To the extent that the nurse is a participant in negligent acts believed to cause harm to clients, he or she shares liability. Proper assignment of total client care is a big step in providing safe care, and it concurrently eliminates the nurse's liability in this matter.

## Accepting Accountability for Assigned Client Care

As mentioned earlier, assigning client care entails designating individual staff members to provide it, within guidelines provided by the agency's formal organization, policies, procedures, position descriptions, and systems of care. When staff nurses assign client care according to the agency's guidelines, they accept responsibility for performing this function. They also accept supervisory responsibility for client care. Staff nurses accept primary responsibility for completing their assignments, however, and expect to answer for their actions. Properly assigned staff nurses are accountable for completing the work allocated to them within the allotted time and for the consequences of their work. They are answerable for completing the assigned client care activities in a safe, efficient, satisfactory manner.

### DELEGATING CLIENT CARE

**Principles for delegating the work of client care managers** differs from those for assigning client care. Assigning client care is a form of delegation. Assigning client care is a required function. It is done regularly to allocate properly the work that staff are employed to do. Client care assigned to others can be reassigned.

Another form of delegating is transferring work to another that is optional, or done by choice of the delegator and delegatee. RNs have the most inclusive legal

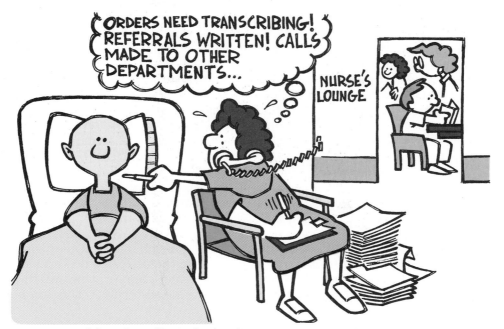

By not delegating effectively, the client care manager takes on extra work.

scope of practice of the various classifications of nursing staff, which permits them to delegate a range of activities to RNs, LPNs, NAs, or other UAP. Client care managers typically have many opportunities to delegate some of their assigned duties and tasks. The primary purpose of delegating client care is to shift some work to another staff member to increase one's own effectiveness and efficiency and improve the skills, effectiveness, and efficiency of those accepting the delegation (Hanston, 1991, p. 126; Sondak, 1991, p. 5). Responsibility for delegated duties and tasks never can be totally delegated, however.

## Process of Delegation

Whether or not client care is delegated is a personal decision of the staff nurse and not a scheduled or clearly defined requirement of the position. To develop skills used in delegating care to increase one's own effectiveness and efficiency and those of coworkers, client care managers need to seek opportunities to delegate constantly. A "Delegation Decision-making Grid" (NCSBN, 1997c, p. 2) may be obtained from the website: http://www.ncsbn.org/public/res/uap/delegationgrid.pdf. This grid provides guidelines and a structured method for delegating to licensed and UAP nursing staff. A score helps the delegator decide whether the nursing activity should be delegated.

Depending on the nature of the client care activities and qualifications of available staff, many characteristics of the process of delegation are similar to those used to assign client care. When assigning client care, the manager needs to know the strengths and weaknesses of the staff to whom the work is allocated. When delegating care, it is also important that the delegator know her or his own personal strengths, likes, dislikes, and vulnerabilities. This helps the nurse to delegate to improve quality of care and staff capabilities rather than seek personal gain or avoid activities that are personally distasteful.

Client care managers can and should delegate direct and indirect client care tasks. The principles delegation to apply to both types. There are several principles for delegating work assigned to client care managers. Box 13-3 lists requirements for properly delegating work to others. The client care manager needs to know what is involved in the activities that are being delegated, within the context of her or his own position description and that of the delegatee. The tasks to be delegated need to be consistent with these position guidelines. In other words, is this work similar in type and complexity (e.g., knowledge, decision making, and technical skills) to that routinely expected of this type of staff member? If the answer is yes, this work could be delegated. In addition, the delegated tasks need to be consistent with the individual's capabilities, interests, and skills because the delegatee needs to accept the additional work voluntarily. Receiving the delegatee's approval ensures that he or she accepts responsibility for completing the specific tasks and accepts accountability for the consequences of actions taken.

---

**BOX 13-3**

## Requirements for Delegating Duties and Tasks

1. Determine the extent and complexity of client needs or the nature of the work to be delegated.
2. Identify the employee to whom tasks or duties are to be delegated.
3. Determine that the work is consistent with the employee's position description and normal duties.
4. Clearly communicate expectations and desired results using concrete, measurable terms; convey trust and sufficient authority. Tell your delegatee what intended outcomes or processes you have in your mind. Discuss these expectations until you believe the delegatee comprehends them.
5. Obtain the employee's voluntary acceptance of the work request.
6. Keep communication lines open while providing needed direction, instruction, and supervision.
7. Compare actual results with desired goals; give constructive feedback and praise to reward the employee's efforts. Seek feedback on your job of delegating.
8. Constantly work toward increased productive use of time and resources and efficiency required to provide cost-effective quality care.
9. Practice, practice, practice!

To delegate client care effectively, the client care manager needs to communicate expectations clearly and completely. The delegatee should be able to describe what results are expected and what types of client responses or variations need to be reported to the client care manager.

Skills needed to delegate effectively are developed through practice, and typically efficiency also increases with practice. Before delegating client care, the desired results must be clear in the manager's own mind and in the mind of the person who will strive to achieve them. The desired results must be described in concrete, descriptive terms so that client outcomes and characteristics can be readily used to determine whether the delegatee was successful. Open discussions help the delegatee to express concerns and questions and agree on mutual expectations of the delegation.

## Barriers to Effective Delegation

Many staff nurses have great difficulty delegating work effectively to available staff (Lane, 1990, p. 46). Often, whether any client care is delegated depends on the norms of a specific work culture. Predominant staff perceptions of the purposes of delegation often condition client care managers (Lawrie, 1990, p. 1). Some cultures encourage delegation, whereas others do not; norms of the work environment, often unspoken, can reinforce or punish individuals who delegate work. For example, a culture's prevailing attitude may be, "We all work together until we're all done," or "Everyone is expected to do a fair share around here." Client care managers in such a culture might hesitate to delegate any client care activities assigned to them, fearing that they might appear incompetent, disorganized, or lazy.

A different work culture might encourage client care managers to delegate in the interests of cost-effectiveness. Managers might hesitate, however, to grant their delegatees decision-making authority consistent with the responsibility needed to follow through efficiently. In such a case, the delegation defeats its purpose because the delegatee spends considerable time and effort relaying information instead of using the delegated authority to make decisions needed to complete activities smoothly and efficiently. Fear of liability for the actions of others is often given as a reason for not delegating (Salmond, 1990, p. 41).

Some nurses might hesitate to delegate client care activities because doing so frees up time for them to do activities that are more complicated or with which they are less familiar. Others believe that because they can perform an activity proficiently, nothing is to be gained by delegating it to other available staff. Other staff members often welcome the challenge of learning new skills or increasing their proficiency in performing them. Some client care managers avoid delegating care for fear of "dumping" extra work on staff. These explanations are invalid in most situations.

## Preparing to Delegate Client Care

The client care manager needs to address several criteria to delegate client care successfully.

### Assess Staff Member Skills

Usually the manager has worked with the delegatee before delegating various activities to him or her. These experiences help the client care manager become familiar with the other staff member's attitudes, knowledge, and skills. They also give the client care manager a chance to evaluate the staff member's skills. Before delegating any client care, the client care manager needs to determine that the staff member has the capacity to complete it.

### Delegate Consistent with Agency Policy

The client care manager needs to ensure that the types of client care delegated are consistent with the agency's policies. That is, the type of work being delegated must be consistent with that normally performed by the delegatee's employee classification. A unit clerk can be asked to requisition supplies, whereas nursing staff can perform various procedures involved in client care. If delegated work is not consistent with agency policy and position descriptions, the employee is less likely to have repeated opportunities to practice new skills to perform them efficiently. The care needs to be delegated to the type of employee who is likely to perform it correctly or who reasonably might be expected to perform this type of work in the future.

### Trust the Delegatee

The client care manager needs to trust the delegatee to complete the delegated work according to established standards or mutual expectations. A positive working relationship reduces any reservation the client care manager might have about granting the subordinate the authority needed to complete the tasks. If the client care manager expresses confidence in the delegatee's capacity to complete the tasks, the delegatee is likely to believe in her or his own abilities. A trusting relationship also promotes open and effective communication, so clear instructions and directions can be given. This increases the chances that the delegatee will accept accountability for the consequences of her or his actions.

### Grant Sufficient Authority

For the delegatee to make decisions to obtain desired client outcomes, the delegator needs to grant sufficient authority. In other words, the person performing the client care activities needs authorization to modify activities to achieve desired results. Requiring the individual to confer repeatedly with the delegator before making necessary decisions is frustrating and inefficient. If the delegatee's decision-making authority is limited, the limits must be clarified at the time the tasks are delegated, not throughout the process of completing them. It is crucial that the manager recognize and praise the coworker for completing delegated care safely and satisfactorily. The manager also should seek feedback to help the coworker and to sharpen delegation skills. With practice, delegation can become an extremely valuable tool for managing time and building effective working relationships. Ultimately, everyone benefits—clients, staff, and the agency.

### Provide Opportunity to Learn and Practice

One purpose of delegation is to help the coworker learn and practice new skills. To be successful, the experience needs to be positive without risking the client's safety.

If the delegatee makes a mistake, the staff nurse, as delegator, needs to explain the error and teach the person how to perform the activity correctly. If too much supervision, humiliation, or frustration is involved in completing the delegated tasks, the delegatee is likely to avoid accepting responsibility for other delegated tasks, and the client care manager is unlikely to use available time and resources more efficiently over the long-term. The client care manager needs to practice delegating activities to improve the quality of care, time management, and development of scarce human resources. Although there are risks involved, if reasonable precautions are taken, delegating client care leads to satisfying work experiences.

## Accepting Accountability for Delegated Tasks

The client care manager accepts primary responsibility for the consequences of delegation and shares accountability for them. These consequences can relate to one's own actions in delegating and to the actions or nonactions taken by the delegatee. If client safety is risked and the individual experiences injury or harm, the client care manager may be liable. When undesired results occur, questions are asked concerning who was responsible for the client's care and why and how the activities were delegated. When reviewing the delegation process, the appropriateness of the delegation and the qualifications of the staff to whom the care was delegated are considered. The client care manager determines the nature of the client's needs and the coworker's capacity to meet them. By including all the components of proper delegation, the client care manager becomes an active participant in the delivery of care with the coworker (Reis, 1991, p. 12). Consequently the client care manager shares liability for the actions or nonactions of the coworker. These legal parameters apply in situations in which the client care manager has delegated care to others or has accepted delegation from others. The client care manager is responsible only when the nurse clearly delegates a task that lies within the professional practice role or scope of practice (Lane, 1990, p. 46).

Authority, responsibility, and accountability for delegation rest primarily in the client care manager's decision-making role. That is, the client care manager has administrative control over the delivery of care and is responsible for "protecting and promoting the common good" (Sullivan and Brown, 1989, p. 563). When delegation is performed properly, no injury or harm occurs, and everyone benefits; only when it is performed improperly does the potential for liability exist. Proper delegation is a skill well worth refining.

### SUMMARY

Staff nurses are expected to assign and delegate client care to available staff while managing care. Assigning client care involves allocating the work to be done and designating who is to do it. To complete this function, work is allocated according to assessed client needs and guided by agency policies, organizational structure, position descriptions, and legal scopes of practice. Responsibility for care assigned to others can be reassigned but not totally delegated. In addition, care assigned directly to the client care manager can be delegated. Client care and nonclinical work can be delegated. Proper delegation of tasks is based on the complexity of the work and the staff member's legal scope of practice, assigned role, attitudes, knowledge, skills, and corresponding position description. The delegatee must accept the work request voluntarily.

When making assignments, the client care manager needs to understand the types of client needs each category of staff member is prepared to meet and the legal limits established for her or his scope of practice. The RN assumes responsibility for assessing client needs and judging the adequacy of available staffing to meet them. Client care is assigned consistent with legal guidelines, agency position descriptions, and established policies and procedures; consequently, each staff member is responsible for her or his own actions and nonactions taken to complete them. The RN is expected to make special provisions for clients with unpredictable, physiologically unstable, infectious, or other complex conditions to ensure that minimum standards of safe care are provided. These standards reflect compliance with established standards of practice, and no exception is made for inadequate staffing. Client care is assigned on the basis of assessed needs and the staff's competence to provide it.

Client care assignments consider continuity of care; geographic location of clients; scheduled treatment programs and related nursing staff demands; and individual staff interests, skills, and talents. Total client care needs to be assigned in such a way as to reduce fragmentation and need for coordination. Assignments include all aspects of client care; focusing on the tasks of care is avoided. RNs need to be assigned with LPNs and UAP to ensure that all nursing functions are included in the work allocation. Staff need respect, recognition, and trust to sustain effective working relationships.

Staff assume primary responsibility for completing the work assigned to them. Consequently, they accept liability for the consequences of their actions. The client care manager shares responsibility with the agency for obtaining staffing adequate to provide minimum standards of safe care. Accordingly the client care manager is accountable for decisions made and actions or nonactions taken to ensure safe care or avoid harm or injury to clients. The client care manager is legally liable for malpractice or negligent acts that result in client injury or harm.

Client care managers may delegate various aspects of their work properly to increase their productivity and to increase the quality of care by developing the skills of other staff. Many nurses hesitate to delegate. Sometimes this reluctance results from characteristics of the work culture or personal fears, but if proper guidelines are followed and preparations are made, delegation can improve the quality of care. The staff nurse is responsible for assessing client needs and matching them to the staff member's nursing skills, attitudes, and qualifications; in addition, expectations and instructions need to be communicated clearly to the delegatee. The delegatee voluntarily accepts the delegated work. The client care manager supervises the staff member's performance and provides feedback to help achieve the desired results. The client care manager grants the delegatee the authority needed to complete the work smoothly; the work relationship is built on trust and confidence in the individual's abilities. The client care manager provides the staff member with corrective feedback to enable her or him to develop nursing skills further. The staff

member needs praise and recognition for accepting and successfully completing delegated care activities.

Client care managers assume primary responsibility for the consequences of delegated work. This responsibility relates to their decision-making role in determining client needs and how to meet them. When client care is delegated properly, no injury or harm is likely to occur. Management skills used to delegate client care properly are well worth nurturing to increase the client care manager's effectiveness and productivity. Use of these skills is instrumental in helping others increase their productivity as well.

## APPLICATION EXERCISES

1. Your nursing work group consists of another staff nurse, two LPNs, and two NAs. Identify the activities that you can assign to each category of nursing staff based on your assigned agency's policies, procedures, and position descriptions.
2. Your group of 20 clients includes some with stable conditions and others who are not physiologically stable. Describe guidelines you would use to assign client care to available staff.
3. Contrast nursing authority with accountability for meeting client needs.
4. Describe which activities and functions an RN can delegate to members of the nursing work group. Give reasons for your answer.
5. Describe approaches you would use to promote positive experiences for your delegatees.

## CRITICAL THINKING SCENARIO

Imagine yourself employed in a home care hospice program. You typically are expected to manage the care of 12 terminally ill clients on your unit and all the associated support of their families and social support groups. Frequently, clients' perspectives change regarding expectations of their families and needs for comfort and hydration. These changes often require major changes in the medical management and prescriptions. Your nursing work group usually includes one RN, one LPN, and two UAP that have completed the agency's 40-hour orientation program. You often feel stretched beyond your limits of energy and time, trying to complete all prescribed treatments and administer intravenous analgesics and prescribed hydration regimens.

1. Describe what you think only you could do for this client group. Give reasons for your answer.
2. How would you assign the nursing care of 12 terminally ill clients with the available staff?
3. In your opinion, what task would be most difficult to perform but needed to ensure that each client/family/social support group received personalized care?
4. What strategies would you use to see that all of the care that you assessed as being needed is assigned? Provided?

# REFERENCES

Ameduri PB: Directing others is a demanding role, *RN 57*(10):21, 23–24, 1994.

Barter M, Furmidge ML: Unlicensed assistive personnel, *J Nurs Admin 24*(4):36–39, 1994.

Bernzweig EP: *The nurse's liability for malpractice*, ed 5, St. Louis, MO, 1990, Mosby.

Calfee BE: Understaffing, *Nurs Life 7*(6):25–29, 1987.

Conger MM: The nursing assessment decision grid: tool for delegation decision, *J Cont Educ Nurs 25*(1):21–27, 1994.

Creighton H: Understaffing, part I, *Nurs Manage 17*(4):24, 27–28, 1986a.

Creighton H: Understaffing, part II, *Nurs Manage 17*(5):14, 16, 1986b.

de Ruiter HP: NAs aid RN retention, *Nurs Manage 32*(11):39–40, 2001.

Evans SA: Delegation: what do we fear? *Heart Lung 20*(1):17A–20A, 1991.

Feutz SA: Nursing work assignments: rights and responsibilities, *J Nurs Admin 18*(4):9–11, 1988.

Fink JLW: Smoothing the transition: use these tips to help agency nurses get up to speed, *Nursing 32*(2):32, 2002.

Habgood CM: Ensuring proper delegation to unlicensed assistive personnel, *AORN J 71*(5):1058–1060, 2000.

Hanston RI: Delegation: learning when and how to let go, *Nurs '91* 21(4):126–133, 1991.

Lane AJ: Nurse extenders: refocusing on the art of delegation, *J Nurs Admin 20*(5): 40–46, 1990.

Lawrie J: Turning around attitudes about delegation, *Supervis Manage 35*(12):1–2, 1990.

Loquist RS: State Boards of Nursing respond to the nurse shortage, *Nurs Admin Q 26*(4):33–39, 2002.

Manthey M: Trust: essential for delegation, *Nurs Manage 21*(11):28–29, 1990.

Murphy EK: RN liability exposure for delegated acts, *AORN J 69*(1):277–279, 1999.

National Council of State Boards of Nursing: *Glossary—delegation terminology*, 1997a, pp. 1–4. http://www.ncsbn.org/public/res/uap/glossary.pdf

National Council of State Boards of Nursing: *Role development: critical components of delegation curriculum outline*, 1997b, pp. 1–15. http://www.ncsbn.org/public/res/uap/roledevelopment.pdf

National Council of State Boards of Nursing: *Delegation decision-making grid*, 1997c, pp. 1–2. http://www.ncsbn.org/public/res/uap/delegationgrid.pdf

Rabinow J: Inadequate staffing? Don't take chances with risky solutions, *Nurs Life 5*(4):28–30, 1985.

Reis DG: Appropriate delegation of activities, *Nurs Manage 22*(1):12, 1991.

Rhodes AM: Liability for the actions of others, *MCN 11*(5):315, 1986.

Salmond SW: Clinical support workers: a help or a hindrance to the shortage crisis? *Orthop Nurs 9*(5):39–46, 1990.

Schaffer RR: Demand better results and get them, *Harv Bus Rev 69*(2):142–149, 1991.

Sheehan JP: Delegating to JAPs—a practical guide, *RN 64*(11):65, 2001.

Sondak A: Delegation: getting to the heart, or gut, of the matter, *Supervis Manage 36*(3):5, 1991.

Sullivan PA, Brown T: Unlicensed persons in patient care settings: administrative, policy, and ethical issues, *Nurs Clin North Am 24*(2):557–569, 1989.

Tremblay LM, Roach J: The patient care manager, *J Nurs Admin 24*(10):5, 47, 1994.

Vernarec E: Just say "No" to mandatory overtime? *RN 63*(12):69–74, 2000.

White GB: Patient safety: an ethical imperative, *Nurs Econ 20*(4):195–197, 2002.

# 14

# *Conducting Client Care Conferences as a Management Tool*

*When you complete this chapter, you should be able to:*

1. State common purposes of client care conferences.
2. Distinguish client care conferences designed primarily to manage care from conferences designed primarily to teach others.
3. Describe the process used to prepare for a client care conference.
4. Describe the process of conducting a client care conference.
5. Describe strategies to increase the effectiveness and efficiency of client care conferences.
6. Describe various methods of evaluating the effectiveness of client care conferences.

## KEY CONCEPTS

conduct a client care conference as a management tool

process of conducting a management conference

identifying clients who could benefit

prepare for and plan

purpose

conduct the meeting

structure

evaluate the effectiveness

## CLIENT CARE CONFERENCES

Entry-level staff nurses are expected to manage client care using a variety of management skills in many different organizational contexts. They are expected to direct, supervise, and coordinate the efforts of nursing and multidisciplinary work groups to enable clients to meet their health needs in a cost-effective manner. In the past, many nurses did not develop the skills needed to participate in or conduct conferences, especially conferences involving multidisciplinary work group members (where roles might overlap) (Coker and Schreiber, 1990, p. 46) as a component of their formal educational preparation. As a consequence, many nurses undervalue their contributions to nursing and multidisciplinary work groups. More recently, the value of group work has been recognized sufficiently to merit educators helping students learn to conduct effective meetings and participate in work group processes (Asselin, 2001, p. 24; Bigelow et al., 1999, p. 355; Godfrey, 1999, p. 363; Winter, 2000, p. 210). Client care managers, similar to other knowledge workers, need and should plan to develop skills needed to work effectively with groups. Conducting client care conferences as described in this chapter helps one to develop this much-needed skill that also benefits client care.

This chapter is designed primarily to help the beginning staff nurse to develop conferencing skills to manage complex client care. This management tool is different from the regularly scheduled conferences held to promote communication between members of a nursing unit's multidisciplinary work group. The regularly scheduled conferences typically are attended by the nurse assuming the lead position for the nursing work group, who provides current information to the multidisciplinary work group members and later provides feedback to various members of the nursing work group. To perform this function satisfactorily, the nurse needs current information about the client's goals, functional abilities, any changes necessitated by the client's responses, and anticipated length of stay, if pertinent. The skills needed to contribute successfully to this type of conference are discussed in detail in Chapter Eleven.

When used selectively and skillfully, the management tool of conducting a client care conference is effective in identifying current client needs in complex situations and matching staff approaches to meet them. It could be considered a "creativity-relevant work group skill" or one strategy for creative problem solving (Gilmartin, 1999, p. 1; Sewell et al., 2002, p. 176). The client care manager can use the lack of client progress as an opportunity to stimulate creative, innovative group work and practice her or his management skills. When selecting this strategy, the nurse believes that the client's care will be improved to justify the expense of conducting the conference.

When a client is not making expected progress, the nurse can **conduct a client care conference as a management tool** to improve the quality of the client's care. A client might not make anticipated progress for many reasons. One reason might be that some of the many people involved in the client's treatment do not share the same client care goals. Another reason might be that the client did not respond to treatment as expected.

Clinical conferences designed to help staff manage a client's care better with available resources are the focus of this chapter. This type of management conference is designed, planned, and implemented at the discretion of the staff nurse or other multidisciplinary work group member to improve the quality of care received by clients at serious risk. Staff nurses conduct management conferences to build staff, client, and family or support group commitment to individualized plans of care; to facilitate desired staff approaches; and to coordinate the various disciplines involved. Conducting a management conference requires distinct nursing skills. Nurses who use these skills regularly refine them with practice, to the benefit of clients.

Management conferences consume agency resources, primarily scarce staff time. Management conferences are used to help staff recognize complex client problems and their possible causes and to identify and evaluate proposed solutions that are acceptable to the client and staff. The client benefits from the care plan adjustment, and staff members gain insight into the individual's situation. Having participated in formulating the plan, staff members increase their commitment to carry it out. Because management conferences use staff time, they are costly, but failing to recognize clients who could benefit from management conferences is more costly in terms of increased lengths of stay or services or ineffective expenditure of staff time, equipment, supplies, and facilities to achieve desired client outcomes.

## Other Types of Conferences

Nursing students usually are familiar with the types of conferences conducted for teaching purposes. A clinical conference (sometimes referred to as a *preconference* or *postconference*) held for teaching purposes usually has as its primary purpose to teach others, including fellow students and staff. The "ground rules" for conducting the meeting reflect its teaching purposes; these conferences include specific categories of information and discussion and are scheduled according to the needs and goals of the learners. They are evaluated in terms of their effectiveness in addressing the learners' needs (Skurski, 1985, pp. 166–168).

Another common type of clinical conference is that which is regularly scheduled for the multidisciplinary work group to help coordinate routine activities and update plans of care. These conferences are organizationally sanctioned and structured to meet the facility's needs for discharge planning. Nursing students often participate in client care conferences while working with psychiatric or chronically ill clients. The work group regularly schedules time to meet to review systematically treatment plans for each client. These conferences increase the effectiveness and efficiency of multidisciplinary work groups by providing regular opportunities for members to express their concerns, share observations, and plan or revise client care plans. These multidisciplinary client care conferences are an integral part of coordinating efforts on the client's behalf.

Change-of-shift reports are another type of clinical conference used to manage care, although they are not the type of conference that staff nurses use at their discretion to manage client care. Rather, these conferences are regularly scheduled sessions that give staff nurses an opportunity to discuss client needs, concerns, and progress to promote continuity of care.

## CONDUCTING A MANAGEMENT CONFERENCE

The **process of conducting a management conference** involves four phases:
1. Identifying clients who could benefit
2. Preparation
3. Implementation
4. Evaluation and follow-up

### Phase One: Identifying Clients Who Could Benefit from a Conference

Client care managers accept responsibility for **identifying clients who could benefit** directly from being the focus of a management conference. Certain characteristics increase a client's risk of responding ineffectively to treatment. These characteristics vary, but they include the following:
1. Language or communication barriers
2. Extremes in chronologic age
3. Complexity of disease processes
4. Staff unfamiliarity with treatment approaches
5. Unusual client coping styles
6. Lack of meaningful or supportive relationships

The client care manager is in a good position to identify clients at special risk, such as clients confronted by complex situations not addressed adequately by agency routines or clients who are not achieving desired outcomes within the anticipated time frames. Accordingly the client care manager can mobilize agency resources in the client's behalf. Consequently, conducting a management conference can lead to more effective use of available resources.

Corkery (1989, p. 21) reported that staff nurses practicing on an orthopedic inpatient unit identified the following client characteristics that complicated discharge planning: (1) one or more functional disabilities, (2) urinary or fecal incontinence, (3) altered mental conditions, and (4) limited social support. Similarly, Bull (1988, p. 418) reported that direct care providers found discharge planning most difficult for clients who (1) required highly skilled care, (2) were without support systems, (3) were confused, (4) had Medicaid health insurance, and (5) were without money. Clients with these characteristics were difficult to place because they often exceeded prescribed lengths of stay. Bull (1988, pp. 418–419) also noted that, with the implementation of DRGs (diagnosis-related group as a basis for estimated cost of care and length of stay) as a reimbursement strategy, professional staff needed to make a deliberate effort to remain focused primarily on client needs rather than on the facility's strategies for educating clients about lengths of stay prescribed by DRGs. As entry-level staff nurses gain experience, they become familiar with common patterns of client response to various health conditions and to typical treatment processes from admission to discharge. Nursing students who choose to develop skills needed to conduct management conferences might turn to their resource persons (e.g., clinical instructors or experienced staff nurses) to help them identify clients who could benefit from such a conference.

As they gain experience, staff nurses learn to differentiate common individual variations from characteristics that indicate that a client is at serious risk for potential complications or is unable to make desired progress to meet care goals. For example, a client might be confronted with language or cultural barriers that complicate her or his ability to understand the purposes of various diagnostic procedures or treatments. This might delay informed consent and active participation based on comprehension of desired behaviors. Or a client experiencing a multiplicity of diseases and complications might perceive treatment goals differently from health-care providers. As a result, there may be conflict instead of a mutually agreed-on program of treatment. Sometimes it is assumed that clients understand disease processes, when in reality they have not received adequate instruction and are unable to carry out the self-care procedures required to manage safely at home. Clients may feel overwhelmed by the many demands placed on them by family and staff and be unable to use coping mechanisms that were effective in the past in enabling them to adjust.

To avoid discharging clients without adequate preparation, the client care manager, as advocate, needs to intervene in a timely manner. By implementing teaching plans or communicating special needs to home care agency staff, workable discharge plans can be implemented that are mutually agreeable to clients, families, and staff.

In some health-care organizations, any member of the health-care team can suggest that a client care conference be held (Jaeger, 1988, p. 62). This approach encourages staff to communicate openly their concerns about client care. The client care manager often determines, however, when a management conference is needed to benefit a specific client (Ceccio, 1986, p. 42). The best time to identify these clients is when the client care manager evaluates an individual's progress in meeting the desired outcomes of a current plan. Does the current plan address the client's problems and needs? If the answer is no, the nurse needs to consider what changes in the client's condition, treatment, or response may indicate serious risks or complications. Does the client's response relate to lack of information or skills or inadequate preparation for discharge? If the answer is yes, a management conference could be an effective strategy for taking action.

Generally a potential candidate for a management conference is (1) a client with complex needs who has been admitted within the last 24 hours and needs a care plan, (2) a client who has developed new problems or needs, or (3) a client who has long-term needs that should be reevaluated. By deliberately concentrating on identifying clients who could benefit and by providing opportunities to practice communication skills, management conferences can be a viable, cost-effective strategy to coordinate team effort (Reed, 1987, p. 66).

## Phase Two: Preparing to Conduct a Management Conference

*Formulate Conference Purpose*

Client care managers **prepare for and plan** management conferences. When a client is identified as being at serious risk or as not making anticipated progress, the nurse begins to formulate the specific **purpose** of the management conference. Management conferences focus on the nature of the client's situation and on finding more effective approaches to priority needs. For the conference to be successful, client needs must be matched accurately with available staff knowledge and skills. For example, if the client's needs relate to physical mobility, physiotherapists likely need to be involved; or if the client's needs are related to unrelieved pain, a pharmacist could provide valuable information. Finding timely answers is crucial; to confer after the client has been discharged from the unit or agency is unlikely to be of much practical use. Box 14-1 lists some common purposes of management conferences. The client care manager continuously evaluates client success in meeting desired outcomes and reacts when clients are identified who could benefit from a management conference.

The purpose or specific objective for holding a meeting must be stated clearly. The purpose must be identified, verbally or in writing, before preparing to conduct the meeting. Frequently, more than one purpose for a management conference can be identified. Sometimes, depending on the client's situation (e.g., rare disease entity), an additional purpose may be to enable staff to gain an accurate perspective. The purpose guides identification of nursing staff and multidisciplinary team members needed to participate in the conference.

Consider a pediatric client suspected of being a victim of child abuse who is experiencing discomfort related to multiple abdominal and skeletal injuries and is exhibiting delayed emotional and social development. This situation would require careful attention to nursing and multidisciplinary staff interactions. The purposes of this conference might be to manage the client's discomfort better and to establish

---

**BOX 14-1**

## COMMON PURPOSES OF MANAGEMENT CONFERENCES

1. To obtain input about the client's responses to treatment
2. To gain insight into the causes of the client's behavior and responses
3. To identify current priorities of client needs
4. To identify and evaluate proposed plans for addressing client needs
5. To build staff commitment for implementing desired approaches to client needs
6. To revise client care plans in a timely manner
7. To promote multidisciplinary work group communication needed to coordinate care
8. To resolve differences in perceptions of client responses needed to guide treatment plans
9. To formulate discharge plans that address complex client needs
10. To promote efficiency and success in satisfying client needs in a cost-effective manner

a discharge plan. The conference participants would include direct nursing staff, family, and involved multidisciplinary team members, such as a clinical pharmacist, social worker, and discharge planner.

Another client might be an anxious, middle-aged adult experiencing a progressive degenerative disease, with serious complications requiring the use of assistive respiratory equipment, oxygen, suctioning, and postural drainage. Family caregivers indicate that they feel tired, frustrated, and apprehensive about providing the needed care at home. The client has not improved noticeably during the first week of treatment. The purposes of the management conference might be to gather information about the client's current health problems and to make plans for long-term care. The conference participants might include direct service staff, client, family, respiratory therapist, physical therapist, and discharge planner.

As these examples show, the client care manager uses the purpose of the staff meeting to guide the selection of conference participants (Palmer and Palmer, 1983, p. 30). Because they need to approve the overall plan, physicians are encouraged to attend conferences. If they cannot, however, the client care manager collaborates with physicians to ensure that they understand staff concerns and recommendations for improving the client's quality of care (Kerstetter, 1990, pp. 216–217). Alternatively the person leading the efforts of the multidisciplinary work group accepts responsibility for obtaining the medical approvals needed to carry out the client's care plan (Herzog, 1985, p. 192).

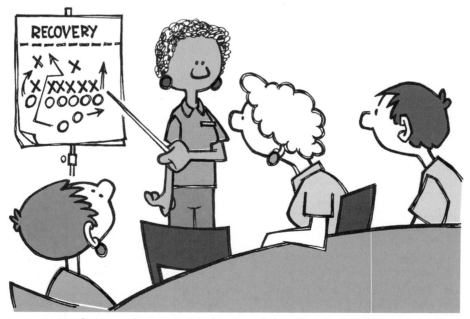

Management conferences focus on the nature of the client's situation and finding more effective approaches to priority needs.

In a similar manner, the client and members of the client's support group need to be involved if possible. The client needs to be involved in making decisions about her or his care when possible (Carroll, 2000, p. 83). This may require special provision to enable the work group to meet in the client's presence so that communication and clarification can occur and questions can be answered. This type of involvement typically results in greater commitment of staff and client to the plan of care.

## Match Purpose with Skills

Matching the purpose with needed skills is essential to increasing staff efficiency and success. The client care manager, who knows the roles and functions of various multidisciplinary staff members, can identify staff members who can contribute by and benefit from attending a management conference. It is important to include staff members who are authorized to make decisions about the client's care, rather than choosing substitutes or subordinates who lack the needed knowledge, skills, or authority. Subordinates benefit from participating in management conferences by learning about the importance of their observations and services (Coker and Schreiber, 1990, pp. 47–48). Their increased awareness helps them to carry out the client's plan of care. They also learn about the contributions made by various members of the multidisciplinary work group. Discussion of the client's situation usually generates additional information that can be used immediately to improve the client's quality of care.

To promote efficiency, duplication of multidisciplinary staff knowledge, skills, and expertise is avoided. As an advocate and coordinator of the client's care, the nurse often expects and agrees to communicate staff concerns to attending physicians who are unable to attend these conferences. Sometimes individual multidisciplinary staff members discuss their specific concerns directly with attending physicians, depending on their preferences and the complexity of the client's needs. These approaches promote the interdisciplinary collaboration and efficient exchange of information required to implement the client's overall treatment plan.

## Address Scheduling Issues and Requirements

Before scheduling a management conference, the client care manager needs to consider whether there is a better method available to address the client's needs. Other agency resources might be used, such as telephone conferencing or computerization of interdepartmental communications. If only one other discipline is involved, a telephone call might suffice to obtain the needed information. If multiple sources of input, discussion, and decisions are involved, however, a face-to-face conference might be most efficient and productive. If the participants are all nursing staff, the management conference might be scheduled to maximize involvement of members on two shifts to increase input and commitment to carrying out the desired approaches.

When the planning is finished, a specific time is set that allows the greatest number of participants in the client's care to attend. To the extent possible, department routines are considered so that key staff members are not asked to leave their work area during periods of peak work activity. Timeliness in addressing the client's needs has high priority, however. Generally, members of the multidisciplinary staff are flexible in planning to participate in management conferences. Being invited to attend implies that their contributions are valued highly.

Each staff member accepts responsibility for using the available time wisely. Consequently, participants use their discretion when deciding to attend a client care conference. Duties and functions of various disciplines may overlap (Gunn et al., 1988, pp. 33–34). The client care manager considers suggestions by staff that other persons might be selected more appropriately as conference participants.

To the greatest extent possible, the participants are asked to meet within or near the clinical area. If the client is asked to attend the conference, the group often meets in the client's room. Sometimes the staff members confer briefly to organize their approach before reporting to the client's room. When staff and family meet, they frequently use the ward conference room, which is near the clinical area but subject to fewer distractions. It is important to note whether other activities are scheduled in the meeting area to avoid last-minute conflicts. When informing participants of the scheduled conference, let each of them know the time and place. Also, let them know the purpose of the conference and the name of the client on whom it focuses. Try to notify participants far enough ahead, preferably 24 hours, so that they can plan and prepare to attend. Let the participants know that the length of the conference will be 30 minutes, maximum, to help them plan for needed clinical "coverage." Ceccio (1986, p. 42) reported from "our experience . . . the most successful conferences last 25 to 30 minutes. Moreover, they begin on time and end on time."

### Gather Current Information About the Client

Before the conference, the nurse needs to gather current information about the client as a person and about her or his health problems and needs. This preparation includes meeting the client (preferably by prior participation in her or his care) and reviewing the clinical record and written plan of care. To increase self-confidence, the client care manager makes a few brief notes about her or his professional perceptions of the client's priority nursing diagnoses or collaborative problems. Ceccio (1986, p. 43) described a "patient care conference format" that might be used or modified to increase the organization of information and efficiency of its presentation for beginning client care managers (Figure 14-1).

## Phase Three: Implementation of the Management Conference

Client care managers **conduct the meeting**. Often, primary nurses, nursing team leaders, or nursing case managers also might use this management strategy; if they are not in a direct caregiving relationship with the selected client on whom the conference is focused, they should defer final clinical decisions to the designated nurses who are in such positions with the client as a matter of professional courtesy.

### Convene the Conference

In contrast to many other types of meetings, the participants already have been informed of the meeting's purpose, time, and place. Formal agendas are not used. It

Client Care Conference Format

Date:_____  Time:_____  Room:_____

Client ID:_____  Age:_____

Staff and client/significant other(s) attending:_____

_____

Conference objectives:_____

Client's health history:_____

Client's current health status:_____

Client's sociocultural background:_____

Client/family/significant other strengths:_____

Client/family/significant other limitations:_____

Client's perception of illness/current health status:_____

Brief summary of nursing plan of care/collaborative problems:_____

_____

Client's progress toward desired outcomes (goals):_____

Other concerns:_____

Submitted by:_____

FIGURE 14-1 Example of a client care conference format. (Adapted from Ceccio CM: Professional development for orthopaedic nurses through patient care conferences, *Orthop Nurs* 5[2]:43, 1986.)

is important to start the conference at the scheduled time and place and to ensure that the participants are reasonably comfortable before beginning the discussion. Distractions such as noise, bright lights, extremes in temperature, or lack of chairs or space need to be addressed to avoid interrupting the conference later to attend to them. This approach conveys a genuine concern for the participants and an interest in their ability to contribute. Unless participants object, try to seat them in a circle or in such a way that they can face each other. Stress informality to the extent that it promotes open communication and encourages self-expression. All participants should introduce themselves if they have not been introduced previously. Familiarity with each other's disciplines helps participants to communicate with each other according to their roles and functions within the agency.

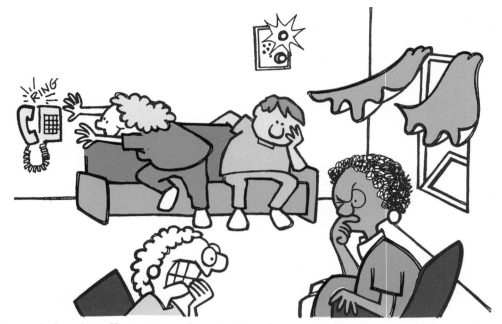

To maximize the effectiveness of a client conference, distractions should be kept to a minimum.

## Take Notes

The client care manager appoints someone to take notes, especially to record priority concerns and proposed solutions. The conference leader refers to these notes to help summarize the discussion. The **structure** or sequencing of components of management conferences may vary. The components usually include background information about the client, discussion of the client's current needs, formulation of the care plan, and a summary. Generally the conference is structured to address one or two (maximum three) top-priority client needs within the allotted time.

## Begin the Discussion

The leader begins by briefly reviewing the client's name, age, health problems, treatment plans, priority nursing diagnosis or collaborative problems, and any other information pertinent to the discussion. If helpful, the leader may note priority needs on an index card to use as a reference. Participants are invited to share concerns and identify their perceptions of the client's priority needs. They are encouraged to discuss their feelings or any problems that they have experienced. Everyone is encouraged to contribute to the discussion.

The leader assumes responsibility for keeping the discussion client-centered. Accordingly the leader minimizes digressions to other topics and avoids hidden agendas by returning the discussion to the client's situation and priority needs. When discussing the client's needs, participants are guided to avoid repetition, but they should take time for clarification. The leader gives participants sufficient time to describe their concerns but discourages lengthy explanations. The leader tries to prioritize the client's needs and address them one at a time.

### *Formulate Possible Solutions*

The leader asks the staff, client, or family members to describe possible solutions and how the client's needs could be met best. Participants are asked to clarify comments that are unclear to others. They are encouraged to make a special effort to identify differences in perception of client needs and their proposed solutions by listening actively to each other. They are asked to describe what each believes should or could be done to address these needs.

### *Summarize and Implement*

To help the recorder, the leader summarizes what the client's priority needs are (one at a time), what revisions are to be made in the care plan, and who is to do what to carry it out to accomplish the desired outcomes. The leader closes the conference on time, even if the discussion is still going. The discussion is closed early if completed ahead of schedule. This enables staff to return to their regular work as anticipated. The leader expresses appreciation for the participants' contributions and willingness to find workable solutions.

As soon as possible, the client care manager enters the revisions in the client's care plan on the appropriate agency form. In many agencies, these entries are documented directly in the client's clinical record or other communication tool used by staff providing the care. A summary of the conference results also might be recorded in the clinical record.

## Phase Four: Evaluation and Follow-up

Client care managers **evaluate the effectiveness** of the meeting, which is influenced by its specific purpose. It is not unusual for conferences to produce additional benefits, such as staff development (or gaining insight into agency policies or procedures that are ineffective or inefficient) and identification of possible improvements in client care. Sometimes conclusions drawn from participating in several conferences stimulate "customer-driven" organizational development. As staff gain experience working together, they are likely to become more efficient at responding to clients with similar needs and in using their conferencing skills.

Evaluation of the effectiveness of the client care conference is important. Lowenstein and Hoff (1994, pp. 47–49) indicated that feedback about the effectiveness of discharge planning (often involving multidisciplinary conferencing) was "limited." They suggested that such information likely would reinforce the value of the nurses' efforts toward effective discharge planning. Nurses were hesitant to replicate potentially flawed plans for other clients without information about effectiveness.

Several criteria can be used to judge the effectiveness of the management conference. Some can be used immediately after the conference, whereas others depend on the client's response to the revisions made in the care plan.

The conference should generate efficiently accurate information useful in planning and coordinating staff effort. The approaches established reasonably can be expected to benefit the client. If participants agree to the revisions, they are likely to follow up on the established care plan.

Figure 14-2 shows a brief conference evaluation form that might be used to help client care managers develop skills in conducting management conferences. Participants should be able to complete it in less than 5 minutes immediately after attending a conference. Sincere verbal feedback to conference participants who provided meaningful input or ideas provides intrinsic satisfaction and promotes future participation (Cisar, 1988, p. 88). After effective management conferences, partici-

---

### EVALUATION OF CLIENT CARE CONFERENCE

1. Did the conference focus on the client?     Yes     No

2. List the main nursing needs of problems that were not discussed and should have been.

3. Did the participants develop a useful plan that you could follow? If not, give reasons.

4. Did you feel comfortable with the staff members' contributions to the discussion? If not please explain.

5. Will the conference improve the client's care?     Yes     No

   In what ways?

About the Leader

1. Did the leader:

   A. Help the group identify client needs?     Yes     No
      What suggestions would you share to help the leader improve?

   B. (Guide discussion) or (control interaction)?   (Circle your response.)

   C. Summarize the care plan?     Yes     No

2. On a scale of 1 to 10 (10 being the highest), rate the conference.

FIGURE 14-2 Client care conference evaluation form.

pants should expect to observe improvements in client care. They also should concur that the cost of the conference is worth the expenditure of agency resources (e.g., the staff time consumed in completing the process). Ultimately, management conferences increase staff effectiveness and the quality of client care. With practice, skills used to conduct management conferences improve as well.

## SUMMARY

Staff nurses are expected to coordinate staff efforts to meet client needs in a cost-effective manner. As client care managers, they can conduct management conferences to increase staff efficiency and effectiveness in providing cost-effective care. They need to develop and practice specific skills to use this management tool effectively.

The purpose of management conferences differs from that of conferences conducted primarily for teaching purposes. The process of conducting management conferences involves four phases: (1) identifying clients who could benefit, (2) planning and preparation, (3) implementation, and (4) evaluation and follow-up. The client care manager needs to attend to various components in each phase to conduct a successful conference.

With experience, staff nurses learn to differentiate common individual variations in client responses from changes that indicate serious risk of complication or inability to progress in achieving desired outcomes. The client care manager is in a strategic position to identify clients at special risk, clients who are confronted by complex situations that are not addressed adequately by agency routines, and clients who are not progressing within reasonable time frames. Although any staff member can identify a need for a management conference, client care managers accept the responsibility and often take initiative for doing so when evaluation of client progress indicates need for more detailed consideration of the client's circumstances.

After identifying a client who could benefit from a management conference, the nurse begins to formulate the specific purpose for conducting one. Next, participants are selected. Selection criteria include knowledge and skills that match the nature of the client's anticipated needs and concerns. In addition, participants need authority to make the clinical decisions inherent in developing or revising care plans. To promote efficiency, duplication of staff expertise is avoided. Conferences are scheduled in or near the clinical area at times that are compatible with the participants' work flow. Participants are informed in advance of the subject, purpose, place, and time of the meeting.

Client care managers often lead management conferences. After completing introductions and ensuring the comfort of the participants, a recorder is appointed. The discussion begins with a brief overview of the client's circumstances, priority needs, and concerns. Informality and open communication are encouraged. All participants are expected to contribute. The leader accepts responsibility for keeping the discussion focused on client needs and the plan of care. The leader also summarizes the discussion to reinforce the expectations of the staff members who will implement the revisions in the client's care plan. Revisions are documented on the appropriate agency forms and communication tools to promote follow-through.

The success of the management conference relates directly to the purpose for which it was held. Although other benefits often are realized as well, results of the conference should improve the quality of care the client receives. Because of their involvement in developing specific approaches to the client's needs, participants expect the plan to benefit the client in a timely manner. Various methods of obtaining feedback from participants might be used to help the leader develop the skills used to conduct successful management conferences.

## APPLICATION EXERCISES

1. Compare the purpose of a management conference with that of a change-of-shift report.
2. Identify one of your assigned clients who could benefit from a client care conference. Confirm the appropriateness of your selection with your instructor or supervisor.
3. Discuss how this type of conference differs from conferences that are regularly scheduled to monitor client progress toward treatment goals and conferences that often are held for discharge planning purposes.
4. Plan and prepare a management conference so that needed participants can attend and contribute.
5. Evaluate the effectiveness of communication techniques you used during the management conference to promote implementation of the treatment plan.

## CRITICAL THINKING SCENARIO

Imagine yourself practicing nursing on a busy extended care unit. Most clients are elderly; fewer than 10% are younger than age 60. The primary purpose of this unit is to provide convalescent, rehabilitative care to clients required to enable them to return to their private homes. On admission, clients know their "allowed" length of stay; however, they are often frail physiologically, fatigue before completing daily therapies, and require environmental adaptations to meet activities of daily living. Their social support systems frequently visit during late afternoons, evenings, and weekends. On a number of occasions, you have heard clients remark, "I'm not sure I can make a go of it before I'll be thrown out." The multidisciplinary work group includes consulting clinical psychologists, consulting dietitians, nurses, occupational therapists, physical therapists, physicians, recreational therapists, social workers, and speech therapists.

**CRITICAL THINKING SCENARIO—cont'd**

1. What would you do first to reduce excessive fears of the clients?
2. Whom would you involve in the "image" issue? How?
3. What strategies would you suggest to fix the focus of treatment and rehabilitation on clients and their support systems?
4. What types of evaluation data would you request that the facility provide? (*Clue:* Review Zarle NC: Continuity of care: balancing care of elders between health care settings, *Nurs Clin North Am 24*[3]: 697–705, 1989.)

## REFERENCES

Asselin M: Time to wear a third hat? *Nurs Manage 32*(3):24–28, 2001.

Bigelow J, Seltzer J, Hall JC, Garcia J: Management skills in action: four teaching models, *Journal of Management Education 23*(4):355–376, 1999.

Bull MJ: Influence of diagnosis-related groups on discharge planning, professional practice, and patient care, *J Prof Nurs 4*(6):415–421, 1988.

Carroll TL: Patient satisfaction with participation in decision making, *Nurs Admin Q 24*(2):83–86, 2000.

Ceccio CM: Professional development for orthopaedic nurses through patient care conferences, *Orthop Nurs 5*(2):40–45, 1986.

Cisar NS: Nursing rounds: a method to facilitate patient care conferences, *Crit Care Nurs Q 11*(2):85–88, 1988.

Coker EB, Schreiber R: The nurse's role in a team conference, *Nurs Manage 21*(3):46–48, 1990.

Corkery E: Discharge planning and home health care: what every staff nurse should know, *Orthop Nurs 8*(6):18–26, 1989.

Gilmartin MJ: Creativity: the fuel of innovation, *Nurs Admin Q 23*(2):1–8, 1999.

Godfrey PC: Service-learning and management education: a call to action, *Journal of Management Inquiry 8*(4):363–378, 1999.

Gunn R, Timms S, Terry J, et al: A communication model in a day hospital, *J Gerontol Nurs 14*(8):30–36, 1988.

Herzog KR: Documentation of hospice care plan development and team meetings, *QRB 11*(2):190–192, 1985.

Jaeger TB: A head nurse's approach to multidisciplinary ethical conferences, *Nurs Manage 19*(1):60, 62, 1988.

Kerstetter NC: A stepwise approach to developing and maintaining an oncology multidisciplinary conference, *Cancer Nurs 13*(4):216–220, 1990.

Lowenstein AJ, Hoff PS: Discharge planning: a study of nursing staff involvement, *J Nurs Admin 24*(4):45–50, 1994.

Palmer BC, Palmer KR: *The successful meeting master guide for business and professional people*, Englewood Cliffs, NJ, 1983, Prentice-Hall.

Reed C: Patient care conferences: 3 fast steps to better patient care plans, *Nurs '87 17*(3):66, 1987.

Sewell AM, Fuller S, Murphy RC, Funnell BH: Creative problem solving: a means to authentic and purposeful social studies, *The Social Studies* July/Aug 2002, pp. 176–179.

Skurski V: Interactive clinical conferences: nursing rounds and education imagery, *J Nurs Educ* 24(4):166–168, 1985.

Winter JK: Student evaluation of a learning exercise designed to develop effective meeting skills, *Journal of Education for Business* March/April 2000, pp. 210–214.

Zarle NC: Continuity of care: balancing care of elders between health care settings, *Nurs Clin North Am* 24(3):697–705, 1989.

# PROFESSIONAL DEVELOPMENT

# 15

# *Addressing Ethical and Legal Issues*

*When you complete this chapter, you should be able to:*

1. Describe fundamental ethical concepts.
2. Distinguish among ethics, spirituality, and law.
3. Describe the consequences of violating codes of conduct.
4. Describe appropriate responses to incompetent colleagues.
5. Describe legal ramifications of life-and-death issues that might stimulate conflict between coworkers.
6. Describe how health-care financing methods might generate conflict.
7. Describe mechanisms used to protect subjects of nursing research.
8. List three emerging ethical issues that affect nursing practice.

## KEY CONCEPTS

values
beliefs
cultural norms
ethics
ethical principles
essential professional values
  altruism
  equality
  esthetics
  freedom
  human dignity
  justice
  truth
common ethical principles of nursing
  autonomy
  beneficence
  nonmaleficence

justice
veracity
confidentiality
fidelity
moral conflicts
moral reasoning process
  moral issue
  moral dilemmas
  moral uncertainty
  moral judgment
  ethical behavior
  ethical nursing practice
  moral distress
spirituality
laws
code of nursing conduct
  legal

ethical
quality of life
living will
advance directive
durable power of attorney
providing aggressive treatment
 extraordinary support
  measures

resuscitative measures
withholding aggressive treatment
 death with dignity
 supportive measures
protecting the rights of human
 subjects
institutional research committees
using new knowledge

## INCORPORATING ETHICAL DECISIONS IN NURSING PRACTICE

All nursing practice entails ethical decision making. Understanding common ethical concepts helps the nurse to practice nursing in accordance with ethical standards established by the profession. This chapter discusses some of the common ethical issues confronting managers of client care.

## Applying Knowledge of Ethical Concepts

Addressing ethical concerns requires application of knowledge of ethical concepts. These concepts frequently concern such topics as client autonomy, client participation in clinical decision making, justice in the context of the health-care setting, and use of scarce available resources. Other common concerns relate to quality-of-life issues, advance directives, living wills, withholding aggressive treatment, and extraordinary means of prolonging life or promoting comfort. The health technology used to diagnose, treat, and substitute for human functions also has created a variety of ethical issues. In the future, the ethical issues inherent in nursing practice, which reflect social and technologic changes, are likely to become increasingly complex and require more complex strategies for addressing them (Martin, 1999, pp. 319–320).

As we make the transition from the industrial era to the informational era and the global economy continues to evolve, American culture is likely to become even more diverse. Increasing cultural diversity is reflected in prevailing societal values, norms, and mores (commonly accepted behaviors). Behaviors considered acceptable to members of one culture may be unacceptable to members of another. A persistent value held by Americans is the ideal of free choice. Each nurse needs to identify and clarify her or his own personal and professional values as a basic requirement for sound ethical reasoning.

## Applying Ethical Principles

The various nursing codes of conduct used to delineate ethical nursing practice are all similar. According to Sawyer (1989, p. 148), who surveyed codes of nursing ethics, there is universal nursing agreement that the nurse should:

1. Accept responsibility for maintaining competence in nursing practice.
2. Strive to maintain "good relations" with coworkers.

3. Respect life.
4. Respect the dignity of every client.
5. Preserve confidentiality.
6. Provide care in a nondiscriminatory manner.

Differences in codes of ethics reflect the cultures of the nurses who adopted them (Sawyer, 1989, pp. 147–148). The American Nurses Association (ANA) Code for Nurses reflects the diversity of American culture and the expectation that the nurse will accept differences in lifestyles, standards of living, and the values of others. The ANA Code for Nurses is presented later in this chapter.

The principle of nondiscrimination prohibits stereotyping clients according to age, gender, race, ethnicity, economic background (including methods of financing care), or disability. How nondiscrimination affects nursing practice is discussed in more detail later. Nondiscrimination is an integral part of the ANA Standards of Practice.

Ethical skills (i.e., applying ethical principles to address ethical conflicts) are the foundation on which the entry-level staff nurse nurtures a sense of professional integrity. Nurturing professional integrity is discussed in more detail in Chapter Sixteen.

## COMPARING COMPONENTS OF CLIENT CARE MANAGEMENT AND ETHICAL NURSING PRACTICE

Although it was not often recognized until more recently, the ethical components of the role of the nurse are integral to core nursing functions (Killeen, 1986, pp. 337–339). Some shared aspects of the nursing process and the ethical reasoning process also have been identified. Box 15-1 compares the phases of the nursing process with those of the ethical reasoning process.

---

**BOX 15-1**

### Comparison of the Nursing and Ethical Reasoning Processes

| Nursing Process | Ethical Reasoning Process |
|---|---|
| 1. Assessing | 1. Recognizing the moral issues |
| 2. Analyzing | 2. Analyzing relevant facts and identifying the moral dilemma |
| 3. Planning | 3. Formulating possible actions |
| 4. Implementing | 4. (a) Selecting the action(s) and (b) Taking the morally right action(s) |
| 5. Evaluating | 5. Evaluating the effectiveness of the moral action(s) taken |

## Values and Beliefs

**Values** are difficult to define. Nursing students usually receive instruction to help them identify and clarify their personal values. They are characterized subjectively by the individual and reflect personal preferences, commitments, and patterns of using resources. The person considers certain beliefs, events, objects, people, places, or goals to have special meaning. An individual's values influence her or his choices, behaviors, and actions. They often serve as motivators. For example, clients who decide not to adhere to prescribed treatments may have decided to spend their money on other basic needs, such as food, housing, education, or clothing.

**Beliefs** are the basic ingredients of values. Beliefs are basic assumptions or personal convictions that the individual perceives as truthful or factual or "takes for granted." Beliefs are not true or false. They frequently are handed down from generation to generation as cultural traditions (Jameton, 1990, p. 444). Cultural beliefs are commonly held by the others in the primary social groups (or subcultures) to which the individual belongs, such as families, work cultures, community interest groups, and church groups. For example, first-generation families of Eastern cultures may not believe in Western medical practices, but instead choose to manage serious diseases by "deep faith" in a Higher Source or Being.

## Cultural Norms

The individual's beliefs and values and those held by others in the same subcultures link the person to **cultural norms**. Predominant cultural norms prescribe expected behavior of clients and staff and provide guidelines for judging its acceptability. They strongly influence the person's actions and behaviors.

Cultural norms are rooted in values held by individuals. Figure 15-1 depicts the interconnectedness of individual values and cultural norms. When an individual accepts the beliefs and values of her or his work group or profession, the person is more likely to follow its code of conduct without experiencing conflict. If the individual does not accept these predominant values or beliefs, potential for conflict exists.

## Ethics

When conflicts occur, ethical principles or guidelines are used to distinguish right from wrong. Broadly defined, **ethics** is the study of rightness of conduct, the processes used to judge moral behavior, and the problems encountered when applying principles of morally correct behavior. As such, it incorporates cultural norms and mores. Ethics involves the study of values held by individuals and groups within social contexts. Nursing ethics reflects values held by members of the nursing profession within the social context of their practice. **Ethical principles** are used to judge right from wrong and good from bad and to identify solutions to problems arising from conflicts (Fowler, 1989, p. 956). The ethical principles that guide the conduct of various disciplines differ according to the basic values espoused by members of the profession (Scanlon and Flemming, 1990, pp. 64–65).

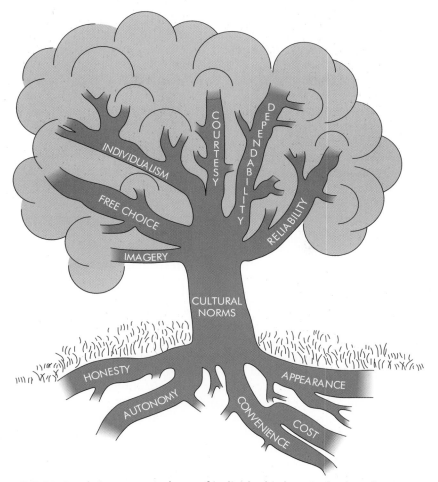

FIGURE 15-1  Interconnectedness of individual values and cultural norms.

Accordingly, the nursing ethics incorporated in codes of conduct may differ from the ethics of other disciplines, including medicine.

As Curtin (1988, p. 7) so aptly stated, "Ethics, as applied to the profession of nursing, is concerned with the duties voluntarily assumed by nurses and with the consequences of nurses' decisions on the lives of patients and their families, on the lives of their colleagues, on the profession itself and on the health care delivery system as a whole." Nursing ethics involves the study of the principles and duties used to judge whether nursing motives and actions are right or wrong or good or bad in a specific client's situation and context of practice. As cultural plurality (diversity of values, norms, and mores) increases, the need to understand ethical principles will increase. Given current societal trends, the need to understand nursing ethics is likely to become more important.

The study of ethics requires a reasoning process using values to guide behavior. **Essential professional values** commonly used to guide staff nurse behaviors include **altruism, equality, esthetics, freedom, human dignity, justice,** and **truth** (American Association of Colleges of Nursing, 1986, pp. 5–7). Within the nursing context, these values reflect **common ethical principles of nursing,** as follows:

1. Promoting **autonomy:** supporting the client's independence in making decisions affecting herself or himself
2. **Beneficence:** doing good for the client
3. **Nonmaleficence:** avoiding harm to the client
4. **Justice:** using available resources fairly and reasonably
5. **Veracity:** communicating truthfully and accurately
6. **Confidentiality:** securing the client's privacy
7. **Fidelity:** following through on one's word by carefully attending to details of the client's care (Gaul, 1989, p. 475)

Essential professional values influence the effectiveness of nurse-client relationships. Ethical nursing practice is guided by professional values and corresponding "correct" behaviors. Nurses study ethics to help them gain insight into how these principles affect practice. Applying ethical principles helps nurses resolve ethical conflicts (disagreement over principles of correct conduct in specific situations) by guiding their moral decisions and taking corresponding moral actions.

Nurses frequently are confronted with **moral conflicts** between loyalties to clients and to employers; loyalties to employers and compliance with regulations of licensing bodies; responsibilities to clients and physicians, peers, or other multidisciplinary work group members; and conflicting responsibilities to clients and their families. With the increasing emphasis on cost containment, nurses frequently have experienced moral conflicts between organizational policies and procedures and complex client needs (Koloroutis and Thorstenson, 1999, p. 13). Both types of needs can and need to be addressed in the resolution of these conflicts. Curtin (2000, pp. 12–13) described 10 principles that could be used by nursing managers to make resolution of ethical conflicts feasible in the modern health care environment.

To resolve moral conflicts, nurses follow a **moral reasoning process** to make value judgments as the basis for ethical nursing actions. Nurses who do not use ethical reasoning skills are likely to respond to moral conflicts intuitively, on the basis of their personal values. Consequently the nurse's behaviors are likely to serve her or his own needs instead of focusing on those of the client. This incorrect focus is even more likely when nurses work in settings that afford themselves and clients little authority to participate in clinical decision-making processes.

## ETHICAL REASONING PROCESS

Client care managers use moral reasoning to resolve moral conflicts. The specific steps in this process might vary, depending on the nurse, the values involved, the client's circumstances, and constraints inherent in the situation or limits of the practice environment. Basically the ethical reasoning process consists of the following phases:

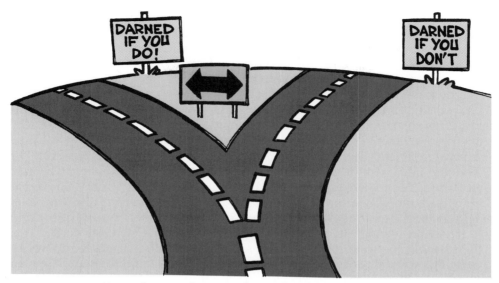

Nurses frequently are confronted with moral conflicts.

1. Recognizing the moral issues
2. Analyzing relevant facts and identifying the moral dilemma
3. Formulating possible actions
4. Selecting the action that best resolves the moral conflict consistent with principles of ethical conduct
5. Taking morally right action
6. Evaluating the effectiveness of the moral action taken

Each phase of the ethical reasoning process needs to be completed to address the dilemma successfully.

## Recognizing Existing Moral Issues

A **moral issue** exists when questions of morals or values arise and seem to conflict or when the consistency of one's actions with ethical principles is questioned. Moral issues frequently present themselves when clients and nurses experience difficulty in decision making (Chia and Swee Mee, 2000, p. 257). Typically the moral issue poses significant consequences for the individuals involved and is intensified by time constraints. Common moral issues often pertain to such issues as quality of life, death, comfort, "to treat or not to treat," and the use of scarce resources to provide extraordinary measures to prolong life.

To recognize a moral issue, the nurse needs to know which essential professional values are involved and how ethical principles can be used to sort out the key values of the nurse and the client. This knowledge is in addition to that needed to perform nursing procedures, communicate and teach clients effectively, and manage client care.

Professional autonomy (nurse's freedom to make clinical nursing decisions) is gaining attention as nursing establishes itself as a profession. It is important that the nurse understand how professional autonomy enhances one's practice and how a lack of autonomy can limit the nurse's effectiveness in making clinical decisions. For example, nurses who have organizational authority to plan and evaluate care can make timely revisions as clients' needs change. Nurses who are limited by the pattern of nursing service delivery, multidisciplinary work group routines, or policies are less likely to exercise professional autonomy. As a result, clients may not receive as effective or efficient care that nurses perceive to be indicated. Consequently, these nurses may experience less satisfaction from the practice of their profession.

The staff nurse also should understand the various strategies that can be used to promote the client's autonomy. Limiting the client's participation in decisions affecting him or her can diminish the quality of care provided and affect the client's perceptions of the quality of care received. Strategies for maintaining client autonomy include protecting the rights of clients who depend on significant others to act on their behalf due to age, illness, or disability. The nurse may need to act as an advocate by providing information about client's rights to families and significant others, communicating client concerns to the multidisciplinary work group, and supporting clients in implementing advance directives (legally binding descriptions of the client's directives regarding treatment).

Similarly the nurse needs to understand how the ethical concepts of beneficence, nonmaleficence, justice, veracity, confidentiality, and fidelity are incorporated in nursing practice (Cassells and Redman, 1989, p. 465). These concepts are incorporated in standards of nursing practice, codes of conduct, and lists of client's rights. The nurse should understand how these concepts guide nursing practice, influence staff perceptions of client's rights, and contribute to the design of strategies to protect them. The concept of justice is incorporated in endeavors to provide quality care, regardless of the source of payment. The concept of veracity is involved in informed consent. The principle of confidentiality protects clients who experience socially isolating or stigmatizing conditions. In actual practice, clinical situations often involve more than one ethical concept.

To resolve these **moral dilemmas** (situations involving undesirable choices for personal behavior), the client care manager needs to decide which value or goal takes precedence. Prioritizing the conflicting values inherent in moral dilemmas requires the nurse to pay specific attention to who has responsibility for what in finding the solution and the extent to which the client and nurse have control over needed moral actions.

Research indicates that some nurses, for reasons not yet clearly identified, have difficulty separating their personal values from those that guide nursing practice. Personal values often change over time as individual circumstances evolve, whereas essential ethical guidelines persist over longer periods. Clarification of personal values is a prerequisite for recognizing moral issues in clinical practice. Not to differentiate personal and professional values leads to difficulty in perceiving moral issues. The client care manager who does not distinguish personal values from professional guidelines is less likely to recognize the need for ethical reasoning. Such a client care manager also is less likely to recognize the need to gather relevant facts.

## Analyzing Relevant Facts to Identify the Moral Dilemma

Several research studies have indicated that many nurses experience difficulty identifying ethical dilemmas in practice (Ketefian, 1989, pp. 518–519). In other words, **moral uncertainty** is common. Nurses are often unsure which essential values are at issue and which values or ethical principles are in conflict in a specific situation. To ensure that the moral dilemma is identified accurately, the nurse needs to decipher the sources of conflict. These may include the client's values, organizational interest in controlling costs, and consumption of scarce resources such as staff time.

For example, a moral dilemma may exist when a client who is a recent immigrant and has trouble communicating with staff due to language barriers and cultural differences is placed in a health-care facility that is rewarded consistently for discharging clients early. The nurse accepts responsibility for gathering information about the client's understanding of available health-care options, their consequences, and the cost of each. Before formulating plans for addressing individual client needs, however, the nurse should be aware of staff perceptions of their obligations in preparing clients for discharge. If staff do not feel responsible for adequately preparing the client for discharge, the client may not receive information about treatment options, supervised practice of self-care activities, or needed referrals. These omissions are likely to jeopardize the client's well-being or may even be life-threatening. This situation involves the ethical concepts of client autonomy, beneficence, nonmaleficence, informed consent, justice, veracity, and fidelity. The nurse encourages the client to participate in selecting available options after receiving truthful and accurate information about them. The client needs information about anticipated outcomes of care and estimated times to reach them. If the client is to leave the hospital early, the nurse explains possible consequences; costs; need for special supplies, equipment, and skilled help associated with private home care services; hospital-based home care services; and other matters (autonomy, veracity). The nurse is mindful that reasonable plans are necessary to provide continuing services to avoid harming the client by early discharge (e.g., risking complications due to lack of follow-up services [nonmaleficence]). In addition, the nurse advocates that sufficient organizational resources be used to implement the plan (justice). Finally, the nurse makes a specific effort to ensure that the details of the client's plan are carried out to enable the client to meet adequately her or his specific health needs (fidelity, nonmaleficence).

The nurse makes a **moral judgment** regarding the rightness or wrongness of the direction that the client's situation is taking. The judgment focuses on whether staff behaviors match standards of ethical conduct. The nurse evaluates the extent to which the client's rights are supported or violated and the extent to which staff behaviors adhere to standards identified in codes of conduct. For example, will the client be harmed by being unprepared for early discharge? By being uninformed of the treatment plan? By not comprehending what she or he needs to do to perform self-care procedures? If the answer to these questions is yes, the client's rights are being violated. The nurse begins prioritizing various activities needed to enable the client to participate in planning treatment, preparing for discharge, and performing self-care procedures.

## Formulating Possible Actions

After the relevant facts are analyzed and the moral dilemma is identified, actions that could contribute to resolving it are considered. Specific actions that could change wrong actions into right actions are described. When first learning to formulate possible actions, the nurse should list the possibilities so that each can be recalled and considered. Each solution needs to be evaluated in terms of the extent that it meets the needs of the client, staff, and organization. The consequences of each possible solution are considered, including demands placed on the client and support systems and use of agency resources and their costs.

For example, the attending physician initially might explain the treatment plan to the client in the presence of the staff nurse. To enable the client to comprehend the plan fully, staff on later shifts might need to explain the plan to the client's family (who, let us suppose, can be available only later in the day due to other commitments). This is done to increase comprehension of the plan and to evaluate its suitability, given the client's needs, options, and financial resources. If language barriers exist, more time is needed to communicate, reinforce, and follow through. The more complicated the plans, the more time it takes to establish them and the more agency resources (e.g., staff time) are consumed in following through. Not to involve the client and staff (within organizational constraints) places the client at increased risk of harm. In addition, client rights are more likely to be violated if the client does not participate in making treatment plans.

If specific effort and time are not taken to formulate all possible actions, the best solution might go unrecognized. Consequently, either the staff could become involved in efficiently providing the wrong services, or the client's needs might be treated as less important than agency efficiency or staff convenience.

## Selecting the Action That Best Resolves the Moral Conflict

The nurse needs to select the action that best resolves the moral conflict consistent with codes of conduct. To select the best solution, the client's priority needs and values and the consequences of these values must be considered. Often the nurse uses advocacy skills to ensure that the client's lack of communication skills, lack of comprehension of important information, or decreased self-esteem or feelings of self-worth do not result in hasty decisions that are not in her or his best interest. Staff working under tight time constraints must avoid nonverbally communicating frustration and impatience to the client who has trouble comprehending information and explanations. The client must receive and comprehend information so that she or he can select the option that best meets her or his needs and can understand possible consequences and demands on the client of the option selected. The client care manager should keep in mind that the client might not select the same solution the manager would select. It is important that the client receive support to select the solution that best addresses the person's health needs and solves the moral dilemma under consideration. All too often the nurse witnesses the signature of a client signing a consent form when it is clear that the client does not understand the nature of the procedure, risks, or consequences. The nurse must notify the attending physician in accordance with codes of conduct to ensure that the client is giving an informed consent.

The client care manager has an obligation to communicate accurately and truthfully. All relevant information should be presented. The client needs information about probable undesired or negative consequences of the options selected as well as positive consequences that are easy to hear. The client needs a realistic perspective to consider various factors that affect the potential success of the plan.

## Taking the Morally Right Action

When the best action is selected, it needs to be carried out. **Ethical behavior** is conduct consistent with the values inherent to the situation. **Ethical nursing practice** involves taking morally right actions within the context of the client's needs and values and the nursing codes of conduct. The client and staff need to know what is expected of them—what they are to do and when. Frequently, solutions to moral dilemmas are not equally acceptable to both parties. The action might be best for the client but complicate demands on the family or staff. Unforeseen responses may occur that might be more or less desirable than anticipated. The client care manager is obligated to follow through on the selected action.

## Evaluating the Effectiveness of the Moral Action Taken

The client care manager needs to focus specific attention on determining what happened after desired actions were taken. Because the client care manager knows the initial moral dilemma that stimulated use of the moral reasoning process, she or he is in a good position to judge whether the moral action taken resolved it. Did the actions help the client progress toward her or his goals? Does the client need further consideration and help to resolve the conflict? For example, did taking more time to communicate effectively with the client with the language barrier help to clarify expectations and enhance the client's dignity and autonomy? Did the client's change in condition require that staff continue to take more time to explain and reinforce expectations related to the selected treatment options?

Reviewing the similarities between the phases of the moral reasoning process and those of the nursing process shows the relative ease with which ethical issues can be incorporated into nursing practice. Noting the similarities between the two processes should help to integrate moral reasoning into nursing practice (Murphy, 1989, p. 74). Considerable attention has been paid to helping nursing students learn to use the nursing process. More effort is needed to help them integrate ethical reasoning while using the nursing process to make clinical decisions. What is important is the nurse's sensitivity and recognition of moral dilemmas as they are evidenced by the client's expressed concerns and the staff's response to identified needs.

As mentioned earlier, health-care settings exist that do not allow or promote ethical nursing practice. Nurses who know the moral values at issue and choose the right courses of action but are not allowed to take action to resolve them experience **moral**

**distress**. Common constraints that cause moral distress include organizations that do not permit nursing autonomy in clinical decision making, policies that limit the nurse's authority, and lack of respect for nursing's ability to respond appropriately to moral issues (Fry, 1989, p. 490; Tiedje, 2000, p. 38). As if the complexity of addressing moral dilemmas is not enough of a challenge to staff nurses, circumstances that cause moral distress complicate nursing practice and the ethical dilemmas confronting clients. Moral distress associated with these constraints can lead to tragic results. It is common and often unrecognized as a contributing factor to the increasing nursing shortage (Erlen, 2001, p. 76). Wilkinson (1987/1988, p. 27) reported, "Those nurses who are unable to cope with moral distress and who leave bedside nursing seem to be those who are most aware of, and sensitive to, moral issues, and who feel a strong sense of responsibility to patients for their own actions." It is critical that moral distress be addressed by moral action individually or collectively. Such moral action might involve "whistle blowing" or collaborative projects that use internal strengths and external resources (e.g., mentors, coaches, and educational programs) (Tiedje, 2000, pp. 40–42). The issue of whistle blowing is discussed further in Chapter Sixteen, as a strategy for maintaining professional integrity.

## DIFFERENTIATING BETWEEN ETHICS AND SPIRITUALITY

Staff nurses need to distinguish a client's spirituality from ethical issues. As discussed earlier, ethics is the study of the rightness or wrongness of behavior. It incorporates an understanding of beliefs and predominant cultural values that guide conduct. It considers variations in personal values, cultural norms and mores, and the context of the specific situations being studied.

**Spirituality** refers to a person's emotional investment, "attaching positive or negative importance to persons, places, objects, events, beliefs, and goals that seem to be relevant to the self" (Salladay and McDonnell, 1989, p. 544). A person's spirit relates to aspects of her or his mind or soul and is distinct from the body. Spirituality refers to the person's search for meaning from individual experiences. It is a basic human need that must be met to sustain a person's well-being. Often spirituality refers to the human spirit's involvement with a greater power or divine spirit. One's spirituality reflects personal beliefs, values, and ethical choices made to realize goals and to make life worth living. Although religious practices rooted in spirituality may differ widely, the spiritual needs of valuing, seeking meaning, and setting personal goals are similar in all religions.

Ethics and spirituality are concerned with values, with good or bad, right or wrong behavior. Although ethics relates to a systematic approach to judging behavior, spirituality refers to the person's individual emotional investment in persons, objects, places, events, beliefs, and goals that make life meaningful. Ethics emphasizes cultural values, whereas spirituality focuses on values of the individual. Ethical and spiritual considerations usually are involved in the moral reasoning inherent in nursing practice. The nurse attempts to adhere to ethical codes of conduct formulated by the profession and to address the spiritual concerns of clients.

## DISTINGUISHING BETWEEN LAW AND ETHICS

As a study of conduct, ethics contributes to guidelines for desired behavior. The ethical behaviors expected of nurses are delineated in various codes of conduct. These codes describe various types of expected behaviors aimed at protecting clients' interests and, indirectly, interests of nurses. They prescribe approaches to moral issues to avoid, reduce, or resolve conflict. Ethical concepts change as cultures, values, and socially accepted patterns of behavior change.

**Laws** are rules for required behavior that define personal and professional relationships. Laws tell people what they may and may not do individually and to or with others. Laws are generated by governments or by government sanction of customs. They change as social issues and concerns change. Various types of laws create different privileges, protections, and responsibilities.

Constitutional law protects individual rights, such as freedom of speech, right to self-determination, and right to refuse treatment. Administrative laws define regulations for agencies, such as the authority of state boards of nursing to define and regulate nursing practice. Other administrative laws direct other agencies, such as those participating in Medicare and Medicaid health insurance programs. Criminal laws define actions such as murder, theft, or illegal possession of drugs. Nurses removing life-support systems, consuming agency supplies for personal use, or abusing chemical substances violate criminal laws. Contract laws refer to legally binding agreements. Nurses may enter into contracts by agreeing to work schedules and job descriptions. Tort laws relate to compensating clients for harm or injury caused by malpractice.

Laws reflect public policy. As such, they reflect society's view of what is good or bad, right or wrong behavior (Kjervik, 1990, p. 138). Good laws reflect desired ethical practices, including predominant cultural beliefs, values, and customs. Ethics and law are not mutually exclusive. Figure 15-2 illustrates how law is conceptualized as being a part of ethical concerns. Ethical guidelines are used by legislators to judge the rightness or wrongness of conduct and might be used in legal courts to determine the extent to which laws were violated. Lawyers often use standards of nursing practice (which incorporate ethics) (i.e., "what a reasonable and prudent nurse would do") to defend the adequacy of services provided to clients.

As ethical issues emerge, professional organizations frequently prepare position papers on issues to guide their members. Ethical guidelines frequently are used to inform policy makers and legislators of the expected behaviors of health-care professionals (Fowler, 1988, p. 104). Laws change as legislators respond to social pressures to regulate behaviors that infringe on the rights, safety, or well-being of the public.

## ADHERING TO NURSING CODES OF CONDUCT

Codes of acceptable conduct change in response to evolving cultural values and beliefs related to primary societal trends. For example, methods of child rearing are changing as increasing numbers of women pursue careers. Explicit guidelines describing expected nursing conduct have been revised to correspond to evolving societal circumstances, economic constraints, and technologic advances. The

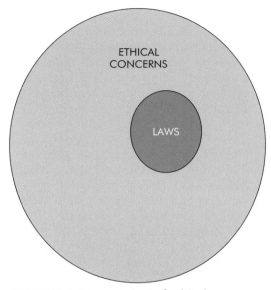

FIGURE 15-2 Law as a part of ethical concerns.

resulting situations are frequently inconsistent with ideal behaviors. Significant differences in values and beliefs frequently give rise to moral conflicts. For example, in American culture, many individuals believe they are entitled to affordable health care. Many employers, who often pay for part of the cost of health insurance, are less willing to do so. Consequently, more Americans seek less health care because of its costs. The ANA nursing code of conduct directs nurses to provide services ". . . unrestricted by consideration of social or economic status . . ." (American Nurses Association, 2001, p. 2).

Entry-level staff nurses are expected to adhere to legal and ethical codes of conduct. A **code of nursing conduct** such as the ANA's Code of Ethics for Nurses is a description of standards of moral behavior required of nurses. Box 15-2 lists these standards. The consequences of violations of these codes depend on which type of code of conduct was violated.

## Legal Codes of Conduct

**Legal** codes of conduct are rooted in specific state Nurse Practice Acts (which often are delineated in state statutes) and ANA Standards of Nursing Practice (established voluntarily by members of the ANA). To be licensed to practice nursing, each nurse is required to meet requirements for licensure and registration. That is, each nurse must present evidence (i.e., credentials, including educational qualifications) of capability to practice nursing safely. Initial licensure often involves meeting educational requirements that ensure the individual has the knowledge and skills deemed critical for safe nursing practice. Registration requirements also include information about the nurse's current name and address.

---

**BOX 15-2**

## American Nurses Association Code of Ethics for Nurses

1. The nurse, in all professional relationships, practices with compassion and respect for the inherent dignity, worth and uniqueness of every individual, unrestricted by considerations of social or economic status, personal attributes, or the nature of health problems.
2. The nurse's primary commitment is to the patient, whether an individual, family, group, or community.
3. The nurse promotes, advocates for, and strives to protect the health, safety, and rights of the patient.
4. The nurse is responsible and accountable for individual nursing practice and determines the appropriate delegation of tasks consistent with the nurse's obligation to provide optimum patient care.
5. The nurse owes the same duties to self as to others, including the responsibility to preserve integrity and safety, to maintain competence, and to continue personal and professional growth.
6. The nurse participates in establishing, maintaining, and improving healthcare environments and conditions of employment conducive to the provision of quality health care and consistent with the values of the profession through individual and collective action.
7. The nurse participates in the advancement of the profession through contributions to practice, education, administration, and knowledge development.
8. The nurse collaborates with other health professionals and the public in promoting community, national, and international efforts to meet health needs.
9. The profession of nursing, as represented by associations and their members, is responsible for articulating nursing values, for maintaining the integrity of the profession and its practice, and for shaping social policy.

From American Nurses Association: *Code of ethics for nurses with interpretive statements*, 2001, Washington, DC, American Nurses Publishing, American Nurses Association.

---

ANA Standards of Nursing Practice often are used in courts of law as minimum standards needed for safe practice. They provide guidelines that often are used to judge the reasonableness of actions taken by an individual nurse in a specific situation. They frequently are used to compare the practices of peers as described by "expert witnesses" in court hearings. Additional institutional standards of care incorporate accepted standards of practice and often are described in policy and procedure manuals and those delineated by quality assurance and improvement processes.

If convicted of violating established standards of practice that result in harm to a client (usually consistent with ANA Standards of Nursing Practice and other organization specific standards), the nurse is legally responsible for the consequences. The nurse is required to compensate injured parties for the damages or injuries resulting from these violations. Because these consequences can be costly, most nurses obtain malpractice insurance to address the risks. In addition, depending on the gravity of the violation, the nurse's license could be suspended or revoked.

## Ethical Codes of Conduct

In contrast to legal requirements, **ethical** codes of conduct are developed by nursing organizations and describe expectations for moral conduct of a nurse. They are designed to protect the rights of all clients and to describe the moral obligations of nurses. They provide guidelines for making appropriate ethical decisions to provide quality care for clients with diverse spiritual, ethnic, racial, age, and gender characteristics, which often differ from those of the nurse. They also provide guidelines for nurses to avoid discriminating behaviors that could decrease the client's dignity or respect.

Violating ethical codes of conduct usually entails interference with the exercise of client rights. Violations of ethical codes of conduct could be described in courts of law as evidence of engaging in less than the minimally accepted standards of practice. Not all violations of ethical codes of conduct result in legal disputes, however; sometimes they simply infringe on client's rights (Kendrick, 1994, pp. 826–829). Depending on the consequences of violations, legal disputes might follow.

To ensure that clients are informed of their rights as patients in acute care facilities or as residents in long-term care facilities, federal regulations require that health-care providers be familiar with these rights. In addition, federal regulations require that clients be informed of their rights on admission to these facilities.

### COMMON VIOLATIONS OF NURSING CODES OF CONDUCT

Entry-level staff nurses are likely to encounter a variety of situations in which violations of codes of nursing conduct could jeopardize client rights and safety. Several of these situations are described to help client care managers promote safe care and protect client rights.

## Identifying Life-and-Death Issues

The media have sensitized the public to many of the technologic advances in health care. Most adults express a desire for "death with dignity" when good quality of life is not possible and the individual perceives the alternative as unacceptable. **Quality of life** is a subjective measure of acceptability of pain and suffering; it is difficult to define on more than an individual basis. Ethical codes of conduct require that the client's expressed desires for "death with dignity" be honored. Difficulties arise when the client has not established her or his wishes legally before the time when such life-and-death decisions need to be made.

Many American adults know that current medical technology sometimes can support physiologic processes indefinitely on a mechanical level. Consistent with the Supreme Court ruling in *Nancy Cruzan vs. State of Missouri*, many individuals have completed living wills. A **living will** is a legal document that indicates individual directives for the care desired and indicates who is authorized to make medical decisions if the person becomes incapacitated. If these documents have been completed satisfactorily with appropriately witnessed signatures, they are legally binding in most states (Lammers, 1986, p. 629). Effective December 1, 1991, hospitals and nursing homes receiving Medicare and Medicaid funds were required to inform patients of their rights under state law to make living wills or other advance directives under the Patient Self-Determination Act (Dolan, 1991, p. 7; Mezey et al., 1994, p. 30). An **advance directive** is a written statement made while an individual is still capable of making decisions that describes her or his treatment preferences in the event of serious illness (Mezey et al., 1994, p. 32; Reigle, 1992, p. 197). Advance directives include designations of persons authorized to make decisions on the client's behalf (e.g., durable power of attorney) should the client be seriously injured, terminally ill, or in a persistent vegetative state and unable to make decisions and communicate them. A person with adequately documented authority to act as **durable power of attorney** is empowered legally to carry out decisions and activities on behalf of the client. In most states (but not the District of Columbia), a person with durable power of attorney can perform all legal actions needed to fulfill the client's wishes as if she or he were the client (Lammers, 1986, pp. 629–630).

Client care managers are expected to adhere to these advance directives. In addition, they are expected to include designated individuals in decision-making processes involved in providing care in accordance with legitimate living wills and related directives. They need to distinguish clearly between measures that prolong life and measures that hasten death. Measures prolonging life would be inconsistent with the goals of a client striving for "death with dignity." Measures that hasten death may be illegal. Nurses need to be prepared to defend their actions if their interventions are questioned. In addition, they need to explain such decisions and subsequent actions taken.

## Distinguishing Treatment from Nontreatment Plans

Client care managers are expected to know the goals of care for each of their clients (Thompson, 1989, p. 344). That is, they need to understand whether the measures taken are to restore health, treat symptoms of a disease, or provide supportive care for "death with dignity." Each type of goal implies different priorities. The nurse's activities and cares are adjusted accordingly. Generally, treatment includes measures taken to restore health or treat disease. Nontreatment plans emphasize measures designed to provide comfort or alleviate suffering. The purpose for which these measures are taken rather than the type of measure is what is paramount. For example, a specific analgesic could be given to treat incisional pain postoperatively or to alleviate the discomfort of a terminally ill client. The nurse's evaluation of its effectiveness, including risks, benefits, and side effects, depends on the purpose for which it was given. In such a situation, the appropriateness of the dose may be a major concern, depending on its purpose: 6 mg intravenously of morphine sulfate is too high for postoperative pain, whereas the same dose is too low for treating pain caused by cancer.

Client care managers need to distinguish between **providing** and withholding **aggressive treatment**. Aggressive treatment usually includes **extraordinary support measures** used to support physiologic processes. One type of extraordinary life-support measure includes any strategy used to maintain or restore a function of a person's vital organs. Another type includes **resuscitative measures** taken to reverse immediate, life-threatening situations, such as cardiopulmonary arrest. Resuscitative measures are performed to prevent death and often are considered heroic. Life-support measures that are unnatural, such as mechanical respirators or enteral tube feedings, often are considered to be extraordinary. Extraordinary life-support measures are used to provide aggressive treatment and are designed to maintain and restore life and health.

When health-care providers are requested to withhold aggressive treatment, they are expected to eliminate all measures designed to maintain body function and restore health. This does not preclude the use of measures designed to promote comfort or alleviate suffering; such comfort measures do not deliberately prolong life or hasten death. Rather, the purpose of **withholding aggressive treatment** is to avoid prolonging life without dignity. A "nontreatment" program is designed to provide supportive care. **"Death with dignity,"** as perceived by the client, is a common goal of "nontreatment" programs. These programs incorporate **supportive measures** that enable the client to achieve "death with dignity." Special consideration is indicated to ensure that the "nontreatment" program is not viewed as a situation in which the client is ignored or rushed toward death; rather, its focus and top priority are the client's comfort and supportive needs.

Many clients are hesitant to complete advance directives and specify their preferences not to be resuscitated, incorrectly believing that staff may interpret these directives as refusing all care and treatment. Consequently, clients often need assistance to help them understand the purpose of advance directives, consequences of choices made, and their implications for the type of care to be provided based on the individual's circumstances. Client care managers must know the agency's policy, procedures, and standards of care that pertain to implementing the Patient Self-Determination Act and advance directives. Client care managers often are asked to collaborate with members of the multidisciplinary work group to educate clients, complete the advance directives, and compile this information appropriately so that it is accessible when needed. This process requires timely communication and follow-up on an individual basis.

## Recognizing Ethical Issues Related to Health Insurance Benefits

As described in Chapter Two, health-care agencies are influenced heavily by mechanisms commonly used to finance various treatment options. Consequently, clients frequently choose options that fit the design of their health insurance benefits.

Clients assume that their insurance benefit programs determine the type of treatment they should receive. The purpose of insurance programs is to help pay for needed health care, not to determine what health care is needed. This fact has been obscured by the preadmission consultations required by many insurance programs.

Entry-level staff nurses as client care managers are expected to be accountable to the clients they serve. Codes of nursing conduct require client care managers to provide care without discrimination on the basis of economic status. That is, providing client care is nursing's primary function, for which nurses are ethically responsible and legally accountable. Financing health care, although important, is secondary. Client care managers need to remain focused on providing care on the basis of their assessments rather than emphasizing economic pressures originating inside or outside their practice settings (Cushing, 1989, pp. 471–472).

This approach does not mean that the high cost of health care can be ignored. Rather, each client is entitled to cost-effective and efficient care, regardless of how it is financed. Client care managers, as advocates, are expected to help clients understand their needs and priorities and the various options available to meet them.

By requesting detailed documentation of the services provided, insurance companies have gained considerable influence over health-care providers, sometimes to the detriment of their beneficiaries (Hines, 1988, p. 586). Insurance companies sometimes have attempted to reduce their costs by denying client benefits, refusing to reimburse clients or agencies for services that the insurance companies decided were documented inadequately or incorrectly. To satisfy the demands of health insurance companies and, more important, to provide a nursing evaluation tool,

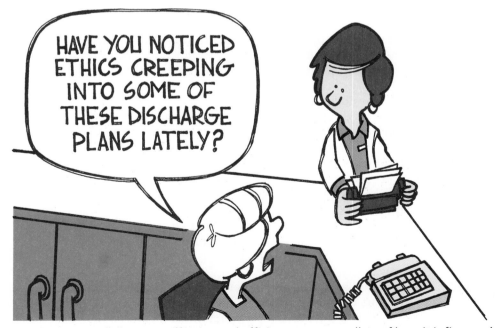

Each client is entitled to cost-effective and efficient care, regardless of how it is financed.

client care managers, as advocates, ensure that client progress and services provided are recorded accurately and reflect that standards of care were maintained (Murphy, 1987, pp. 537–538, 540).

## Responding to an Incompetent Colleague

To succeed as a member of a work group, everyone must work together cooperatively and with mutual respect. From time to time, every nurse encounters situations in which the safety of clients is endangered by the conduct of colleagues. When circumstances evolve in which a colleague's behavior is questioned, tension associated with intrapersonal and interpersonal conflict is likely. Specific steps for resolving conflicts are detailed in Chapter Seven. The unacceptable conduct of colleagues also may lead to intergroup conflicts. The differences causing the tension may relate to variations in perceptions of acceptability of personal behaviors, to lack of adherence to agency's standards of care, or to noncompliance with the specified multidisciplinary treatment plan. Coping with a colleague whose conduct and competence are under question always produces anxiety. Although entry-level nurses may lack self-confidence due to lack of experience, they are expected to evaluate the competence of their peers, especially if suspicious behaviors place client safety at risk. Codes of nursing conduct require the nurse to respond to colleagues whose behavior places the clients they care for at risk.

First, the nurse must become familiar with the agency's policy for the management of unsafe practice (Rushton and Hogue, 1993, p. 285). Usually the nurse is expected to discuss her or his concerns with the colleague in question, noting whether it is the behavior or the outcomes of care that are problematic. Has the conduct resulted in harm to a client? Do client outcomes of care change under different workers? For example, is relief from narcotic analgesia reduced when the colleague is present, suggesting that she or he might not have administered the drug? Or is the client's response a reflection of the difference in the nurse's clinical decision making based on the client's pain rating (i.e., one nurse medicates a pain rating of "2," whereas another does not)?

Do policies or procedures run contrary to the colleague's typical pattern of behavior? For example, is there a need to countersign for "wasted" controlled substances, or are alcoholic beverages prohibited before or during scheduled work hours? The more endangered the client's safety and well-being, the greater the pressure on the nurse to respond to the colleague's conduct. In any event, the nurse needs to follow the agency's policy, if one exists.

Second, when the nurse approaches the colleague, she or he should follow the steps of conflict resolution. The colleague may agree with the nurse or deny the problem. If the nurse participates in a cover-up of the colleague's behavior, she or he is ethically and legally accountable for the problem and its consequences (Rushton and Hogue, 1993, p. 286).

Third, if the nurse believes there is evidence of drug or alcohol abuse, the nurse needs to write a report outlining concerns and evidence to the supervisor. If the supervisor is unresponsive, the nurse reports her or his concerns to the supervisor's supervisor, often the director of nursing.

Fourth, the nurse might want to seek guidance from unbiased sources, such as other client advocates, clergy, ombudsmen personnel, or the "employee directives committee" or a representative of the Employee Assistance Program (EAP). The nurse may be protected from reprisal by state laws or administrative rules. The nurse's primary responsibility is the client's safety and well-being, for which the nurse is ethically and legally accountable.

The presence of an incompetent colleague engages the nurse in conflict resolution on behalf of client safety. The nurse is expected to comply with agency policies related to unsafe, illegal, or unethical conduct. Failure to do so makes the nurse accountable for the consequences of the conduct in question. The nurse should use communication skills to resolve conflict and ethical issues and report concerns in writing to her or his supervisor.

## PROTECTING THE RIGHTS OF HUMAN SUBJECTS

Entry-level staff nurses may be expected to participate in research activities involving clients assigned to their care. Several important ethical concerns need to be addressed adequately, including **protecting the rights of human subjects,** protecting nurses as employees, and protecting the integrity of the specific research study. For example, staff nurses are asked to witness client signatures verifying informed consent for surgical or invasive procedures. Similarly, staff nurses might be asked to witness client signatures on "informed consent" forms or to collect data consistent with the purposes of the study. If the staff nurse questions the adequacy of the protection afforded the human subjects, the nurse needs to confer with her or his immediate supervisor to ensure that the activities adhere to the agency's policies and procedures in addition to rights of human research subjects, who have rights for equitable access to the benefits of experimental treatments (Kahn et al., 1998). Nurses share responsibility for ensuring that the research purposes and methodology preserve the dignity and rights of the individuals and social groups they are intended to serve in the variety of settings that they practice (Davis, 1991, p. 652). Each consent form indicates whom to contact for questions and concerns about injury or adverse effects.

Wilson (1989) delineated guidelines for ensuring ethical research practices using the acronym *SCIENTIFIC*. Box 15-3 describes these guidelines. If a research project satisfactorily addresses the criteria set forth in these guidelines, the integrity and the rights of the human subjects and nurses involved are likely to be protected.

While participating in research projects, nurses need to make a special effort to protect the rights of clients serving as human subjects. Clients must comprehend when the nurse is providing care and when her or his activities are primarily of a research nature. The distinction is necessary to prevent clients from assuming that the nurse is acting in their best interests when clients may be taking risks while participating in specific research activities (Davis, 1989, pp. 450–452). For example, a nurse might administer prescribed experimental drug treatments that pose potential risks to assigned clients. The clients may believe the nurses are providing prescribed treatment, when the participation in research protocols may place the clients at significant risk (Davis, 1989, p. 451).

BOX 15-3

## Guidelines for SCIENTIFIC and Ethical Research Practices

*Scientific objectivity.* The investigator includes all data points, including those that are unsupportive; tries to be aware of personal values and biases; and doesn't preconceive a study's outcome or engage in any misconduct, fraud, or acts of bad faith in connection with the research.

*Cooperation with duly authorized review groups, agencies, and institutional review boards.* This means that you submit your proposed research to the appropriate committee in charge of reviewing provisions for the protection of subjects' rights and are willing to comply with their recommendations. Many journals require that study reports contain a statement that the research was approved from an ethical standpoint by the appropriate institutional committee.

*Integrity in representing the research enterprise.* This means that you do not withhold information about the possible risks, discomforts, or benefits of your study, nor do you intentionally deceive study subjects on these matters.

*Equitability in acknowledging the contributions of others.* This means that you give credit where credit is due in publications by listing coauthors, or in speeches and presentations by acknowledging the work of others.

*Nobility in the application of processes and procedures to protect the rights of human subjects.* This means that you actively assume responsibility for protecting subjects from harm, deceit, coercion, and invasions of privacy, even when your own study may be inconvenienced.

*Truthfulness about a study's purpose, procedure, methods, and findings.* You do not attempt to disguise your research or conduct it "under cover."

*Impeccability in use of any privileges that may be associated with the researcher's role.* The investigator keeps data anonymous and confidential. The investigator is discreet about what is learned about people.

*Forthrightness about a study's funding sources and sponsorship.* You disclose all sources of financial support, as well as any special relationship between a study and its sponsors in publications and presentations of research findings.

*Illumination brought to the discipline's body of scientific knowledge through publications and presentations of research findings.* Research should yield fruitful results.

*Courage to publicly clarify any distortion that others make of your research findings.*

From Wilson HS: *Research in nursing*, ed 2, Redwood City, CA, 1989, Addison-Wesley, pp. 67–69.

BOX 15-4

## Rights of Human Subjects

1. Right to freedom from intrinsic risk of injury
2. Right to privacy and dignity
3. Right to anonymity

From American Nurses Association: *Human rights guidelines for nurses in clinical and other research*, Publication D-46 5M 2/85. Kansas City, MO, 1985, American Nurses Association, pp. 6–7.

Before implementation, all research projects in which clients participate as human subjects need to be approved by the organization's designated institutional board. These groups often are known as the **institutional research committees** or human subjects committees and are responsible for ensuring that the purposes and procedures adequately protect the rights of the human subjects. Institutional research committees typically have multidisciplinary representation, consult with the researchers, and oversee research processes within the organization to ensure that standards for ethical research are met. Box 15-4 lists the rights of human subjects as participants in research, as delineated by the ANA.

Nurses need to know that clients as human subjects participate voluntarily after the risks and benefits of involvement are disclosed truthfully to them. Clients can end their participation at any time without fear of punishment or reprisal. In addition, the nurse needs to know the specific plans to protect the subjects' anonymity and confidentiality and to ensure that the researchers adhere to them.

Concurrently, while clients participate in research projects, staff nurses provide nursing care to them in accordance with established standards of care. Protecting the rights of human subjects is undertaken in addition to providing established standards of care, not instead of it.

Evaluating research reports and **using new knowledge** are integral to sound nursing practice. Entry-level staff nurses are expected to review current literature and determine whether the findings have implications for their practice. Typically, staff nurses are required to comprehend the rationale underlying new policies, procedures, and techniques that incorporate research findings. Employers make resource persons available, often through committees and in-service programs, to help nurses maintain competencies based on evolving nursing knowledge.

## BLENDING PRESENT AND FUTURE NURSING ETHICAL ISSUES

At the risk of overwhelming the entry-level staff nurse with a wide variety of moral issues currently confronting client care managers, some future concerns merit a brief introduction. Anticipating potential moral dilemmas may help to prevent them or reduce their seriousness. Recognizing patterns of persistent moral issues focuses emphasis to help resolve them in a positive manner.

## Violations of Client's Rights

Regardless of the context in which care is provided, violations of client's rights will continue to be a common ethical concern of the public and, it is hoped, of the nursing profession. If the public does not perceive that progress is being made in protecting human dignity, for whatever reasons, codes of conduct guiding ethical practice may be accorded less credence. Their value to the profession and their effectiveness in ensuring the common good are likely to be questioned more frequently and seriously. Consequently, political effort will be made to legislate proper behavior. The emerging political debates over nurse staffing ratios and mandatory overtime concurrent with increased concern for client safety reflect such public concern.

## Controlling Health-Care Costs

Ethical issues related to controlling health-care costs, to the constraining effects of costs on clinical decision making, and to the design of the technology that underlies health systems are likely to continue (Moczygemba and Hewitt, 2001, p. 33). The Health Insurance Portability and Accountability Act of 1996 is directed at retaining clients' privacy rights and requires specific actions of all providers (Frank-Stromborg and Ganschow, 2002, pp. 55–57). Controlling cost at the expense of client well-being and satisfaction is likely to cause the public to question whether current laws regulating professional practice are adequate to protect the public. Is peer review of professional practice effectively addressing increasing complaints of unsafe, harmful, or insensitive care? Is the current system, which relies on nurses to practice ethically, working? If it is not, do solutions lie in changing ethical principles or laws?

Considerable evidence exists that, until more recently, principles of ethical nursing practice have been neglected in educational programs (Cassells and Redman, 1989, p. 463; Fry, 1989, pp. 485–497; Gaul, 1989, pp. 476–477; Killeen, 1986, pp. 334–340). The nursing profession is faced with many questions. Will including ethics in nursing curricula ensure ethical nursing practice? How can health-care organizations contribute toward creating work environments that promote ethical nursing practice? What can individual nurses do to protect client rights?

## Commitment to Health-Care Goals

Are ethical issues related to the individual nurse's commitment to health-care goals? As members of the nursing profession and members of larger communities, are nurses showing their commitment to health in their individual lifestyles and interactions with individual clients and community-interest groups by promoting health and reducing the need for expensive illness care? If not, does their behavior reflect persistent personal values or incomplete preparation for professional nursing practice?

The interconnectedness of the global economy and its increasing complexity seem to indicate that economic constraints on the costs of care are likely to continue. As financing mechanisms continue to evolve, they may be allowed to usurp clinical decision-making authority in the guise of "managing care" for the purpose of reducing financial liabilities. Providers may be led to believe mistakenly that payers also voluntarily assume legal liabilities for the consequences of unsafe treatment decisions and ineffective services. Nurses need to continue to protect their legal authority, responsibility, and accountability for their professional practice and its consequences for clients served. Nursing interests need protection in political arenas and in organizational settings through responsible use of power and client advocacy.

Closely related to moral issues affecting ethical nursing practice are issues that challenge the individual client's right to body integrity, which are nurtured by technology that has an increased capacity to substitute for bodily functions and parts. Increasing sophistication in successfully transplanting organs and inserting artificial body parts will require that individuals prepare advance directives to ensure that their desires are addressed as their health conditions change. Moral dilemmas surrounding intergenerational donation of body parts are likely to become more common as advances in the life sciences continue. Questions concerning who can and should be authorized to permit donation of her or his body or any of its organs are likely to arise more frequently.

The staff nurse's involvement in nursing research is likely to expand as the management of data and information becomes easier and more efficient. Nurses need to develop creative methods of extracting the data used to evaluate nursing practice. Although data collected for clinical decision-making purposes are likely to differ from data gathered for research and evaluation purposes, nurses are likely to be asked to help collect data of both kinds. Both types of data must be managed so as to maintain confidentiality. As client advocates, they will be required to ensure that the rights of clients as subjects of research studies are protected, in addition to clients' rights as recipients of nursing care. To maintain competencies, staff nurses will need to evaluate research reports as to the soundness of their findings and recommendations to determine whether following them is likely to improve the effectiveness of nursing care.

Special consideration is required to ensure that research designed to improve practice is distinguished from research designed to decrease costs. Another way to look at a research problem is to analyze whether its top priority is increasing economies in health care or designing more effective nursing strategies.

## SUMMARY

All nursing practice involves ethical decision making. Client care managers, as members of the discipline of nursing, need to incorporate ethics in clinical decision making. Understanding common ethical concepts helps the nurse to practice in accordance with the ethical standards and codes of conduct established by the profession.

One's personal beliefs and values are rooted in cultural norms. These norms provide broad guidelines for judging whether one's conduct is right or wrong.

Ethics is the study of rightness of conduct, the processes used to judge moral behavior, and the problems encountered when applying principles of morally correct behavior.

Ignoring moral conflicts does not cause them to cease to exist. Nurses need to develop sensitivity to moral issues and dilemmas. These moral conflicts usually involve misaligned personal and professional values that adversely affect clients and staff. Essential professional values include altruism, equality, esthetics, freedom, human dignity, justice, and truth. Translated into the nursing context, these concepts reflect commitment to promoting client participation in clinical decisions, doing good for the client, avoiding doing the client harm, using available resources fairly and reasonably, communicating truthfully and accurately, securing the client's privacy, and following through on treatment by carefully attending to details of the client's care. When an existing moral issue is recognized, nurses use a moral reasoning process to seek appropriate solutions to resolve the conflict.

Ethical nursing practice involves taking morally correct actions within the context of the client's needs and values and nursing codes of conduct. Nurses suffer from moral distress when they know what moral values are at issue and choose the right courses of action but are not able to take action to resolve them. Excessive moral distress causes some nurses to leave nursing.

Ethics differs from spirituality. Spirituality reflects personal beliefs, values, and ethical choices made to realize goals and make life meaningful. Religious practices are rooted in spirituality, whereas ethics places more emphasis on cultural values.

Laws are rules for required behaviors that define personal and professional relationships. Laws reflect public policy. Good laws reflect desired ethical practices. Ethical guidelines are used to inform policy makers, legislators, health-care professionals, and the public about desired behaviors.

The consequences of violating ethical and legal codes of conduct vary, depending on their effects on client safety and well-being, institutional standards, and state laws. Client care managers are expected to adhere to directives described in living wills or provided by legally authorized persons. In addition, they are expected to distinguish between providing aggressive treatment and "nontreatment" and among extraordinary life-support measures, resuscitative measures, and supportive care measures.

Nurses focus on providing for client needs and documenting progress; they record client responses to treatment in a way that reflects that standards of care were maintained. Every client is entitled to efficient, cost-effective care. Similarly, nurses are expected to protect client safety by responding in an accountable manner to the conduct of incompetent colleagues. This response entails adhering to agency policies and following through with the steps of conflict resolution.

Nurses might be able to prevent future moral dilemmas and conflicts by learning about ethical nursing practice. By resolving current moral conflicts, health-care organizations can develop mechanisms that more effectively address client needs and concerns. They also can participate in systematic studies designed to devise more effective nursing strategies using available technology.

## APPLICATION EXERCISES

1. One of your peers believes that each individual has an inherent right to make as many choices as possible affecting one's lifestyle. Identify the nursing value reflected in this behavior. Discuss whether this value can be overemphasized to the detriment of other professional values. Give examples.

2. One of your assigned clients repeatedly refuses to adhere to prescribed treatment. He has suffered several serious complications. Some staff have expressed frustration with the client's behavior, which they attribute to "not having to pay for it," because the client's care is funded by government programs. identify which ethical nursing concepts are involved in this moral conflict.

3. Describe how the moral reasoning process could be used to address the following moral issue. Your client has been ventilator dependent for 2 years and has expressed his wish to die on several occasions because his "life is no longer worth the effort." He also has asked several members of his immediate family to disconnect his respiratory equipment. Some nursing staff "don't think he really means it" and consequently have ignored his request.

4. Discuss practical strategies that nurses might use to reduce moral distress.

5. Your client is a subject in a research project. He has suffered two serious setbacks since beginning his participation and now says he "wants out." The investigator is intent on retaining the client in the study for as long as possible, stating that the complications are not related to participation in the project. State whether you think the client's rights as a human subject are being violated. Give reasons for your answer.

## CRITICAL THINKING SCENARIO

Imagine yourself employed by a long-term care agency that does not have an Ethics Committee or Institutional Research Review Board. It is closely aligned with a local medical school that has such committees, however. These committees have one nurse member on the Ethics Committee and none on the Institutional Research Review Board. While caring for your assigned clients, you become aware of two clients whose condition has deteriorated, and you question whether the deterioration may be related to their participation as research subjects. The nurse researcher wants to retain these clients as subjects for as long as possible until the study is complete. You are unclear whether the subjects or their legal guardians have been informed of the potential risks of participating in the research.

1. What would you do first? Give reasons.
2. How would you ensure that the subjects were informed appropriately to sign the research subject consent form voluntarily?
3. Whom would you involve in resolving the ethical dilemma?
4. What organizational channels of communication would you use to do so?

## REFERENCES

American Association of Colleges of Nursing: *Essentials of college and university education for professional nursing*, Washington, DC, 1986, American Association of Colleges of Nursing, pp. 5–7.

American Nurses Association: *Code of ethics for nurses with interpretive statements*, Washington, DC, 2001, American Nurses Association.

American Nurses Association: *Human rights guidelines for nurses in clinical and other research*, Publication No. D-46 5M 2/85. Kansas City, MO, 1985, American Nurses Association.

Cassells JM, Redman BK: Preparing students to be moral agents in clinical nursing practice, *Nurs Clin North Am 24*(2):464–473, 1989.

Chia A, Swee Mee L: The effects of issue characteristics on the recognition of moral issues, *Journal of Business Ethics 27*:255–269, 2000.

Curtin L: Ethics in nursing practice, *Nurs Manage 19*(5):7–9, 1988.

Curtin LL: The first ten principles for the ethical administration of nursing services, *Nurs Admin Q 25*(1):7–13, 2000.

Cushing M: Who's responsible for too early discharge? *Am J Nurs 89*(4):471–472, 1989.

Davis AJ: Informed consent process in research protocols: dilemmas for clinical nurses, *West J Nurs Res 11*(4):448–457, 1989.

Davis AJ: Ethical issues in nursing research: dilemmas in alternative care settings, *West J Nurs Res 13*(5):650–652, 1991.

Dolan JF: Mounting interest in right to die issue, *AARP Bulletin 32*(2):7, 1991.

Erlen JA: Moral distress: a pervasive problem, *Orthop Nurs 20*(2):76–80, 2001.

Fowler MDM: Ethical guidelines, *Heart Lung 17*(1):103–104, 1988.

Fowler MDM: Ethical decision making in clinical practice, *Nurs Clin North Am 24*(4):955–965, 1989.

Frank-Stromborg M, Ganschow JR: How HIPAA will change your practice, *Nursing 32*(9):54–57, 2002.

Fry ST: Teaching ethics in nursing curricula, *Nurs Clin North Am 24*(2):485–497, 1989.

Gaul ALV: Ethics content in baccalaureate degree curricula: clarifying the issues, *Nurs Clin North Am 24*(2):475–483, 1989.

Hines GL: DRGs: nursing documentation contributes to the bottom line, *Nurs Clin North Am 23*(3):579–586, 1988.

Jameton A: Culture, morality, and ethics: twirling the spindle, *Crit Care Nurs Clin N Am 2*(3):443–451, 1990.

Kahn JP, Mastroianni AC, Sugarman J: *Beyond consent: seeking justice in research*, New York, NY, 1998, Oxford University Press.

Kendrick K: An advocate for whom—doctor or patient? *Prof Nurs 9*(12):826–829, 1994.

Ketefian S: Moral reasoning and ethical practice in nursing: measurement issues, *Nurs Clin North Am 24*(2):509–521, 1989.

Killeen ML: Nursing fundamentals texts: where's the ethics? *J Nurs Educ 25*(8): 334–340, 1986.

Kjervik DK: The connection between law and ethics, *J Prof Nurs* 6(3):138, 185, 1990.

Koloroutis M, Thorstenson T: An ethics framework for organizational change, *Nurs Admin Q* 23(2):9–18, 1999.

Lammers P: Ethics euthanasia, suicide focus of ethics conference, *AORN J* 44(4): 626–630, 1986.

Martin PA: Bioethics and the whole: pluralism, consensus, and the transmutation of bioethical methods into gold, *J Law Med Ethics* 27:316–327, 1999.

Mezey M, Evans LK, Golub ZD, et al: The Patient Self-Determination Act: sources of concern for nurses, *Nurs Out* 42(1):30–37, 1994.

Moczygemba J, Hewitt B: Managing clinical data in an electronic environment, *Health Care Manager* 19(4):33–38, 2001.

Murphy CP: Integration of diagnostic and ethical reasoning in clinical practice: teaching and evaluation. In Carroll-Johnson RM (editor): *Classification of nursing diagnoses: proceedings of the eighth conference*, Philadelphia, PA, 1989, JB Lippincott, pp. 73–76.

Murphy EK: Undocumented nursing care does not always indicate liability, *AORN J* 46(3):537–538, 540, 1987.

Reigle J: Preserving patient self-determination through advance directives, *Heart Lung* 21(2):196–198, 1992.

Rushton CH, Hogue EE: Confronting unsafe practice: ethical and legal issues, *Pediatr Nurs* 19(3):284–288, 1993.

Salladay SA, McDonnell MM: Spiritual care, ethical choices, and patient advocacy, *Nurs Clin North Am* 24(2):543–549, 1989.

Sawyer LM: Nursing code of ethics: an international comparison, *Int Nurs Rev* 36(5):145–148, 1989.

Scanlon D, Flemming C: Confronting ethical issues: a nursing survey, *Nurs Manage* 21(5):63–65, 1990.

Thompson TC: Rehabilitation: option or requirement? *Rehabil Nurs* 14(6):344, 1989.

Tiedje LB: Moral distress in perinatal nursing, *J Perinat Neonat Nurs* 14(2):36–43, 2000.

Wilkinson JM: Moral distress in nursing practice: experience and effect, *Nurs Forum* 23(1):16–29, 1987/1988.

Wilson HS: *Research in nursing*, ed 2, Redwood City, CA, 1989, Addison-Wesley, pp. 67–69.

# 16

# Nurturing Professional Integrity

*When you complete this chapter, you should be able to:*

1. Discuss ethical issues related to accepting personal responsibility for self-management.
2. Describe a nurse's responsibility for lifelong learning.
3. Discuss common ethical issues associated with contributing to the nursing profession.
4. Describe adaptive attitudes used to cope and adjust to change.
5. Describe ethical issues related to meeting employee obligations.

## KEY CONCEPTS

personal responsibility for
 self-management
advocates for the nursing
 profession

ethical obligations as an employee
 of a health-care agency
loyalty

The ethical concepts related to managing client care discussed in this chapter were selected to help the beginning staff nurse nurture a sense of professional integrity. These concepts concern personal and professional obligations.

## ACCEPTING PERSONAL RESPONSIBILITY FOR SELF-MANAGEMENT

As a member of the discipline of nursing, client care managers are expected to accept **personal responsibility for self-management**. They make a special effort to ensure that their practice is characterized by the values accepted by nursing as a profession. Altruism—unselfish concern for the welfare of others—is one of those values. Being committed to altruism, client care managers accept obligations and rely on inner motivations to ensure that they practice nursing safely on their clients' behalf. Rather than waiting for others to request specific changes in their behavior, they are motivated by their inner desire to do what is right for clients.

Accepting altruism as a professional value carries the potential for serious personal risk. Placing the needs of others before one's own on a regular basis is stressful. One study found that "focusing on the needs of others, often to the exclusion of meeting personal needs, contributes to addiction" (Gelfand et al., 1990, p. 76). Nurses who have not incorporated these demands into their lifestyles may pay a high cost in terms of poor health and ethically questionable nursing practice.

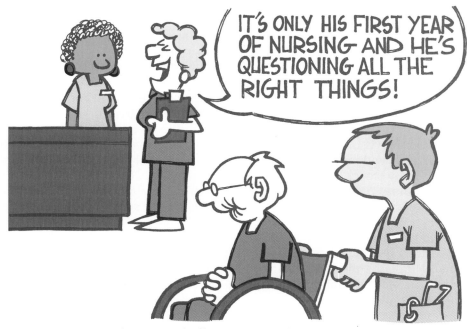

Client care managers make a special effort to ensure that their practice is characterized by the values accepted by nursing as a profession.

# Requirements of Professional Autonomy and Critical Thinking

As Holden (1991, p. 400) stated, "Effective emotional self-management as a health professional demands a clear conception of: (a) the limits and extent of one's responsibility towards the recipient of care; (b) establishing limits on the intensity of one's emotional involvement in the delivery of that care; and (c) being clear about whose problems belong to whom." As professionals, nurses accept responsibility for their interventions, actions, and nonactions in each clinical circumstance. This type of acceptance of responsibility requires freedom to act, or professional autonomy. Making choices among various possible courses of action requires critical rather than ritualistic thinking. This pattern of behavior may not be well received in some nursing practice settings that reward compliance with nursing unit–centered routines versus client-centered routines; impulsive or compulsive nursing actions often indicate abandonment of professional responsibility. Critical thinking followed by conscientious actions on behalf of clients need to be combined with a strong, discernible sense of purpose. All of these criteria depend on the client care manager's integrity and sense of self-respect and worth. To maintain a sense of professional integrity is demanding and energy-consuming. Client care managers may feel the need for a "professional skin" similar to that of the thick, leathery posterior of a wombat (Curtin, 1995, p. 7).

## Promote Client Safety

As professionals, nurses share responsibility for the safety of clients consistent with the principle of nonmaleficence. They are expected to recognize unsafe practice and monitor the practice of peers. Meeting this ethical and legal obligation requires the nurse to collaborate with peers to develop mechanisms (if none exist within the practice setting) for monitoring practice and making timely responses to unsafe practice (Rushton and Hogue, 1993, p. 284). In addition, depending on current state law, nurses may be required to collaborate with state licensing boards designed to protect the public.

Although easily said, ensuring client safety in the modern health-care environment is a complex issue and places significant demands on the involved professionals. Client safety will remain in the public awareness until multiple ethical conflicts are addressed by stakeholders (Gilmartin and Freeman, 2002, p. 52; Gostin, 2000, pp. 27–28; Leape, 2001, p. 145). Staff nurses will be challenged to develop leadership skills consistent with societal trends and the need to sustain autonomy in practice (Gatzke, 2001, p. 13; George et al., 2002, p. 44). Client care managers as knowledge workers who have been known and trusted to provide compassionate care need to sort ethical principles so that fair allocation of health-care resources occurs and that the demands (chronic and increasing staff shortages) placed on them by their professional lives do not prohibit healthy personal lives. Ultimately, external (accreditation requirements, growing political pressure, and system reform) and internal (personal and professional values and commitments) forces will need to be harnessed to stimulate meaningful health-care reform legislation that addresses safety concerns of clients and providers.

## Promote Quality of Life and Practice

Client care managers are individually responsible for the quality of their own lives and that of nursing practice. Each nurse is responsible for making the lifestyle changes needed to reduce the consequences of stress. Stress management can include a wide variety of relaxation techniques; physical exercise; and various diversional, recreational, and leisure activities. Effective stress management helps ensure that the demands of nursing practice do not destroy one's dignity and personal livelihood. Making the lifestyle changes required to manage stress effectively is challenging but crucial to enjoying a successful career. Neglecting to manage stress increases the nurse's vulnerability to "burnout" (Holden, 1991, p. 400). *Burnout* is a term commonly used to describe behaviors that reflect lower levels of physiologic, psychological, and emotional functioning. Nurses experiencing "burnout" might feel increasingly pessimistic and dissatisfied, chronically fatigued, frustrated, and irritable.

Successful staff nurses use several common strategies to maintain a sense of dignity. First, the nurse's appearance must convey the image of a mature adult. Although one may consider as fashionable tee shirts with various pop slogans or crop tops that show one's abdomen, they are inappropriate attire for a professional person. The nurse should wear attire suitable for meeting the public and adapted to the diversity of activities that nurses perform as part of their routine duties (e.g., walking, reaching, bending, stooping, and stretching). The nurse's clothing needs to be clean, comfortable, neat, and becoming.

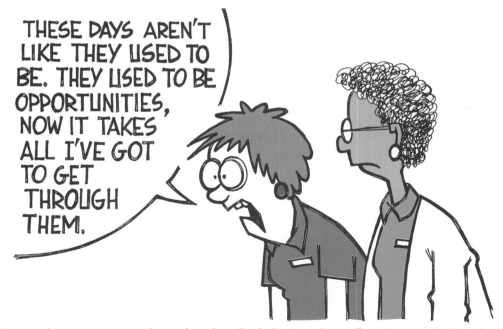

*Burnout* is a term commonly used to describe behaviors that reflect decreased physiologic, psychological, and emotional functioning.

Second, a person's demeanor—tone of voice, facial expressions, and body movements—contributes to her or his public image and needs regular attention. Focusing on others requires the nurse to separate home and work concerns. Clients expect to be the focus of the nurse's attention; they should not need to console or empathize with their nurse.

By attending to the public image projected by one's appearance and demeanor, the nurse can convey a positive attitude about nursing and display confidence when approaching others. Client care managers are amply aware of the widespread anxiety among clients and understand the need to display confidence in the clinical area. To do otherwise increases client anxiety about their safety.

## Identify Strengths and Limitations

Nurses committed to the essential values of their profession take the initiative in identifying their individual strengths and limitations. Accordingly, they strive to develop their strengths as a means of creatively diminishing the influence of their limitations. It is impossible to know and do everything. When effective nurses lack knowledge or skills needed to address client needs, they do not perceive the limitation as a personal inadequacy. Rather, they appropriately admit their limitations so that they can obtain resources to ensure that the quality of care received by clients is not affected adversely. Seeking to address one's limitations on behalf of clients is an ethical requirement and professional strength. They also accept constructive criticism. When strategies, procedures, or techniques exceed their capabilities, nurses seek help to develop knowledge, skills, and assistance with giving care. As knowledge workers, nurses need to know that such learning is a social process that occurs in a "community of practitioners" (Brown and Duguid, 2002, p. 135).

## Maintain Nursing Competencies and Commit to Lifelong Learning

The nurse has a responsibility to maintain nursing competencies. Client care managers are required to possess the attitudes, knowledge, and skills needed to provide safe and effective care for one's assigned clients (versus those needed for all types of clients anywhere). Staff nurses accept responsibility for lifelong learning by maintaining a positive attitude toward gaining insights from experience and participating in structured learning activities, such as regularly reading professional journals, participating in systematic studies designed by others, and using research findings to improve nursing practice. Many nurses contribute to the evolving knowledge base of the nursing profession, while implementing personal strategies for self-management.

In the informational era, nurses need to be personally committed to lifelong learning. They need to maintain openness toward possible solutions to clinical problems and possible sources of related information that might be used to resolve them. Nurses who adopt a positive attitude toward lifelong learning typically actively participate in professional organizations and seminars, informally review current professional and related scientific literature, and share new ideas and concepts with peers. Current nursing knowledge is useful only when it is integrated in nursing standards of practice and care. That is, as a profession, nurses need to integrate current professional knowledge and skills directly in the processes of client care. To succeed, the profession depends on nurses who maintain currency of nursing knowledge and competencies to participate in nursing practice, staff development, and quality improvement committees. Client care managers who participate on these committees will find that they have an opportunity to share their professional knowledge and to learn from others with similar concerns on a regular basis. The financial cost of this type of learning is typically low, but time and energy required to meet these professional demands are high; however, they are well worth the efforts expended. Learning, when defined as a change in behavior, is usually demanding, but nonetheless necessary. Lifelong learning is essential to a successful, enjoyable nursing career.

Formal educational programs also can be used to contribute to one's lifelong learning and professional advancement. Each nurse needs to make such decisions as they fit personal and professional goals. Typically, nurses have many educational opportunities, some of which may be financed partially by one's employer. Information about these programs is available from nursing education departments, human resource management personnel, and colleagues who have completed similar programs. Because educational endeavors are investments in one's self, one's career, and one's future, individuals who decide to pursue higher education generally are encouraged and supported organizationally and financially. The crucial components are the nurse's decision to pursue and commit resources to this avenue of career advancement.

## SERVING AS AN ADVOCATE FOR THE PROFESSION

Although all nurses should serve as **advocates for the nursing profession**, not all do. It is reasonable to understand this lack of advocacy because it can be difficult to do, often causes nurses to feel vulnerable, and requires valuing one's profession (Maier-Lorentz, 2000, p. 25; Ulmer, 2000, p. 9). Advocacy requires a time commitment, and when combined with mandatory overtime and other work-related ad hoc committees or task forces, time can become an issue as well. Professional advocacy is critical in these uncertain times, however. Individuals who do believe that they can should offer their contributions to nursing's evolving knowledge base without apology for credentials or professional stature. Accordingly, they belong to nursing organizations that advance their interests and, indirectly, the interests of the various client populations they serve. They accept change as a challenge and understand that it is essential to the viability of nursing. They actively develop and maintain organized groups, such as local nursing specialty groups, to sustain the nursing profession as a valued component of society. Without continued support from special nursing interest groups, member socialization, advocacy, and development of meaningful relationships with other groups are not feasible. Nurses who do not belong to professional organizations (and some do not for a variety of reasons) limit their potential influence and contributions to society as members of their discipline. Their interests and concerns are more likely to be unrecognized, underrepresented, and unmet because they lack strength through numbers. It behooves every nurse to join one or more nursing organizations and actively participate in special interest groups. Although organizational activities exact personal costs in terms of time, effort, and money, many nurses use this approach to address actively their obligations to the profession.

American society is politically pluralistic. That is, it incorporates many different, often conflicting views. These different views often are reflected in organized special interest groups. To ensure that the nursing profession's interests are expressed and responded to by policy makers, special organizations are necessary. In addition to the American Nurses Association (ANA), many other nursing speciality groups have been formed to represent diverse nursing interests and concerns. When elected officials are informed of their constituents' concerns, they are in a better position to act on them. If they are not informed, concerns expressed by other vested interest groups are likely to take precedence. For example, the public, through the mass media, has expressed distress about the increasing costs of health care and consequent decrease in accessibility. Although the special interests of nursing might provide some solutions to these problems, nurses compete for the attention and resources of public policy makers and elected officials. To be successful, nursing interests must be articulated in such a way as to promote the public good. Frequently, information sharing by nursing groups enables legislators to fashion and approve legislation to address expressed concerns. In addition, nurses might participate on task forces to help governments initiate legislation to prevent or address emerging social problems (e.g., advocating nutrition programs for preschool children or the elderly). The opportunities for nurse involvement in organizations for the common good are limitless and considered by some to be a part of professional practice (Jardin, 2001, p. 618).

Nurses also can contribute to public education through active involvement in local community activities. For example, by participating in recreational, volunteer, or religious groups, nurses frequently provide health education. They often participate in programs designed to prevent diseases, promote health, and provide support for those with diagnosed diseases.

## MANAGING INFORMATION

As discussed in Chapter Two, societal trends affect nursing practice. Evolving technology has made it possible to handle more information and manage it such that people who are in decision-making positions have access to it. Several important ethical issues are emerging as a result of this trend.

### Using Computer Literacy Skills to Influence Organizational Decision Making

People who have the skills to use technology to acquire information are more likely to participate in organizational decision making than those people who do not. To sustain autonomy in clinical decision making, nurses need computer literacy and database management skills. Increased access to information about clients helps

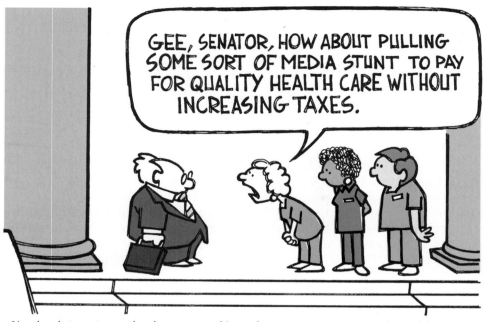

GEE, SENATOR, HOW ABOUT PULLING SOME SORT OF MEDIA STUNT TO PAY FOR QUALITY HEALTH CARE WITHOUT INCREASING TAXES.

Nursing interests need to be conveyed in such a way as to promote the public good.

nurses use knowledge more efficiently to benefit clients. Processing detailed information more efficiently saves time to provide care. Evidence indicates, however, that nurses have not considered carefully how best to use their time and skills to manage the data needed to enhance their nursing practice. Rather, nurses often spend considerable time and effort making detailed observations and entering data for other disciplines (Woolery, 1990, pp. 50–51). Using available technology is integral to nursing practice. In the future, the quality of client care will depend on the extent to which nurses efficiently manage data in accordance with established standards of care and nursing practice. These standards represent common nursing strategies and outcomes designed to guide the services provided to individual clients.

Closely associated with the benefits of information technology are the ethical and legal issues of protecting every client's personal privacy and maintaining confidentiality. Information systems provide easy accessibility to large amounts of data about individual clients; to respect client privacy, nurses keep this information secure to prevent its use for other than its intended purposes (Rittman and Gorman, 1992, p. 16) with the aid of the Health Insurance Portability and Privacy Act. Whenever the entrusted information is used for other than authorized purposes (e.g., care and treatment versus research and marketing), the client's explicit permission is needed. This is no less important with integrated systems that link information from several different agencies or health-care organizations (Romano, 1987, pp. 101–103).

Similarly, the information systems need to control user access by tracing all users and their actions to maintain security and ensure legitimate use. Correspondingly, nurses do not have a right to access information about persons with whom they have no professional relationship, and they breach confidentiality if this information is used for other than providing care and treatment (e.g., inquiry about relatives or friends).

## Participating in Designing and Using Available Technology Wisely

The nurse's effective use of technology and input into its system design are rapidly growing, interrelated concerns (McConnell and Murphy, 1990, p. 333). Nurses need to accept responsibility for maintaining nursing standards by using available technology wisely on their clients' behalf. Not to assert nursing interests when information systems are developed and rented or purchased often results in decreasing the availability of the system and its usefulness to nursing staff. In addition, nurses should expect to evaluate software and recommend changes that will increase their effectiveness and efficiency.

Information management systems are evolving to address outcome criteria (individual client care goals) and to gather the data needed to evaluate the quality of care provided. This technology can be used to collect, store, and retrieve accurate, current information needed to formulate nursing diagnoses. The design of information systems can influence what data are collected and who uses various databases. Taking initiative in expressing concerns about information systems and how they help or hinder client care can save nursing time and effort. Computerized information systems must incorporate nursing's needs for accurate, current data to use in making clinical decisions in a timely manner. This often includes nurses' need to have access to the information system "at the point of care" to promote accuracy and efficiency. Nursing diagnoses of client needs must be incorporated into healthcare systems to guide planning, implementing, and evaluating the effectiveness of services provided. Nonnursing activities, such as requesting and distributing equipment and supplies, compiling client charge lists, and staffing, also can be done efficiently with available information technology. In the past, many nurses feared that information technology would consume scarce time and resources and detract from client care. These fears have proved to be unfounded if the system was well designed.

## COORDINATING CLIENT CARE

Despite revolutionary technology, nurses will continue to coordinate client care. Careful consideration is needed to ensure that nursing skills and time are used efficiently so that the resources of support staff also are used wisely. For example, rather than doing work themselves that can be performed safely and efficiently by support staff, client care managers can serve as resource persons helping other staff find ways to serve clients better.

It is crucial that nurses maintain autonomy if they are to be accountable for their own actions and those of staff working under their direction. Nurses can maintain autonomy while delegating nursing tasks to others but not nursing responsibilities for client care. Each nurse shares the obligation of ensuring that available technology and equipment are used properly to adhere to established standards of nursing practice.

As the complexity of client care, integrated health systems, and nursing practice increases, the need for specialized nursing knowledge also increases. To ensure the public of quality care, continuing efforts are being made to establish practice guidelines (standards of providing care established by the agency's multidisciplinary staff) using national standards and federal laws specifically adapted to the agency to help nurses manage the client care process (Sharp, 1990, p. 22). These guidelines need to be written carefully and clearly (Feutz, 1989, p. 5). These guidelines are another way to resolve issues related to transforming scientific knowledge into clinical judgments, treatment effectiveness, and health-care cost controls. Use of these practice guidelines may help to develop more efficient and economical health-care systems that will improve nursing practice. Nursing practice strategies and organizational factors that contribute to or interfere with client care need continuous study. Each nurse shares responsibility for nursing research designed to improve nursing practice (Titler et al., 1994, p. 312). This approach promotes critical thinking and continuous improvement in the delivery of cost-effective quality care. Accordingly, each nursing research project should answer the following questions: How will the results of this study serve clients? How will it contribute to nursing knowledge?

Complexity also increases the demand for nurses with credentials for advanced practice beyond the competencies of beginning nurses to maintain safe, effective, efficient, and often specialized standards of care. The qualifications of such nurses are determined best by nurses practicing in similar specialized settings. For the credentialing processes to be successful, nursing peer involvement is essential. Providing for this involvement is usually one of the functions of specialty nursing organizations. Although this is not often articulated, ethical nursing practice includes taking actions that support the profession in addition to those taken to provide quality care needed by clients. Ultimately, efforts directly made to enhance the profession indirectly benefit clients.

## MEETING PROFESSIONAL RESPONSIBILITIES AS AN EMPLOYEE

In addition to her or his other responsibilities, each nurse has several **ethical obligations as an employee of a health-care agency**. At times in the past, nursing loyalty to the employer took precedence over client needs (Curtin, 1993a, pp. 26–28; Kendrick, 1994, pp. 826–828). Nurses continue to experience ethical conflicts when addressing client needs as their top priority. The client's ability to pay for services received also is a growing concern.

## Identifying Moral Dilemmas Related to Health-Care Financing

The code of nursing ethics requires the nurse to provide quality care without regard for the method of payment used. The current health-care system and financing mechanisms are forcing many clients to accept, and nurses to provide, only the care that individual clients can afford. In an era when health-care costs are spiraling upward, insurance mechanisms are designed to limit costs rather than satisfy client needs. If providing care according to parameters defined by insurers were acceptable, nurses would need to be prepared as insurance agents to assess and design insurance benefit programs, not as nurses who assess client conditions as the basis for care. When current health-care insurers try to control costs by interpreting benefits on a case-by-case basis, the situation begins to resemble that of the proverbial "tail wagging the dog." Nurses need to strive to be cost-effective, but not to the detriment of clients (Smeltzer, 1990, p. 5). Cost-effectiveness is a component of quality care. Strategies for promoting cost-effectiveness are integrated throughout the process of care. Cost-effectiveness is not the primary focus or desired outcome of care.

Legal responsibility and accountability for the consequences of services provided continue to rest primarily with health-care providers, not with health-care insurers. Liability for the consequences of early discharge or selection of treatment options is likely to continue to rest with providers of care. Accordingly, nurses will serve clients well by expanding rather than limiting the accessibility and quality of health care. Nurses need to assess client needs accurately and plan to provide nursing services based on individual responses and anticipated client recovery patterns. For staff nurses, consideration of the methods of financing care is secondary to determining client needs and how they can be addressed by nursing staff. To align priorities in accordance with health-care financing instead of client needs is unlikely to serve either the client's or the health care agency's interests.

Health-care financing mechanisms often cause agency constraints that prevent client care managers from providing quality care. Nurses who understand what clients need but are prevented from providing quality care are likely to suffer moral distress. Complying with various administrative strategies to reduce expenses and increase revenue without acknowledging the consequences can require staff to neglect important details of quality client care. Common results are ineffective treatment, complications, or delayed client recovery. Rather than focusing on client needs, employees devise documentation strategies designed to obtain maximum reimbursement. These operational strategies condition staff to ignore expressed client concerns or "cover up" inadequacies. Slowly, and often unnoticeably, the focus of staff efforts shifts from consumer satisfaction and quality client care to profit making. These regressive shifts in organizational focus interfere with sustaining satisfying work cultures. Instead, employees devalue their work and find it difficult or impossible to remain committed to it. Staff members encounter increasingly complicated moral dilemmas and legal difficulties (Hogue, 1990, pp. 317–318;

Mallison, 1990, p. 25). Ethical solutions lie in administrative and nursing staff sensitivity to the specific moral dilemmas involved in current methods of discharge planning and their selection of available options. Considerable effort will be needed to realize this potential (Lovell, 2002, p. 158). There continues to be strong evidence that clinical staff experience considerable pressure to comply with organizational decisions rather than what they believe as individuals to be appropriate responses to moral issues.

## Maintaining Loyalties

Loyal employees support the agency's philosophy, policies, and procedures. **Loyalty** to the employer involves commitment. It should not require submissive obedience or compromised values (Curtin, 1993b, p. 20).

Loyalty does not include the obligation to provide unlimited overtime and effort without compensation or unceasing moral distress. Taking into account the different circumstances causing the nurse to work overtime, the nurse has a moral obligation to determine which actions are in the best interest of clients, the self, and the employer. To continue to work extended hours without compensation or acknowledgment by the employer is likely to lead to more overtime work. This moral dilemma is similar to many others that result from the expectation that the nurse will manage unreasonable conflicts, inconsistencies, and demands as an employee (e.g., lack of supplies, malfunctioning equipment, or inadequate staffing). Short staffing should be reported to higher levels of management as soon as possible, with clear documentation of the impact that the inadequate staffing has on client care and safety (Fiesta, 1990a, pp. 22–23). This documentation should occur within the management reporting system; it should not be recorded in a client's clinical record. As a matter of professional judgment, it is sound practice to keep a copy of written reports of inadequate staffing, equipment, or supplies to management that are signed and dated for one's personal records.

Collective bargaining, often referred to as *labor relations*, is a legitimate process of joining together of employees to increase their influence on their employer to improve working conditions. It was legally defined and legitimized by the National Labor Relations Act in 1962 and by subsequent amendments (i.e., Wagner Act in 1974). The ANA has supported the concept of collective bargaining as a power strategy to increase influence by increasing numbers since 1946 through its organizations at the state level, but many nurses are reluctant to participate and support collective bargaining activities.

Client care managers may or may not belong (pay dues) to their specific professional collective bargaining unit, depending on whether membership is required ("closed shop") or optional ("open shop"). Because the collective bargaining unit is associated closely with working conditions, salary, and benefits, information about it can be obtained when seeking employment at a specific agency. Although complex processes are involved, collective bargaining has helped nurses successfully to resolve critical issues affecting their capacity to provide quality care and formalized the conflict resolution processes (i.e., negotiations) needed to do so.

## Promoting Client Interests While Communicating with Multidisciplinary Work Group Members

As the coordinator of client care, the nurse frequently becomes aware of multidisciplinary disagreements and role conflicts. Sometimes the nurse seeks to resolve these conflicts in an effort to serve the client's best interest. Some role conflicts relate to overlaps or gaps in the responsibilities involved in providing care over a 24-hour period on a daily basis. Nurses working during the evening and night shifts often are expected to "cover" for other disciplines in the interest of cost-effectiveness. Consequently, they are asked to provide physical therapy, respiratory therapy, or pharmaceutical or social services, in addition to fulfilling nursing responsibilities. Nurses need to articulate their concerns about these situations so that more effective approaches to quality client care can be devised. In addition, their need for adequate preparation to perform such services skillfully and safely must be made clear to the administration. The specific sources of each moral dilemma require analysis, and the options of ethical action to resolve the conflict need to be identified.

Another type of moral dilemma presents itself when multidisciplinary communication patterns evolve into bureaucratic maneuvering for status instead of focusing on client care. High-quality care requires that multidisciplinary staff members communicate effectively with each other in a spirit of collaboration. Among the universally accepted ethical behaviors are effective (open, direct, and flexible communication) working relationships with coworkers (Sawyer, 1989, p. 145). Communication "games" do not serve clients or staff (Marsden, 1990, pp. 422–424). They typically increase stress, conflict, and potential for verbal abuse. Nurses have established a history of seeking autonomy in clinical decision making. What is important is that an environment be created and sustained in which multidisciplinary staff members focus on client needs as their top priority. Multidisciplinary staff members need to feel safe enough to communicate concerns and needs openly to each other. Open communication among multidisciplinary staff members serves to address client needs. This atmosphere is likely to promote effective communication with clients as well. Sensitivity to patterns of communication among staff members helps nurses identify the communication patterns that detract from client care. A spirit of collaboration promotes quality client care by mobilizing costly human resources instead of allowing moral dilemmas to erode them.

## Maintaining Confidentiality

Nurses have an obligation to maintain confidentiality about private and intimate client matters. As members of the larger society, nurses are affected by society's predominant anxieties and stereotypes. To practice ethically, the nurse must become sensitive to keeping clinical information about individual clients private or secret from individuals not directly involved in providing their care. Indiscreet social interactions in nonclinical areas, or "shop talk," can be overheard or misinterpreted and result in considerable damage to clients, without the nurses ever being aware of it (Glinsky, 1987, p. 24). Accordingly, shop talk is unethical because of its potential for violating client rights. Every nurse has a moral duty not to engage in "shop talk."

Nurses need to sort out the nature of the legal relationships of the client's family and significant others before sharing confidential information. Given the many variations in the composition of American families, this is no small achievement. To do otherwise poses serious risk of violating the client's rights, morally and legally (Pinch, 2000, p. 14). It is essential to abide by clients' expressed directions and limitations for communicating information to family members or friends except for legal exclusions, legal guardians, or parents in the case of minors.

Nurses are obligated to provide services to clients in a nondiscriminatory manner. Expression of personal prejudices, evidenced by refusal to provide care or showing disrespect for the individual's characteristics or appearance, is prohibited. One form of discrimination is stereotyping clients on the basis of their diseases or clinical symptoms. Symptoms or diseases such as AIDS, malignancies, or genetic disorders frequently contribute to social isolation or stigmatization of clients. These consequences present moral dilemmas and create the potential for violating client rights. Depending on the severity of the negative stereotypes and the public's concern for the common good, laws usually are passed to protect the individuals who are victims of the disease and to protect the public from contracting the dreaded diseases. For example, many states have laws concerning who is required to be tested for AIDS. In addition, many states have laws dictating how information about persons with the disease is to be handled to ensure the privacy of individual clients (Grady, 1989, pp. 529–531). Associated with the issue of confidentiality are concerns for protecting the client's autonomy (beneficence, nonmalificence) and equal access to health care (justice).

Closely related to client rights to privacy are moral dilemmas associated with a person's right to bodily integrity. Nurses are involved in performing treatment programs in which tissue or organs are transplanted or artificial body parts are inserted. In addition to performing related nursing procedures correctly, nurses need to be sensitive to client responses and know what the selection criteria are for these procedures. What basic values are inherent in the ethical guidelines used? Is the client's autonomy protected, or do financial considerations predominate? Nurses need to be aware of which professional values and ethical principles are involved in protecting client rights and how they are prioritized in individual client circumstances.

## Protecting One's Rights as a Provider of Health Care

Nurses obtain the privilege of practicing nursing after meeting specific licensure requirements. Nurses also have rights related to the practice of their chosen profession. These rights are recognized and protected by position statements formulated by representative nursing organizations. Such position statements are written from time to time to inform the public and guide nurses in selecting moral actions inherent in ethical practice. The ANA Committee on Ethics (1986) issued a "Statement Regarding Risk Versus Responsibility in Providing Nursing Care" to clarify parameters of nursing obligations and options in providing care involving risks to the nurse's life or well-being.

Nurses can morally justify refusal to participate in client care in some circumstances and need to be aware of the conditions required for doing so. The ANA statement delineated four basic requirements for determining the difference between doing good for another as a moral duty and doing so as a moral option. According to the ANA, the nurse is ethically required to provide care when:

1. The client is at significant risk of harm, loss, or damage if the nurse does not help.
2. The nurse's action or care directly prevents harm to the client.
3. The nurse's action will probably prevent harm, loss, or damage to the client.
4. The benefit the client will gain outweighs any harm the nurse might bring on herself or himself and does not present more than minimal risk to the nurse (ANA Committee on Ethics, 1986).

To refuse to provide care for a client requires that the nurse understand the nature of the client's condition, the urgency of the need, and the likelihood that the nurse's help will make a significant difference. Ethical decisions require that the nurse make use of current and accurate information about client conditions, knowledge of the professional values involved, and understanding of the priorities in the nurse's personal values.

The nurse needs to make reasonable efforts to use available technology to process information accurately and efficiently on clients' behalf. Information technology is an agency resource that all personnel need to use appropriately. To sabotage or undermine the use of the agency's technology for any reason (e.g., fear, lack of information or skills) by omitting data or not using the system at all is ethically irresponsible when the quality of client care depends on it. This behavior could jeopardize client well-being, result in lack of follow-through, or cause system inadequacies in meeting standards of quality care. As information technology develops, nurses need to be aware of their moral responsibility to use it for the purposes for which it was intended, which includes using security mechanisms for maintaining confidentiality as described earlier in this chapter.

## Serving as a Role Model

As mentioned in Chapter Ten, nurses can lead and teach others about desired behaviors by modeling desired actions. Nurses' attitudes need to reflect their personal values and commitment to the values espoused by the profession in its ethical codes of behavior. This does not mean that individuals should expect others to mimic their behavior. Rather, functioning as a role model is a teaching strategy used to help coworkers learn about moral issues and acceptable methods of resolving them in the interests of all concerned. Coworkers are encouraged to learn how to solve ethical issues to improve work performance and quality of client care. This approach reinforces respect for individual differences and the dignity of others. It also encourages employees to accept accountability for their actions.

The respect of others is earned, not given. Coworkers might indicate in several different ways that a nurse has earned their respect. One common indicator of respect is the nature of the communication patterns between coworkers, including demeanor and tone of voice. The rights to privacy and to participate in clinical decision making are fundamental to meaningful relationships with peers, as they are to relationships with clients. Patterns of staff interactions can reflect positive attitudes toward clients. For example, staff nurses convey respect for peers and coworkers by using language that is commonly understood, incorporating accepted health-care terminology, and avoiding offensive expressions.

Another common indicator that coworkers respect a nurse is their responsiveness to supervision and instruction. Coworkers tend to seek guidance and direction actively from the nurse to help them complete their work assignments. They effectively communicate their concerns, acknowledge their limitations, and express the need for help or support when it arises. They do not delay such requests until the difficulties are unavoidable or overwhelming.

Another way to show respect for others might involve consulting with the agency's ethics committee to demonstrate the attitude that differing points of view are acceptable. The recommendations of such a committee can be incorporated in making appropriate clinical decisions for clients and staff when the situations encountered are difficult to manage using typical approaches. One suggested strategy is to consult with a mentor or supervisor to discuss moral dilemmas. Another fairly common approach is to use an ethics committee to help fulfill obligations of client advocacy, to clarify facts, and to improve communication (Murphy, 1989, p. 554). Respect for differences requires that differences be acknowledged in the effort to find solutions, rather than suppressed or ignored. After the entry-level staff nurse gains work experience and develops a special interest in addressing moral dilemmas, he or she might seek membership on such a committee.

Finally, coworkers who respect each other tend to use similar approaches to their work. Although they do not agree on many issues, their approaches to meeting diverse client needs become more similar than different. Respect for oneself and others creates work cultures designed to provide high-quality care and reinforces coworker adherence to codes of ethical conduct.

## Preventing Sexual Harassment

Sexual harassment is an area of increasing concern in the work environment. Its definition was broadened by the Civil Rights Act, which became law in 1991. Generally, sexual harassment is defined as behavior that offends (i.e. "unwelcome sexual advances, requests for sexual favors and other verbal and physical contact of a sexual nature that are connected to decisions about employment or that create an intimidating, hostile, or offensive work environment") (Elgin, 1993, p. 207). Complaints of this nature are handled by the Equal Employment Opportunity Commission (EEOC). The nurse, as employee (of employers with 15 or more employees), needs to know who the EEOC officer is and how complaints are processed. Whenever feasible, client care managers try to prevent employees from harassing each other or clients from harassing employees. If sexual harassment cannot be prevented, guidance for implementing sexual harassment policies and procedures should be sought.

Generally clues to sexual harassment are found in mismatches between what is said verbally and body language (Elgin, 1993, p. 210). For example, changes in the tone of voice from what is characteristic for the individual (e.g., higher pitch and courtesy) and gestures that convey hostility or aggression may be warning signs. The tone of voice more than the words used indicates aggression (Elgin, 1993, pp. 73, 220). When the recipient of the verbal or behavioral messages is offended, he or she needs to respond assertively to inform the offender. If a pattern of offensive mismatches develops and the offender does not respond to corrective feedback, formal processing of complaints is in order. Using critical thinking skills, the client care manager determines whether her or his own patterns of verbal and behavioral communication are part of the evolving problem or its solution. Then hard choices need to be made.

## Making Hard Choices

Nurses are required to make hard choices to maintain their personal livelihoods and nursing competencies, support the nursing profession, and remain loyal to their employers. Similar to many ethical issues in nursing practice, situations causing moral dilemmas are usually complex. Solutions require careful attention to the identified differences and persistent commitment to resolving them. For example, making specific changes in one's lifestyle to manage stress effectively is usually difficult due to personal goals, time limitations, family needs, work schedules, commitment to various community groups, and recreational interests. These difficulties do not make the need to manage stress less critical, however. Similarly, societal trends (e.g., the increasing influence of the global economy) continue to influence nursing as a profession and require individual nurses to support creatively its evolution as a science and dynamic force in society. As economic constraints continue to influence the health-care system (requiring more collaboration among various disciplines), the autonomy of all health-care providers is likely to be affected, which probably will stimulate change in the role of nurses as employees.

As members of the nursing profession, entry-level staff nurses are likely to be confronted with difficult choices. Their decisions will affect significantly the quality of their lives, nursing practice, and employment. The best decisions for the involved individuals usually incorporate personal and professional values. For example, a nurse's commitment to providing quality care may lead her or him to "bend the rules for the sake of the patient" (Hutchinson, 1990, p. 3). Doing so carries considerable risk to a nurse functioning as an autonomous professional and participant in a formal organizational system. The positive consequences of the actions taken are likely to be used to justify bending the rules, even though there is no legal or organizational basis for doing so. For example, the client care manager might become aware of another nursing work group member's nonadherence to policy in administering PRN (as needed) medicines (i.e., "bending" the rules in response to multiple requests from a manipulative client and avoiding the need to set limits and the potential of being perceived as less than a caring nurse). The client, encouraged by such responses, makes even more unreasonable requests, however, that require the nurse to "bend the rules" further, resulting in unsafe practice (i.e., giving more drugs than prescribed medically). The client hoards the medicine, combining it with drugs acquired illegitimately, and overdoses. "Responsible rule bending" may produce negative consequences and cause client injury or harm. Legal difficulties may arise when the situation is disclosed. The client care manager, working within the system to meet client needs in a timely manner, has a responsibility to recognize and respond to such conflicts in the interest of client well-being.

The term *whistle-blowing* is becoming common (Jubb, 1999, p. 77). It refers to an employee's voluntary disclosure of information about an organization's wrongdoing that becomes part of a public record (external to the organization) that is intended to effect remedial action (Jubb, 1999, p. 84). Employees who participate in whistle-blowing or criticize an agency's questionable practices accept the positive and the negative consequences of reporting situations that endanger client well-being (Fiesta, 1990b, p. 38; Kiely and Kiely, 1987, p. 42). The positive consequences are the satisfactions and comforts of adherence with the nurses' professional code of ethics. The negative consequences are the lack of organizational or legal support for doing so, which ultimately may result in dismissal, career disruptions, license revocation, malpractice, and possible criminal charge (Adams, 2002, pp. 218–223). Whistle-blowing can imperil a career. Such risks do not reduce the need to disclose unsafe practices, however. As a standard for sound practice, the nurse needs to make an earnest effort to resolve these conflicts within the organization before considering external disclosure. It is hoped that employers of nurses will become increasingly responsive to employee concerns about quality of care. Instead of firing concerned employees for disclosing questionable practices, administrative policies could provide alternatives to public disclosure, such as organizational

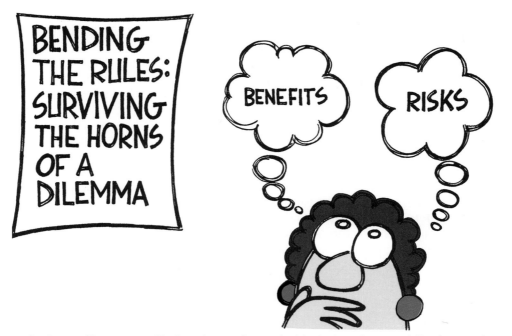

Beginning staff nurses are likely to be confronted with choices that are difficult to make.

communication systems and reporting procedures (Pinch, 1990, pp. 60–61). Some states have laws that protect employees from being fired for disclosing unsafe practices.

Nurses need to remember that the ANA Code of Ethics for Nurses is not law or public policy. Rather, it is "a policy document that constitutes the expression of principles that are geared to the enhancement of health care in general" (Blum, 1984, p. 150). Because it does not have legal status, ethical conduct consistent with established codes may not prevent an employer from dismissing an employee. By following nursing codes of conduct that support the public interest, staff nurses may benefit from societal support for needed legislation that currently does not exist (Fiesta, 1990b, p. 38). Accordingly, the nurse needs to proceed with caution with whistle-blowing (Sloan, 2002, p. 67). It is critical to know what is at stake professionally, what are effective and ineffective responses, what is involved, and what if any support is available for taking such action (McDonald and Ahern, 1999, p. 12).

## SUMMARY

Client care managers accept responsibility for self-management by participating in continued learning experiences to maintain nursing competencies. They are motivated to do what is right for the public and for their clients. They use several common strategies to maintain their health and sense of self-dignity, and they accept responsibility for managing their own individual strengths and limitations. They seek help to develop the knowledge and skills needed to provide care when the necessary strategies, procedures, or techniques exceed their capabilities.

Many nurses also participate in activities advocating the interests of the nursing profession. They join and become actively involved in nursing and special interest organizations. They participate in health education programs with community groups. In addition, nurses make a special effort to learn to use available technology, to maintain nursing standards, and to participate in research endeavors aimed at increasing nursing knowledge.

Client care managers also accept ethical obligations as employees of health-care agencies. They support their agencies' philosophies and policies. They strive to maintain effective communication patterns with health-care work group members to coordinate client care. They are expected to protect clients' rights as well as their own. They take the initiative to teach others about quality care and to demonstrate desired approaches. From time to time, client care managers make hard choices to resolve conflicts regarding the ethical priorities of clients and their employers. They need to distinguish behaviors advocated by ethical codes of conduct from behaviors required by existing laws.

## APPLICATION EXERCISES

1. Interview three staff nurses about their self-management strategies. Ask them to discuss the methods they use to manage stress and set priorities. Compare your findings with peers. Identify predominant strategies and reasons for their popularity.

2. List 10 different ways that nurses participate in lifelong learning. Rate them according to your personal preferences.

3. Your agency uses several different computer networks to store, retrieve, and access client information in an efficient and timely manner. One of your neighbors asks you about the recovery of a mutual friend, knowing that you have access to confidential information. List ethical alternative responses. Select the best option. Give reasons for your selection.

4. A colleague tells you that "things are getting worse instead of better since decentralization." You are new to the organization. When employed, you were informed of administrative plans for promoting professional autonomy and accountability. Describe how you would remain loyal to the organization and support your colleague's need for change.

5. While administering medications during the evening shift, you overhear a client verbally abusing a nursing staff member under your supervision. Describe criteria you would use to determine whether the nursing staff member can refuse to provide further care to the client.

## CRITICAL THINKING SCENARIO

Imagine that you are a recently employed graduate nurse joining a work group in a busy outpatient clinic setting. Most of the staff have worked together for more than 5 years. You observe that the physicians (all but one of whom are men) dominate social conversations, often in sports terminology, using words and tones of voice that are sexually offensive to you. Your nursing colleagues listen quietly in their presence, but describe feelings of embarrassment and fear behind closed doors. The nurses have informed you that the nurse you replaced was "finished" after she asserted herself after being offended by the repeated sexual innuendos in the work setting.

1. Would you seek guidance of your nurse colleagues? Why?
2. What strategies are available to identify the problem?
3. What strategies are available for reducing the sexual harassment? Which would best suit you?
4. Since the employer is covered under the 1991 Civil Rights Act, what would you do? Give reasons for your answer.

# REFERENCES

Adams B: Accountable but powerless, *Health Affairs 21*(1):218–223, 2002.

American Nurses Association Committee on Ethics: *Statement regarding risk versus responsibility in providing nursing care*, Kansas City, MO, 1986, American Nurses Association.

Blum JD: The code of nurses and wrongful discharge, *Nurs Forum 21*(4):149–150, 1984.

Brown JS, Duguid P: *The social life of information*, Boston, MA, 2002, Harvard Business School Press.

Curtin LL: Conscience and clinical care, *Nurs Manage 24*(8):26–28, 1993a.

Curtin LL: When virtue becomes vice, *Nurs Manage 24*(9):20–26, 1993b.

Curtin LL: When the going gets tough, the tough . . . , *Nurs Manage 26*(11):7–8, 1995.

Elgin SH: *Genderspeak: men, women, and the gentle art of verbal self-defense*, New York, 1993, John Wiley & Sons.

Fiesta J: The nursing shortage: whose liability problem? *Nurs Manage 21*(2):22–23, 1990a.

Fiesta J: Whistleblowers: retaliation or protection? Part II, *Nurs Manage 21*(7):38, 1990b.

Feutz SA: Legal implications of institutional standards for nurses, *J Nurs Admin 19*(7):4–7, 1989.

Gatzke H: New skills for a new age: preparing nurses for the 21st century, *Nurs Forum 36*(3):13–17, 2001.

Gelfand G, Long P, McGill D, et al: Prevention of chemically impaired nursing practice, *Nurs Manage 21*(7):76–78, 1990.

George V, Burke LJ, Rodgers B, et al: Developing staff nurse shared leadership behavior in professional nursing practice, *Nurs Admin Q 26*(3):44–59, 2002.

Gilmartin MJ, Freeman RE: Business ethics and health care: a stakeholder perspective, *Health Care Manage Rev 27*(2):52–65, 2002.

Glinsky J: The perils of "shop talk," *Nurs Life 7*(6):24, 1987.

Gostin LO: Managed care, conflicts of interest, and quality, *Hastings Center Rep* Sept/Oct 2000, pp. 27–28.

Grady C: Ethical issues in providing nursing care to human immunodeficiency virus-infected populations, *Nurs Clin North Am 24*(2):523–534, 1989.

Hogue EE: The liability of payors and providers in health care treatment decisions, *Pediatr Nurs 16*(3):317–318, 1990.

Holden RJ: Responsibility and autonomous nursing practice, *J Adv Nurs 16*(4): 398–403, 1991.

Hutchinson SA: Responsible subversion: a study of rule-bending among nurses, *Scholar Inq Nurs Pract 4*(1):3–17, 1990.

Jardin D: Political involvement in nursing—politics, ethics, and strategic action, *AORN J 74*(5):614–628, 2001.

Jubb PB: Whistleblowing: a restrictive definition and interpretation, *Journal of Business Ethics 21*:77–94, 1999.

Kendrick K: An advocate for whom—doctor or patient? *Prof Nurs 9*(12):826–828, 1994.

Kiely MA, Kiely DC: Whistleblowing: disclosure and its consequences for the professional nurse and management, *Nurs Manage 18*(5):41–45, 1987.

Leape LL: Foreword: preventing medical accidents: is "systems analysis" the answer? *Am J Law Med 27:*145–148, 2001.

Lovell A: Ethics as a dependent variable in individual and organizational decision making, *Journal of Business Ethics 37*:145–163, 2002.

Maier-Lorentz MM: Invest in yourself: creating your own ethical environment, *Nurs Forum 35*(3):25–28, 2000.

Mallison MB: Controversies in care: a jury defines "neglect" in nursing homes, *Am J Nurs 90*(9):25, 1990.

Marsden C: Ethics of the "doctor-nurse game," *Heart Lung 19*(4):422–424, 1990.

McConnell EA, Murphy EK: Nurses' use of technology: an international concern, *Int Nurs Rev 37*(5):331–334, 1990.

McDonald S, Ahern K: Whistleblowing: effective and ineffective coping responses, *Nurs Forum 34*(4):5–13, 1999.

Murphy P: The role of the nurse on hospital ethics committees, *Nurs Clin North Am 24*(2):551–556, 1989.

Pinch WJ: Nursing ethics: is "covering-up" ever "harmless"? *Nurs Manage 21*(9):60–62, 1990.

Pinch WJE: Confidentiality: concept analysis and clinical application, *Nurs Forum 35*(2):5–16, 2000.

Rittman MR, Gorman RH: Computerized databases: privacy issues in the development of the nursing minimum data set, *Comput Nurs 10*(1):14–18, 1992.

Romano CA: Privacy, confidentiality, and security of computerized systems, *Comput Nurs 5*(3):99–104, 1987.

Rushton CH, Hogue EE: Confronting unsafe practice: ethical and legal issues, *Pediatr Nurs 19*(3):284–288, 1993.

Sawyer LM: Nursing code of ethics: an international comparison, *Int Nurs Rev 36*(5):145–148, 1989.

Sharp N: National practice guidelines: what do they mean for nurses? *Nurs Manage 21*(11):22, 24, 1990.

Sloan AJ: Whistleblowing: proceed with caution, *RN 65*(1):67–81, 2002.

Smeltzer CH: The impact of prospective payment on the economics, ethics, and quality of nursing, *Nurs Admin Q 14*(3):1–10, 1990.

Titler MG, Kleiber C, Steelman V, et al: Infusing research into practice to promote quality care, *Nurs Res 43*(5):307–312, 1994.

Ulmer BC: Professional advocacy, *AORN J 72*(1):9–11, 2000.

Woolery LK: Professional standards and ethical dilemmas in nursing information systems, *J Nurs Admin 20*(10):50–53, 1990.

# Epilogue

## *Managing Your Career*

*When you complete this chapter, you should be able to:*

1. Refine your personal nursing philosophy, interests, and talents.
2. Identify 5-year personal and career goals.
3. Seek employment corresponding to your personal career goals.
4. Organize information about your qualifications and nursing credentials.
5. Determine the need for malpractice insurance.
6. Use available support systems to promote personal growth.
7. Establish licensure and maintain your registration as a registered nurse.
8. Write a letter notifying your employer of a desire to change or terminate employment.
9. Nurture an indefatigable sense of humor!

**KEY CONCEPTS**

nursing philosophies
  personal values
  beliefs
characteristics of nursing as a
  profession
  maintain nursing competencies
  need for continued self-development
  personal life goals
5-year goals

nursing employment
  qualifications and requirements
  credentials
licensure
registration
malpractice insurance
support systems
changing an employment status
humor

## BLAZING A PERSONAL CAREER PATH

In addition to managing client care, successful staff nurses manage their careers to ensure that they meet their personal goals. Managing a career is not the same as having a series of jobs (Crawford, 1993, p. 337). Neglecting personal goals contributes to personal frustration, which can diminish the quality of client care management. This epilogue is designed to help entry-level staff nurses gain perspective on their personal needs as a professional person and begin to make choices and decisions conducive to a fulfilling career. To manage other resources well, client care managers first need to manage themselves (Levenstein, 1983, p. 22).

New graduates often have opportunities to select one of a variety of potential employers. They are challenged not so much by getting a job, but by identifying the best employer. To make the best choice, new graduates need to determine what employer characteristics and types of health-care organizations best match their personal and career interests. By making this effort, entry-level staff nurses can match the desired characteristics of potential employers with their individual needs. Subsequently, new graduates can take the initiative to gain satisfaction from their employment and nursing practice.

The entry-level staff nurse realizes that (1) the employer will invest considerable resources to help the recent graduate succeed as an employee, and (2) in return, the employer expects the new graduate to remain employed long enough to obtain a reasonable return on such an investment. Many employers expect new graduates to remain employed for 1 year or longer to adjust to the varied demands of nursing practice and gain the experience required to develop confidence in their application of nursing knowledge and skills. Findings of at least one study indicated that new graduates had a higher probability of staying employed for 1 year than did experienced nurses (Prior et al., 1990, p. 27). To remain with one's first employer for less than 1 year may invite questions from subsequent employers as to the reasons for such a short term of employment. To avoid mismatches between individual goals and needs and the interests of the employer, each nurse needs to identify personal nursing beliefs and career goals as well as special interests and skills.

## REFINING PERSONAL PHILOSOPHY, INTERESTS, AND TALENTS

With the evolution of an increasing variety of health-care settings, recent graduates benefit from clarifying their personal **nursing philosophies** before seeking employment. Each nurse needs to identify and clarify his or her **personal values, beliefs,** and assumptions about basic truths. Each nurse should know what he or she believes about human nature: what she or he believes about societal needs; and what she or he believes nursing has to offer society, particularly as this relates to personal goals, interests, and talents. A balanced appraisal of one's personal nursing philosophy also includes an assessment of what nursing is not. This entails considering one's biases, limitations, and vulnerabilities. For example, a nursing philosophy typically includes beliefs about people's basic needs and the extent to which the **characteristics of nursing as a profession** address them. If the nurse's personal belief is that people are inherently good and may be forced to change due to

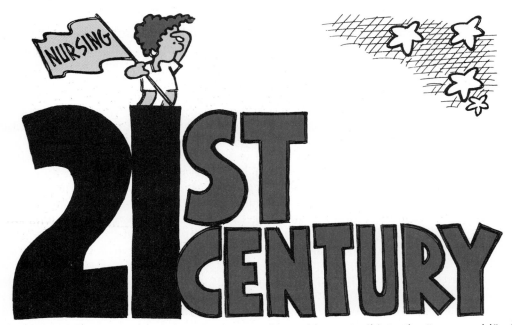

Managing a nursing career today means preparing to blaze a trail into the "new world" of 21st-century nursing.

external circumstances, her or his nursing philosophy might include a commitment to altering external factors that interfere with satisfying basic human needs. If the nurse's personal belief is that people are neither inherently good nor bad and that a person's features depends on the individual's inner resources and personality, her or his nursing philosophy is less likely to express as much commitment to altering external factors to satisfy basic human needs. Another nurse's personal belief might be that whether people are good or bad depends on internal and external factors that need to be addressed. This person's nursing philosophy probably would include a commitment to altering external and internal factors that interfere with satisfying basic human needs.

A nurse's basic beliefs also affect her or his nursing philosophy and involvement in interest groups and professional organizations and activities consistent with it. One's personal nursing philosophy also reflects beliefs about each nurse's responsibility for contributing to the profession's knowledge base. Closely related to this responsibility is the moral obligation to **maintain nursing competencies** required to apply current nursing knowledge and skills to provide safe, high-quality client care.

With the evolving health-care scene, the nursing student needs to appreciate that many of the nursing positions he or she will hold in the course of a career will not exist at graduation time. What is critical is that one develops a commitment or, even better, a passion for serving clients in accordance with one's nursing philosophy. A professional open mind is conducive to caring for clients effectively in the sometimes harsh "modern business" health-care settings. In hasty cost-effective journeys to cure, nurses need to acknowledge the persistence of human suffering and nursing's commitment to care about the people they serve (Muff, 1994, p. 36). Although specific outcomes of cure are sought and sometimes quantified, caring may be more intangible, less readily measured, but no less valued. As has been said, people are not dissatisfied with health care as much as with the care they do not receive (Muff, 1994, p. 34). Nurses can and do contribute to situations in which such caring takes place.

One's nursing philosophy guides one's beliefs about the **need for continued self-development** and growth, which enable the nurse to practice effectively and efficiently. One's nursing philosophy also guides one's selection of an area of practice and settings that match one's values, beliefs, interests, and talents. Often nursing students are asked to write brief descriptions of their individual nursing philosophies to help clarify beliefs about nursing, related values and assumptions, and **personal life goals**. Successfully completing this assignment helps the student identify the characteristics of potential employers that match the individual's personal values, goals, and needs. Box E-1 lists characteristics of potential employers that staff nurses might consider when trying to identify those that best match their individual nursing philosophies, values, beliefs, nursing interests, and goals.

## Critical Thinking

Developing a personal nursing philosophy entails critical thinking throughout one's career. Choice of philosophy has been termed one of the "big decisions" to learn to watch for in one's life (Paul and Elder, 2001, p. 185). The process of critical thinking requires an open mind and the ability to question basic "facts" (which may prove to be inaccurate), beliefs, and assumptions. The critical thinker accepts ideas, facts, and beliefs only after giving them careful thought, rather than casually accepting them as a matter of convenience. Critical thinking also involves elaborate problem solving, beginning with carefully identifying the problem or central issue, selecting the best available option, acting on it, and evaluating the outcomes. Often one learns to identify cues to underlying assumptions that bias thinking and related problem identification and resolution. When identified, these cues require the nurse to use facts in new ways that enhance what and when interventions are made or actions taken.

The process of critical thinking is important in providing and managing client care because the client care manager does more than perform caregiving activities. The effective client care manager constantly evaluates the outcomes of care and, using the processes involved in critical thinking, makes decisions regarding future care planning.

## IDENTIFYING 5-YEAR GOALS

Each nurse has personal and career goals, whether he or she is aware of them or not. Williams (1990, p. 104D) reported that nurses ranked pay, autonomy, professional status, and interaction with other nurses as very important contributors to "job satisfaction." More recently, as the nursing shortage increases, Magnet hospitals

BOX E-1

## Characteristics of Potential Employers of Staff Nurses

### Facility Type
Episodic (acute) care/long-term (residential) care
Profit/nonprofit
Private/public
Rural/urban community
Community-based/teaching/university

### Agency Image
Fast-paced/relaxed atmosphere
Organized/unorganized
Businesslike/friendly

### Organizational Culture
Reward innovation/maintain status quo
Opportunistic/ethical
High-tech/hands-on
Medical model/interdisciplinary health maintenance

### Management Style
Participatory/autocratic
Well-established/flexible/evolving
Short-term/long-term focus
Task-oriented/people-oriented
Centralized/decentralized

### Physical Appearance
Meticulous/casually maintained
Old/new physical plant
High/low security
High/low safety concerns

### Financial Goals
Profit/avoiding loss
Private/publicly financed
Cost controls/creative spending
Survival/expansion plan

have increased in popularity as employers of registered nurses. Fourteen *forces of magnetism* have been identified that are believed to attract and retain nurses. These forces, which are likely to interest graduates of nursing programs, include (1) quality of nursing leadership, (2) organizational structure, (3) management style, (4) personnel policies and programs, (5) professional models of care, (6) quality of care, (7) quality improvement, (8) consultation and resources, (9) autonomy, (10) community and hospital, (11) nurses as leaders, (12) image of nursing, (13)

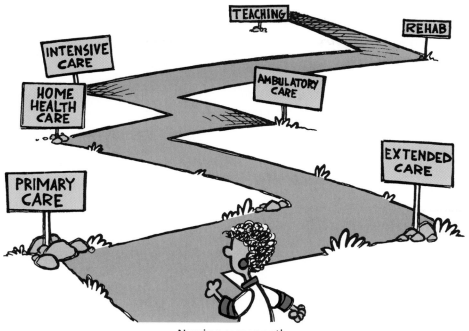

Nursing career path.

interdisciplinary relationships, and (14) professional development (Domrose, 2002, p. 19). This list of forces is intended to provide an example to help nurses think about the desired characteristics of potential employers known to have a strong commitment to nursing. An updated list of Magnet hospitals can be accessed at http://www.nursingworld.org/ancc/Magnet/facilities.html. If one clarifies personal and career goals, progress toward meeting them contributes to a sense of success and can be used to guide choices that increase the probability of reaching them.

Entry-level staff nurses experience difficulty designing a lifelong career plan before they have experience practicing nursing in the areas of their choice. Each nurse enters the profession at a specific point in her or his life, however. For example, unmarried nurses who have no dependents and who hope to combine marriage, family, and career often have different personal goals from those who are married, rearing children of varying ages, and involved in various community groups. Personal needs for satisfactory child care, transportation, housing, and related community resources are likely to influence the nurse's selection of potential employers. Personal goals, such as finding a spouse or enabling children to obtain a particular type of education, influence where some nurses choose to live and practice.

To ensure that their personal goals are met, nurses need to assess the requirements of potential employers and the extent to which the work environment and community characteristics match the nurse's goals, needs, and lifestyle, including recreational and family activities. Box E-2 lists common employer characteristics that affect personal and career goals.

## Matching Employers with Personal Career Goals

1. *Location:* How do you plan to get to work? What are the anticipated transportation costs? Is the job convenient to grocery stores, restaurants, the school you plan to attend? How much security is needed to ensure your safety?
2. *Variety in work activities:* Are you looking for employment that will provide opportunity to perform a variety of tasks and develop new skills, or would you rather become an expert at a few specific skills? Will completing the work require well-developed organizational skills?
3. *Stress:* Do you prefer a fast or slow pace? Do you enjoy change from day to day or a more steady, stable work environment? What are your preferences for shift and type of work schedule? Do you have work schedule requirements due to family or other commitments? How much advance scheduling is done? How many holidays and weekends will you be required to work?
4. *Autonomy versus authority:* Do you prefer to be self-directed or have procedures established in detail? Do you prefer to take the initiative in problem solving, identifying solutions and carrying them out, or to hand over the responsibility for solving problems to others?
5. *Benefits:* How important is the amount of money you make? Would you prefer a full-time position with a predictable income or a part-time position with a fluctuating paycheck?
   *Expendable income:* Get an idea of the income you will require, based on a realistic budget. Allow extra money for expenses that crop up unexpectedly.
   *Insurance benefits:* What kind of coverage do you and your family need? In addition to health and life insurance, are malpractice and disability benefits included? Can you participate in retirement and pension plans? How soon?
   *Vacation and sick pay:* What are the eligibility requirements?
   *Support of professional growth:* Will the employer reimburse some or all costs of continuing education or degree programs? Will further education help you climb this employer's career ladder?
6. *Opportunities for choice of clinical area of practice:* Are clinical interests distinct specialties or are they integrated within the larger nursing practice group? How will the facility support your clinical interest? Are entry-level staff nurses permitted direct entry into a specialty area of practice, or is experience required?
7. *Recognition and advancement:* How does the facility reward individual excellence and dedication? Do you expect a monetary reward? What are the opportunities for advancement? Are you locked into an entry-level position, or could you be promoted based on good work? Where do you want to be in 5 years? Will this employer help you get there? How?
8. *Human relationships:* How important to you are positive relationships among staff, management, and clients? How does this organization promote open communication and continuous problem solving? Does the culture encourage employees to make time-limited or lifelong commitments?

Individual nursing goals also must be considered. As stated by Manthey (1990, p. 17), "Once a nurse has become a member of the profession . . . career choices begin to appear almost immediately." Each staff nurse needs to match carefully beliefs about continuing education and personal growth with opportunities for meeting them, with or without the support and financial assistance of an employer. Personal and professional goals will not be realized unless they are identified, analyzed, and pursued with realistic plans that correspond to the availability of resources. Given the constant, rapid change in nursing and in life experiences, planning for **5-year goals** (rather than an entire lifetime) may be realistic. Such 5-year plans might be compared with the building blocks of a personal career path.

Careers predictably rest on commitment to worthy common goals and ability to articulate them to others. New graduates in nursing need to be mindful of the changing norms in the work culture that emphasize collaboration with other employees (Marshall, 1995, p. 3). In addition to promoting professional autonomy, nurses need to combine efforts with those of others to provide the complex services needed in the competitive health-care arena. As Marshall (1995, p. 3) stated, "Leadership in the new workplace must be seen, not as a job, based on power and authority, but as a function based on principles, new people skills, and the ability to engage others in coming to consensus around critical decisions and problem solving. The resulting trust and productivity will provide the enterprise a clear, competitive advantage." Nursing leaders/managers and staff nurses need to work together to develop cultures (i.e., work environments) that meet needs of both types of nursing personnel (Brown, 2002, p. 15).

The entry-level staff nurse needs to differentiate the career ladders often delineated by employers and the ladders based on one's own nursing interests and talents. Many nursing career models exist. The Dalton/Thompson model (Myers Schim, 1990, p. 96FF) (Figure E-1) is a good example. It provides an overview of the common stages of professional development of nurses and describes achievements during each phase and various choices made in pursuit of personal interests and goals. Usually the employer's career ladder is only one of many available nursing career opportunities. Identification of goals for the next 5 years of one's career is paramount to determining how to achieve them. Personal growth depends on choices among nursing practice opportunities, personal development activities, and involvement in professional organizations that contribute to reaching individual career goals.

## SEEKING EMPLOYMENT CORRESPONDING TO IDENTIFIED GOALS

After the entry-level staff nurse clarifies her or his personal nursing philosophy and has identified personal and career goals, she or he can seek **nursing employment** to match them. Before contacting a potential employer, the nurse needs to learn about the agency's characteristics. Because nursing students frequently begin seeking employment while completing required courses, they can use services available in the student affairs or placement offices. These services can help identify specific types of employers and employment opportunities in desired

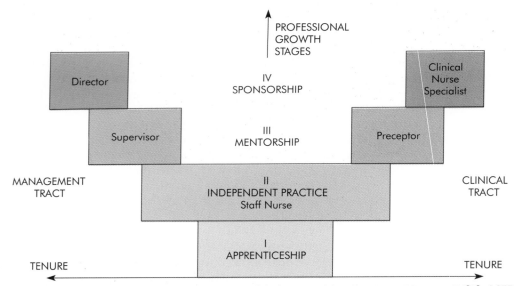

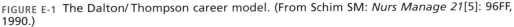

FIGURE E-1 The Dalton/Thompson career model. (From Schim SM: *Nurs Manage 21*[5]: 96FF, 1990.)

locations. In addition, employment opportunities often are posted on bulletin boards. Information about "career days" and other recruitment events is posted routinely. One might inquire about special programs and positions available to new graduates.

When leads about employers of interest have been identified, the nurse can contact specific facilities and request information to compare potential employers. It is helpful to keep track of the names, addresses, and telephone numbers of those you contact to assist with follow-through on subsequent contacts. Keep copies of letters sent in the event that a potential employer contacts you about one of them.

Depending on the nature of the nursing employment desired, the nurse might compile a resumé or marketing letter or complete an application form. A sample cover letter and resumé appear in Boxes E-3 and E-4. Some information should not be included in your resume (e.g., age or marital status, high school attended, work generalities, or salary history) (Cardillo, 2000, p. 40). All correspondence must be neat and accurate. Correspondence needs to project a professional image and show attention to details.

Organize information about your credentials and related experiences to match the employer's **qualifications and requirements** for the desired position. Usually your **credentials** include a brief description of your educational background and previous employment, emphasizing pertinent accomplishments that contribute to the qualifications desired by the potential employer. Accurately communicate achievements and accomplishments that illustrate your qualifications for the desired position. Pertinent personal information on such topics as hobbies, spe-

**BOX E-3**

## Sample Cover Letter

1234 B Busy Lane
Somewhere, USA 58931
January 6, 2002

Director of Nursing
Grand Care Health Center
874 Quiet Street
Fun Spot, WI 53000

Dear Director of Nursing:

Attached is a copy of my resumé. You will note that I have begun to gain experience working with people and have completed requirements for my B.S. degree with a major in nursing. I am interested in obtaining an entry-level staff nurse position on a general medical surgical unit at Grand Care Health Center because of the information I received about it from the Placement Office at Up-to-Date University.

I am interested in gaining nursing experience in an innovative organization that enables nurses to provide high-quality care and grow professionally. I strongly believe that I could become a contributing member of your nursing staff.

Please contact me by telephone before 2:00 pm weekdays to schedule an interview. I look forward to hearing from you.

Sincerely,

Alyce R. Nurse, RN

cial interests, awards, and organizational activities also can be included. Make sure to include your name, address, and telephone number.

It is as important that one's appearance communicate a positive professional image during employment interviews as it is while on duty. Before the interview, you need to learn about the agency and plan to ask at least two or three questions to help you determine whether to accept an employment offer. It is a good idea to follow-up an interview with a brief letter thanking the agency staff for giving you an additional opportunity to express your interest in the position. If you

BOX E-4

# Sample Resumé

Alyce R. Nurse
1234B Busy Lane
Somewhere, USA 58931
(555) 987-6543

**Position objective**

To obtain an entry-level staff nurse position that would provide opportunities to gain experience and further develop my nursing interests, talents, and skills in general medical-surgical nursing.

**Educational background**

Graduated with honors from Middleton High School, in Elsewhere, MA, in May 1996.

Received an associate degree in nursing, graduating cum laude, from Elsewhere Community College in Blue Skies, MA, in December 1998.

Received a B.S. with a major in nursing from Up-to-Date University's College of Nursing located in Rolling Meadows, WI., in January 2002.

While enrolled in nursing courses at Up-to-Date University's College of Nursing, I attended continuing education programs sponsored by the American Heart Association, American Cancer Society, and the University. Topics included "Managing a Heart-Healthy Lifestyle," "Detecting and Treating Breast Cancer," and "Using Nursing Diagnoses to Steer Nursing Practice."

**Work experience**

Employed part-time as a registered nurse at the Golden Gate Residential Center, in Rolling Meadows, WI., since February 2001. I am typically assigned as a team leader, working with 1 to 2 LPNs and 3 to 4 NAs to provide care for 42 residents during the afternoon shift.

Employed part-time as waitress at Sizzling Pizza House in Blue Skies, MA, from September 1997 until December 1999. I waited on customers from 5 to 10 pm 5 to 6 days per week.

Employed part-time as counter help at MacConald's Quick Burgers in Blue Skies, MA, from September 1995 to May 1997. I took customer orders at the counter from 4:30 to 8:30 pm 4 to 5 days each week.

Was a volunteer Candy Striper to deliver newspapers during the evenings at Blue Skies Memorial Hospital from September 1993 to August 1995.

**Professional organizations**

Currently an active member of the National Association of Nursing Students. I served on the local chapter's Membership Committee from September 2000 until December 2001.

Served as student representative of my college class to the Student Government Association from September 1997 to September 1999.

**References**

Available upon request.

make tentative plans to accept employment but later are unable to do so, common courtesy requires that you inform the agency of your changed plans at the earliest possible date. These efforts typically distinguish applicants by showing consideration for the employer's needs. They also reflect professional integrity.

## ESTABLISHING LICENSURE AND MAINTAINING REGISTRATION

While completing the curriculum requirements for graduation from a nursing program, nursing students receive assistance in compiling the credentials needed to obtain **licensure** as registered nurses. Each applicant accepts responsibility for becoming licensed and maintaining **registration** when practicing nursing for compensation. State nurse practice acts not only broadly define the legal scope of practice, but also establish requirements for obtaining and maintaining a nursing license. Although these requirements vary from state to state, the agency authorized to regulate nursing practice also carries out the activities involved in licensing nurses. These activities include implementing plans for administering licensure examinations by screening applicants and carrying out the testing program, compiling educational records, and maintaining records of candidates who satisfactorily complete the licensure examination.

When nurses wish to practice in another state, they need to contact the agency regulating nursing practice in that state. These agencies provide information about the requirements and process involved in becoming licensed and maintaining registration as a registered nurse in that state.

Through Nurse Licensure Compacts between states, a nurse licensed in one's state of residence can practice in other states (physically [e.g., being physically present] and electronically [transmitting information, documentation, and interventions]), subject to each state's practice law and regulation. This has become known as the *mutual recognition model*. A nurse wishing to pursue such licensure should visit the National Council of State Boards of Nursing web site (http://www.ncsb.org) to determine whether the states in question have enacted the Nurse Licensure Compact. A "Nurse Licensure Compact Map" listing the states that have enacted the Nurse Licensure Compact can be viewed at http://www.ncsbn.org/public/nurselicensurecompact/mutual_recognition_state.htm.

Employers verify the licensure and registration status of nurses on initial employment and at regular intervals thereafter. If any questions arise about the veracity of a nurse's license and registration status, they usually can be answered by the state agency regulating the individual nurse's practice.

## DETERMINING THE NEED FOR MALPRACTICE INSURANCE

Licensure laws specify standards for practice necessary to protect the public, define entry-level scope of practice, and provide for disciplinary actions against practitioners who do not comply. New graduates need to know that practicing nursing without a license (or temporary permit) is one basis for disciplinary action.

As mentioned earlier, licensure procedures correspond with each state's established qualification requirements. On completion of educational programs, graduates receive assistance in compiling their credentials with the appropriate regulatory state agency. Often new graduates can obtain a temporary permit to practice nursing until they have completed licensure examinations successfully. After compiling credentials, each nurse obtains a license to practice. Often the state administrative agency is known as a *Board of Nursing* or *Board of Nurse Examiners*. The nurse accepts responsibility for maintaining licensure to practice according to the state laws within which the nurse practices and renewing registration at specified intervals. Renewal of registration entails paying a fee and keeping identifying information current. Practicing according to Nurse Practice Acts usually does not limit the nurse's practice needed to serve clients based on nursing knowledge and skills because such laws are written to provide flexibility to allow for changes and growth within the nursing profession (Fiesta, 1990, p. 20).

A physician or hospital cannot insist that a nurse perform an activity that is contraindicated by the particular state's Nurse Practice Act: ". . . no one profession normally possesses authority to mandate what any other profession is obligated to do" (Fiesta, 1990, p. 21). Similarly, if the health-care agency authorizes the procedure or intervention to be within the scope of nursing practice, the agency insures the nurse's performance of the activity against malpractice claims (Fiesta, 1990, p. 21).

Significant personal and financial risks are inherent in practicing nursing as a career. Purchasing **malpractice insurance** is one strategy for managing these risks. Responding to legal accusations entails psychological and emotional costs as well as financial ones. Strategies for preventing malpractice claims should be incorporated in every nurse's practice (Bernzweig, 1990, pp. 317–355; Luquire, 1988, pp. 61–62; Maher, 1989, pp. 34–41; Showers, 2000, p. 48). Principal among these strategies are communicating effectively with clients and taking an active role in reducing their dissatisfaction as consumers. Another strategy is referring the clients (with dissatisfactions that you cannot resolve) to the health-care agency's "patient representative" or client representative from the public relations department. These interventions may lower the risk for clients taking legal actions. Such efforts do not eliminate completely, however, the potential for legal actions against the nurse.

As discussed in Chapter Thirteen, liability refers to legal accountability for client risks, danger, and injury caused by the nurse's negligent acts. Negligence entails actions or nonactions that the nurse could or should have taken to prevent harm or injury to the client. Malpractice involves nursing actions that are inconsistent with established standards and that are believed by peers to be unsafe or to place the recipient of such care at risk.

Every nurse decides whether to purchase and maintain personal malpractice insurance protection against the financial costs of legal accusations associated with nursing practice. The need for malpractice insurance is based on several factors, including the degree of legal accountability or responsibility for one's actions and nonactions and the associated risks to personal potential or actual assets. Morris, as quoted in Sandroff (1983, p. 29), warned, "With the current legal climate, it's downright foolish to practice in any profession today without professional malpractice insurance." Others have agreed (Showers, 2000, p. 48). Some nurses decide that the malpractice insurance protection provided by their employers is sufficient. This insurance has limits (Varga, 1990, p. 36). It might not cover financial costs of legal defense for actions taken outside of a job description; circumstances in which the employer decides not to defend you or, in some states, decides to sue you for your actions or nonactions that resulted in a successful suit of your employer; or actions taken that were presumed to be protected by "Good Samaritan acts" (state laws providing protection from liability associated with helping accident victims). Every nurse needs to know the protection afforded nurses providing emergency care as "Good Samaritans" in the state in which she or he practices (Northrop, 1990, pp. 50–51). In addition, consideration needs to be given to the liabilities involved in nursing activities performed as a volunteer.

Jane Greenlaw, a nurse and lawyer, offered a rational approach to using one's resources wisely: "I, myself, would not practice nursing without my own coverage" (Sandroff, 1983, p. 29). Several trends make such a decision appropriate, including (1) the increasing public perception of nurses as professionals, who are accountable for their own actions instead of being protected by their employers (Godkin et al., 1987, p. 74); (2) the increasing complexity of skills nurses use when practicing in expanded roles (Bailey-Allen, 1990, p. 14); (3) changes in patterns of documentation to reflect actual care provided and client responses to treatment (Bailey-Allen, 1990, p. 15); and (4) the fact that nurses, as professionals, may have assets that could make a successful suit worthwhile.

Purchasing malpractice insurance is only one way to manage the financial costs of legal disputes. It does not eliminate the need to practice nursing in accordance with established standards to prevent clients and their families and employers or physicians from making legal accusations. Employers or physicians may make legal accusations against nurses in an attempt to recover financial losses arising out of the process of settling legal disputes. Responding to a legal complaint made by others involved in the client's care typically requires considerable legal counsel and costs.

## USING AVAILABLE SUPPORT SYSTEMS TO HELP YOU GROW

Entry-level staff nurses use many different strategies to grow professionally. To increase the likelihood of success, they need to use the **support systems** available at the agency and in their personal social circles. As mentioned in Chapter Fifteen, nurses participate in various structured learning programs while enrolled in nursing courses and in continuing education programs. In addition, they often actively seek learning opportunities to ensure that their nursing knowledge and skills remain current.

Frequently, nursing students participate in preceptorships during advanced nursing courses. Such a one-to-one relationship with a more experienced nurse helps the student practice nursing skills acquired in previous courses (Goldenberg, 1987/1988, p. 11). Under close supervision, the student gains practical nursing experience. Preceptors provide regular feedback to guide learning. These experiences are usually limited, however, by the time allotted for the course. Results of preceptorships indicate that these experiences increase the preceptee's effectiveness (Scales et al., 1993, pp. 45–48).

In addition to providing typical in-service orientation programs and financial support to participate in continuing education programs, many employers develop strategies that encourage nurse retention. These strategies are designed to help nurses develop their professional potential. On the basis of individual career goals, nurses are expected to use this agency support to the advantage of the individual and the benefit of the agency. For example, staff nurses typically share information gained during continuing education programs with other interested agency staff as a stipulation for receiving financial support.

Another strategy used by an increasing number of nursing employers is a dynamic mentorship program. Mentorships are structured nurturing programs involving one-to-one relationships between inexperienced and experienced nurses. Preceptorships are typically part of a formal instructional program, whereas structured mentorships frequently are offered as part of an employer's in-service program. There is some evidence that mentorships for ethnic minority nursing students may increase their retention in instructional programs and contribute to meeting the needs of a culturally diverse community (Alvarez and Abriam-Yago, 1993, p. 230). There is a need to use creative approaches to promote the development of a culturally diverse profession that is prepared to meet the needs of a culturally diverse clientele.

Agencies that offer a structured mentorship program to new employees will be eager to inform nurses of its availability as a recruitment strategy. Employers have learned that mentorship enhances career development and retention of competent nurses (Caracuzzo-Kinsey, 1990, p. 45). Typically the agency uses resources to prepare mentors and implement mentorship programs to nurture entry-level staff nurses during their initial employment and in-service programs (Beeman et al., 1999, p. 91). These programs are designed to build supportive and meaningful relationships between new and more experienced nurses. By being a mentor, staff nurses gain satisfaction from teaching and feeling valued by peers (Law et al., 1989, p. 65). Mentors generally are viewed as respected role models who provide feedback to novices. Although mentorships are not for everybody, many nurses who worked with a mentor recalled positive learning experiences. Caracuzzo-Kinsey (1990, p. 45) reported that "proteges often report feeling replenished, refueled and inspired to make a significant contribution to their field or discipline." Mentorships are gaining popularity among nurses who strive to influence their profession. Mentoring, although arising from different sources throughout one's career, has become known as a valuable strategy for success (Peluchette and Jeanquart, 2000, p. 549).

Depending on the nature of the community and its relationship with the health-care agency, many other resources may be available. These resources often involve opportunities to work with groups of people with interests similar to those of nurses. Common interest groups include local chapters of the American Heart Association; American Cancer Society; and groups involved in caring for disaster victims, controlling communicable diseases, or assisting the homeless. Nurses frequently are invited to participate in efforts to solve the many complex problems affecting the health of a neighborhood or community. They are asked to share their knowledge of desired health practices and teach techniques for adopting them. Ultimately, such experiences help the nurse to develop further personal talents, self-confidence, knowledge, and skills. Similarly the nurse may develop career skills within the organization, increasing her or his visibility and career marketability (Manion, 2001, p. 5).

## NOTIFYING EMPLOYERS ABOUT CHANGING OR TERMINATING EMPLOYMENT

Most new graduates focus attention on various strategies that might be used to seek employment. To establish a reputable work record, however, they also need to know how to notify an employer of a desire to change positions or terminate employment. Whenever feasible, the employee is asked to adhere to the agency's established personnel policy when **changing an employment status.**

Box E-5 lists several guidelines for writing a letter regarding changing positions or terminating a relationship with an employer. The letter must be addressed to the person responsible for managing personnel changes within the agency. You also must notify your immediate supervisor. Giving sufficient advance notice allows time for the employer to change work schedules and plan for adequate staffing.

When composing the letter, the nurse should be mindful that it may be used by the employer to provide future reference information. The letter likely will become part of the individual's personnel file with the employer. The content of the letter should state clearly the position that the nurse is leaving. When possible, the nurse should include a brief, accurate, positive statement about the employment relationship. If appropriate, the notification letter should include reasons the employee is requesting the change. These reasons should be given in such a way that they reflect positively on the employee. Reasons might include career advancement, evolving family needs, or relocation.

It is important for the nurse to project a positive image as a valued employee who consistently shows desired qualities of neatness and attention to detail. This attention includes accurate spelling and proper grammar and punctuation. It also is

---

**BOX E-5**

## Guidelines for Changing Positions or Terminating Employment

1. Adhere to the employer's agency personnel policy when specifying the date the resignation or change is effective.
2. State your reasons, if appropriate.
3. When composing the body of the letter, remember that the letter is likely to become part of your personnel file with this employer and may be used to provide reference information.
4. State the name of the position you are leaving.
5. Project a positive image and desired qualities of clarity and neatness in person and on paper.
6. Use quality paper for the written notification.

important that the letter be written on quality paper—not on notebook paper or dinner napkins! The overall appearance of the letter reflects the character of the employee.

Perhaps the real issue in notifying an employer of a desire to change or terminate a relationship rests with the employee's attitude toward managing her or his career. Obtaining and maintaining the credentials required for the practice of nursing as a registered nurse involves a large investment of time, effort, and money. Careful attention to preserving and increasing the value of this investment reflects an appreciation of sound career management principles.

## USING HUMOR AS AN INTEGRAL NURSING MANAGEMENT STRATEGY

Client care management is often stressful. Although its importance frequently is unrecognized, **humor** can be used as a deliberate strategy to elicit favorable responses from others in the work environment. As Lee (1990, p. 86) so aptly stated, "The positive physiological and psychological benefits of laughter cannot be overestimated." She emphasized that humor as a management tool needs to be positive instead of negative. Positive humor stimulates laughter as a favorable response from an individual or group. As psychologist William James (1948) related, "We don't laugh because we're happy, we're happy because we laugh." Negative humor deliberately attempts to elicit a destructive reaction from an individual or group, leading the individuals

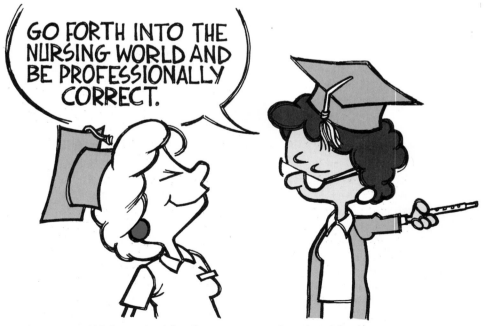

It is important for the nurse to project a positive image.

involved to engage in "put-downs" or self-deprecation. Insensitive, inappropriate joking can diminish effective working relationships. Positive humor promotes effective working relationships or "lightens the load" (Porter O'Grady, 2000, p. 6).

The aim of humor is to increase laughter, get in touch with one's feelings, and increase the acceptance of others. When positive humor is used, staff morale increases, as does the work group's cohesiveness. Because positive humor reflects a healthy attitude, it can be nurtured and rewarded. It is not used so much to reduce stress as to maintain vitality. There is truth to the belief common among direct nursing staff that if you don't laugh, you don't survive! Accordingly, it behooves every nurse, beginning and experienced, to nurse an enjoyable sense of humor.

## SUMMARY

Successful staff nurses manage their careers to ensure that personal goals are met. To do so, each nurse needs to clarify her or his personal and nursing philosophy. Each entry-level staff nurse is encouraged to identify 5-year plans as steps toward meeting career goals. Completing these requirements helps to establish a career foundation and prepare the nurse to seek employment. Successful staff nurses match their goals with the characteristics of potential employers. In addition, they organize and communicate their credentials in such a manner as to reflect a positive image.

Each nurse decides whether to purchase and maintain personal malpractice insurance protection against the financial costs of legal accusations associated with nursing practice. This is only one of several methods of managing the financial costs of legal disputes.

Effective staff nurses use support systems available through their employing agencies and social circles to help them grow. One common method is participation in dynamic mentoring programs. In addition, they accept responsibility for obtaining licensure and maintaining registration while practicing nursing. This responsibility continues throughout the nurse's career. Employers verify that every employed nurse is licensed and registered.

## APPLICATION EXERCISES

1. Write a description of your nursing philosophy, including your beliefs about caring. Compare it with the beliefs and goals you aspired to when you applied for admission to a nursing program.
2. Daydream about your career. List your 5-year goals. Rank their importance to you.
3. Write a resumé for a position as a staff nurse in a long-term care agency. Include your nursing career goals, qualifications, credentials, and personal interests. Match them with the characteristics of your assigned agency as a potential employer.
4. Debate the pros and cons of malpractice insurance. Identify other methods of managing the risks inherent in practicing nursing.
5. Laugh a lot!

CRITICAL THINKING SCENARIO

Relax and imagine yourself successfully practicing nursing for 3 years in a busy primary care clinic located in a rural community. Compared with your colleagues practicing in suburban settings, you are expected to provide a broader range of services, referring clients with more complex needs to specialty agencies in suburban settings. You are the sole provider and a single parent of two school-age children. As the cost and complexity of technology and health-care competition increases, your employer requests that you broaden your assessment skills and instruct clients regarding the results of clinical laboratory studies. In addition, you coordinate the care provided by three health-care technicians. You are concerned that your employer's requests exceed your legal scope of practice.

1. What would you do first? Why?
2. If your first action leads you to believe that you are exceeding your scope of practice, to whom would you talk? Give reasons for your decision.
3. If your employer downsizes, asking you to authorize health-care technicians under your direction to perform tasks beyond their credentials, what would you do?
4. What types of technology might you use to enhance your performance of nursing functions involved in caring for your clients?

Humor is a skill worth nurturing. It helps to increase staff morale and develop coping skills used to manage the diverse stresses inherent in a nursing career. One's nursing livelihood depends on it!

## REFERENCES

Alvarez A, Abriam-Yago K: Mentoring undergraduate ethnic-minority: a strategy for retention, *J Nurs Educ* 32(5):230–232, 1993.

Bailey-Allen AM: Changing liability of the nurse over the past decade, *Orthop Nurs* 9(2):13–15, 1990.

Beeman KL, Jernigan AC, Hensley PD: Employing new grads: a plan for success, *Nurs Econ* 17(2):91–95, 1999.

Bernzweig EP: *The nurse's liability for malpractice: a programmed course*, ed 5, St. Louis, MO, 1990, Mosby, pp. 317–355.

Brown CL: A theory of the process of creating power in relationships, *Nurs Admin Q* 26(2):15–33, 2002.

Caracuzzo-Kinsey D: Mentorship and influence in nursing, *Nurs Manage* 21(5):45–46, 1990.

Cardillo D: What not to put on your resume, *Nursing Spectrum* 13(22IL):40, 2000.

Crawford DL: The glass ceiling in nursing management, *Nurs Econ* 11(6):335–341, 1993.

Domrose C: The rules of attraction, *Nurse Week* 3(6):18–20, 2002.

Fiesta J: Safeguarding your nursing license, *Nurs Manage 21*(8):20–21, 1990.

Godkin L, Wooten B, Godkin J: The jury decides: are registered nurses legally liable for their job-related actions? *Nurs Manage 18*(5):73–74, 76, 79, 1987.

Goldenberg D: Preceptorship: a one-to-one relationship with a triple "p" rating (preceptor, preceptee, patient), *Nurs Forum 23*(1):10–15, 1987/1988.

James W: *Psychology*, New York, NY, 1948, World Publishing.

Law MS, Smith MO, Igoe SN, et al: Nurses helping nurses, *Imprint 36*(2):65, 67–68, 71–72, 1989.

Lee BS: "Humor relations" for nurse managers, *Nurs Manage 21*(5):86, 88, 90, 92, 1990.

Levenstein A: Toward creative self-management, *Nurs Manage 14*(1):22–23, 1983.

Luquire R: 6 common causes of nursing liability, *Nurs 18*(11):61–62, 1988.

Maher VF: Your legal guide to safe nursing practice, *Nurs 19*(11):34–42, 1989.

Manion J: Enhancing career marketability through intrapreneurship, *Nurs Admin Q 25*(2):5–10, 2001.

Manthey M: 1990 nursing: a profession of choice, *Nurs Manage 21*(9):17–18, 1990.

Marshall EM: *Transforming the way we work: the power of the collaborative workplace*, New York, NY, 1995, AMACOM, a division of American Management Association, pp. 1–11.

Muff J: Curing vs. caring: a blessing or curse? *Perspect Psychiatr Care 30*(3):34–36, 1994.

Myers Schim S: Nursing career management: the Dalton/Thompson model, *Nurs Manage 21*(5):96FF, 1990.

Northrop CE: How Good Samaritan laws do and don't protect you, *Nurs '90 13*(2):50–51, 1990.

Paul R, Elder L: *Critical thinking: tools for taking charge of your learning and your life*, Upper Saddle River, NJ, 2001, Prentice Hall.

Peluchette JVE, Jeanquart S: Professionals' use of different mentor sources at various career stages: implications for career success, *J Soc Psychol 140*(5):549–564, 2000.

Porter O'Grady T: Laughter lightens our load, *Nursing 30*(7):6, 2000.

Prior MM, Cottingbam EM, Kolski BJ, et al: Nurse turnover as a function of employment, experience and unit, *Nurs Manage 21*(7):27–28, 1990.

Sandroff R: Why you really ought to have your own malpractice policy, *RN 46*(3):29–33, 1983.

Scales FS, Alverson E, Harder DL: The effect of a preceptorship on nursing performance, *Nurs Connect 6*(2):45–54, 1993.

Showers JL: What you need to know about negligence law suits, *Nursing 30*(2):45–48, 2000.

Varga K: How to protect yourself against malpractice, *Imprint 36*(5):33–34, 36–37, 1990.

Williams C: Job satisfaction: comparing cc and med/surg nurses, *Nurs Manage 21*(7):104A-104H, 1990.

# Index